LIGAMENT INJURIES
and their Treatment

LIGAMENT INJURIES
and their Treatment

Edited by

D. H. R. Jenkins MB, ChB, ChM, FRCS

Consultant Orthopaedic Surgeon
Cardiff Royal Infirmary

LONDON
CHAPMAN AND HALL

First published in 1985 by Chapman and Hall Ltd,
11 New Fetter Lane, London EC4P 4EE

© 1985 Chapman and Hall Ltd

Printed in Great Britain at the
University Press, Cambridge

ISBN 0 412 25470 0

British Library Cataloguing in Publication Data

Ligament injuries and their treatment.
1. Ligament——Wounds and injuries
I. Jenkins, D.H.R.
616.7'706   RD688

ISBN 0–412–25470–0

Contents

Contents

Contents

Contents

Preface

The continued popularity of sporting activities and the concomitant intensity of training and participation has resulted in higher incidences of ligament injuries. This book, written by an international team of specialists, brings together recent advances in treatment. It deals mainly with injuries of the knee joint, but the ankle and elbow are also covered.

The book is divided into three parts. Part One on structure and function, deals with the biomechanical aspects of ligaments. The structure of ligaments and anchorages, together with comments on the mechanical properties and actions of ligaments and joints, are also discussed. These topics are followed by a chapter on collagen metabolism and healing.

Part Two forms the main part of the book and is concerned with treatment. It is well recognized that in 1985 the major interest in the ligament field concerns the knee. It is, however, relevant to have comments on other joints, and for these reasons the elbow and ankle are also included.

Part Three is on the use of graft materials and deals primarily with carbon fibre, although there is one chapter on the use of bovine xenografts.

Collectively, this book presents a view of ligament problems from both sides of the Atlantic. It is aimed at the surgeon who is interested in ligamentous instability, and sets out to present the current view of those who are active in this field.

List of Contributors

Andrew A. Amis, PhD C Eng, M I Mech E
Department of Mechanical Engineering, Imperial College of Science and Technology, London, England.

Priv. Doz. Dr Lutz Claes
Head of Experimental Traumatology Department, Universität Ulm, West Germany.

R. A. Denham, FRCS
Consultant Orthopaedic Surgeon, Portsmouth Group Hospitals, England.

A. E. Ellison, MD
Director of Sports Medicine Division, Department of Orthopaedic Surgery, North Adams Hospital, Massachusetts, USA.

J. F. Fetto, MD
Associate Professor and Assistant Director of Sports Medicine, New York University Medical Centre, Suite 5B, 530 First Avenue, New York, New York 10016, USA.

Gerd Helbing, MD
Assistant Professor of Traumatology, Universität Ulm, West Germany.

Jack C. Hughston, MD
Clinical Professor of Orthopaedics, Tulane University, New Orleans, USA.

Peter A. N. Hutton, MB, BS, FRCS
Consultant Orthopaedic Surgeon, Queen Mary's Hospital, Roehampton and St. Steven's Hospital, London, England.

Frank M. Ivey Jr, MD
Assistant Professor of Surgery, University of Texas Medical Branch, Galveston, USA.

List of Contributors

David H. R. Jenkins, MB, ChB, ChM, FRCS
Consultant Orthopaedic Surgeon, Cardiff Royal Infirmary, Wales.

Norman R. Jaffee, PhD
Xenotech Laboratories Inc, Irvine, California, USA.

J. B. King, MB, FRCS
Clinical Director Diploma Course in Sports Medicine, London Hospital
Medical School, England.

Marcel Lemaire
Groupe de Chirurgie Orthopédique et Sportive de Paris, Clinique de
Maussins, Paris.

William C. McMaster, MD
Adjunct Professor, Division of Orthopaedic Surgery, University of California, Irvine, USA.

J. H. Miller, MB, ChB, FRCS (Glas. et Ed.)
Consultant Orthopaedic Surgeon, The Royal Infirmary, Glasgow,
Scotland.

Priv. Doz. Dr Rainer Neugebauer
Chururgie III, Universität Ulm, West Germany.

Lyle A. Noorwood, MD
Assistant Clinical Professor of Orthopaedics, Tulane University, New
Orleans, Louisiana, USA.

A. E. Strover, MB, ChB, FRCS
Orthopaedic Surgeon, The School House, Belbroughton, England.

Isabel F. Williams, BA, MSc, PhD
Department of Pathology, University of Bristol, England.

PART ONE
Structure and Function

---

1 *Biomechanics of ligaments*

ANDREW A. AMIS

1.1 Introduction

The purpose of this chapter is to examine the behaviour of ligaments in a
wide-ranging and fundamental manner, which should help to explain
many of the clinical details in subsequent chapters. This applies particularly to aspects such as the function of ligaments, their failure or disruption, and attempts to repair them or simulate their structures by artificial
replacements. The basis of a sound understanding of all these aspects lies
in an appreciation of their mechanical characteristics. A surgeon reading
this might be tempted to think that mechanics is not really important
when faced by clinical reality. However, patients with a ligament problem
are in that position primarily because they have contrived to overload
their complex musculoskeletal mechanisms, and an understanding of the
mechanism of injury will often provide the guidelines for a surgical
reversal of the disruption.

Subsequent discussion will deal with ligaments on two levels: a review
of the properties of isolated specimens of ligamentous tissue, then a
review of how bundles of this tissue act to control the motion or stability
of joints.

1.2 The structure of ligaments

The structure of any ligament is basically that of a bundle of fibres which
link two bones. This structure normally functions to control the relative
motions of the two bones, the most common mode of action being that the
ligament inhibits the separation of two points on the bones by providing a
tensile restraint to that motion. Any further excursion may be accomplished only by exerting sufficient force to extend the ligamentous structure. The ligaments function in a passive manner – if the bones approach
each other, then the ligaments slacken and have no influence on the

3

relative movements of the bones. This mechanism is demonstrated by rheumatoid disease, for example, which shortens the bone ends spanned by ligaments by a process of erosion, so that the ligaments are then powerless to prevent the occurrence of subluxation or other deformity – an abnormal relative motion of the bone ends. Conversely, if the bones try to move apart, the restraining forces exerted by the ligaments are determined solely by the tensile (extension versus force) characteristics of their structures.

For this biomechanical review, the functional characteristics described above should be borne in mind as a means of elucidating the significance of the detailed features of the structure of ligaments.

Atomic and microscopic details of the structure of ligamentous tissue have been published by various authors (Viidik, 1966; Tkaczuk, 1968), whose descriptions may be summarized as follows: the basic structural material is collagen. This is a high molecular weight protein, whose long chain molecules arrange themselves along protofibrils. The protofibrils group together to form fibrils, which themselves group together into the bundles which make up the ligament. The essential structural feature of this hierarchy is that the smaller elements always arrange themselves parallel to the major axis of the larger structure in which they are incorporated. This means that the structural protein molecules are arranged along the length of the ligament, adapting it perfectly to resist tension. Trapped within the fibrillar collagen structure are small volumes of other materials: fibroblasts, or fibrocytes, which provide the cellular origin of collagen protein; some elastic fibres (principally in postural ligaments); and an intercellular ground substance. The latter is a viscous hydrophilic material, containing mucopolysaccharides, which can trap or contain water. This viscous medium is believed to control the ease with which collagen fibrils may rearrange themselves. Thus, although it is not itself structural, the ground substance does affect the response of the structure to loads, as will be discussed later.

Although collagen structural fibres surrounded by a ground substance are common both to ligaments and bones, the ground substance of bone contains inorganic material – hydroxyapatite crystals. These crystals give bone its rigidity, and may well have a bearing on the tendency of bones to fail in tension. The structural problem for ligaments is that an anchorage to bone involves bridging a transition from the soft ligament material to the relatively rigid bone. Fortunately, histological examination shows that there is a gradual transition of material types at the interface, thus avoiding stress concentrations which would weaken the structure.

The insertions of ligaments into bones may be classified roughly into two types, depending on whether the ligament approaches the bone surface at a large angle (for example, the cruciate ligaments of the knee), or tangentially (for example, the tibial insertion of the medial collateral knee ligament). If the ligament approaches at a large angle, its collagen fibres continue on into the bone structure, as Sharpey's fibres (Viidik, 1966). The cellular material between the fibres transforms from fibrocytes to a 'chondrocyte' appearance, and then to osteocytes (Ham, 1953). These cellular changes reflect the material types, which have been classified as four layers: ligament, fibrocartilage, mineralized fibrocartilage, then bone, which has a hard cortical shell overlaying a trabecular structure (Noyes, DeLucas and Torvik, 1974). The fibrocartilagenous layers provide a zone of mechanical property transition, thereby avoiding stress concentrations at the interface.

When a ligament meets the bone surface tangentially, however, most of its fibres do not penetrate deeply into the bone, but dissipate themselves into the fibrous periosteal layers, normally over a large area (Laros, Tipton and Cooper, 1971; Noyes *et al.*, 1974). Although the cellular material goes through a chondrocyte transition at the interface, there is no fibrocartilage zone, so that fibrous tissue lays directly on the bone cortex. This difference in anchorage morphology causes a differing response to exercise or immobilization – the relatively vascular fibrous tissue anchorages being more susceptible to deterious changes.

Although it is generally accepted that ligaments have a very low rate of metabolism, their tissues do contain an adequate vascular supply to enable slow healing to occur, and nerve fibres are associated with the blood vessels. This is so even within the mid-substance of the cruciate ligaments, which is probably the site most remote from well-vascularized surroundings (Kennedy, Weinberg and Wilson, 1974). The paravascular nerve fibres probably provide a sensory feedback to warn when joints are reaching their limits of motion – a function which an artificial ligament could not duplicate.

1.3 The mechanical properties of ligament tissue and isolated ligament specimens

Many people have published the results of studies of the strength of ligaments, yet, as will be shown later, very little of the material is of use for providing surgeons with data which may be used as guidelines for reconstructive procedures. A major barrier between laboratory work and realism is the complex nature of real injury mechanisms, few of which have been recorded (for example, when a football player's injury has been televised). Analysis of falling and twisting movements requires films shot simultaneously from two directions, so perhaps it is not surprising that such data is not available. Studies of ligament strength have therefore

Ligament Injuries and their Treatment

confined themselves to relatively simple tests, in which bones are clamped into machines and pulled apart in a particular direction. Even on this simpler level, however, there is great scope for error, so results must be viewed critically.

1.3.1 TYPICAL TENSILE BEHAVIOUR

Typical tensile behaviour of ligament material is shown in Fig. 1.1. The initial extension, into region 1 on the graph, from the origin, occurs for a very small load. The upward curve of the graph indicates that the ligament becomes progressively stiffer as it is stretched through region 1, until the slope of the graph reaches a maximum gradient, which is maintained through region 2, indicating a constant stiffness (amount of force per extension).

Constant stiffness is a feature of normal Hookean elastic behaviour, but the elastic line should pass through the origin, as shown. There are two main reasons why this does not happen for ligaments. Firstly, the fibrous structure of a relaxed ligament does not have all the collagen fibres pulled straight and parallel – they buckle into a wavy configuration – so the initial extension, for a low load, is pulling the fibres straight rather than stretching them. Once straight, their elongation is of an elastic nature (region 2). This mechanism was shown by Rigby *et al.* (1959), using a polarizing microscope. The second reason is that ligaments originate or insert over areas of bone, rather than at points, so there will be a range of fibre lengths within each ligament. Since, also, ligament fibres are not arranged as regularly as in a tendon, for example (Viikik, 1966), it seems

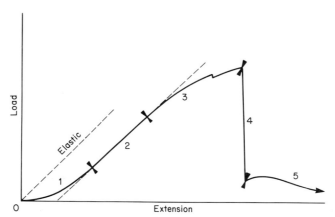

Fig. 1.1 Typical tensile load versus extension behaviour of a ligament; regions 1–5 are explained in text.

inevitable that fibres will tighten at different extensions, thus progress-ively contributing to the stiffness transition seen through region 1.

In region 3, the load line starts to drop away from the linear behaviour of region 2. Although the exact mechanisms are unknown, something akin to shearing or other movement of the collagen fibrils must occur within the viscous ground substance, because the ligament will not now return to its original length when the load is released. This deformation is not due to rupture of the collagen fibres (Smith, 1954). Further extension causes the ligament to rupture, and the load which it can sustain falls dramatically (region 4). Despite the fact that the ligament is now useless, it may still appear to be intact. This is because the collagen fibres have lost their origin-to-insertion continuity, but still lie alongside each other. Further extension (region 5) will cause the fibres to slide apart under a low load. Microscopic examination will reveal the disruption of the collagen matrix (Kennedy *et al.*, 1976, 1980) but a functionless cruciate, for example, might look intact when seen through an arthroscope.

1.3.2 TIME DEPENDENT EFFECTS

Although the above description fits in with the findings of many previous workers, the reader should realize that it fails to mention the complexities of ligament behaviour under load. One effect which cannot be ignored is time dependence, which implies that loads applied for different times will produce different elongations. This behaviour has been hinted at above, when it was suggested that permanent elongations derived from viscous flow phenomena. In basic terms, it is difficult to move quickly through a viscous medium, so it is not surprising that a tensile test done slowly allows the specimen to 'flow' to a greater extent than if the load were applied quickly. This time-dependent behaviour is only of practical significance at higher loads, particularly if they are sustained. Since ligaments do not slacken progressively with exercise, it seems that normal working loads and extensions operate into region 2 (see Fig. 1.1), but not into region 3. The ultimate properties, which are affected signifi-cantly by the rate of load application, or extension, are of interest with respect to injuries, or reconstruction procedures.

The effects of testing speed are shown in Fig. 1.2, for a tensile test on an intact bone–ligament–bone specimen. Failure occurs at both a higher load and a greater extension if the test is done at high speed. The amount of energy or work needed to produce failure is represented by the area beneath each of the load curves, so it is apparent that more energy is needed to rupture the specimen at high speed. When testing specimens consisting of the femur, anterior cruciate ligament, and tibia, Noyes, DeLucas and Torvik (1974) found that the failure load increased 21%, the

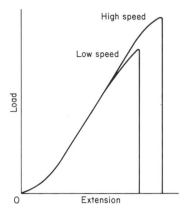

Fig. 1.2 The effect of extension speed on the tensile behaviour of a ligament; The energy needed to produce failure is represented by the area under each loading curve.

extension to failure by 15%, and the energy to failure by 31% for a hundred-fold increase in test speed – the higher speed being similar to that encountered during trauma. It was shown that test speed effects only become significant at high loads by Dorlot *et al.* (1980), who found no changes for a wide range of test speeds if they extended (strained) their anterior cruciate specimens less than 14%. An investigation of the canine medial collateral ligament by Woo, Gomez and Akeson (1981) did show stiffening with strain rate even at low loads. They found that 2.5% extension needed 56 N force at an extension speed of 0.5 mm/min, or 67 N at 50 mm/min – a 20% stiffness increase for a hundred-fold speed increase.

One side-effect of variation of the rate of elongation of a ligament is that the failure mode changes with speed. It has been shown that bone–ligament–bone specimens tend to fail by avulsion of a bone fragment if extended slowly, while a similar specimen extended rapidly will fail by rupture of the ligament itself. The significant change in failure mode found by Noyes, DeLucas and Torvik (1974) for the anterior cruciate ligament is illustrated by Fig. 1.3, with tibial fractures being replaced by ligament ruptures as the speed increased. Testing at a higher speed (a strain rate of 100% per second), Cabaud *et al.* (1980) produced interstitial ligamentous ruptures in 119 of 121 rat anterior cruciate specimens. Since the clinical picture is one of ligamentous ruptures, rather than avulsion of anchorages, this evidence confirms the commonsense impression that joint injuries occur rapidly.

Both the increased strength of the bone–ligament–bone unit with speed and the change in failure mode can be explained by a single factor: the

8

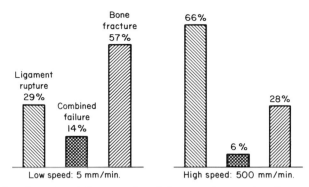

Fig. 1.3 The changing failure mode of the anterior cruciate ligament between slow and physiological test speeds, as reported by Noyes, DeLucas and Torvik (1974).

strength of bone increases with testing speed. It is difficult to apply the published results of tests of bone strength (mostly on cortical bone) to the ligament anchorages, which are normally a thin cortical shell over trabeculae, because the properties of bones vary greatly at different positions (Pope and Outwater, 1974), but the results must provide guidelines relevant to our situation. The ultimate tensile strength of bovine cortical bone has been shown to double for a hundred-fold increase in loading rate (Wright and Hayes, 1976), while both deformation prior to failure and energy absorption were shown by Panjabi, White and Southwick (1973) to increase with loading rate when twisting whole bones. Thus the bone itself may be the weakest point when the load is applied slowly, causing avulsion of ligament anchorages, but becomes stronger with speed, so that the ligament becomes the weakest part during rapid trauma.

A further manifestation of 'viscosity' effects in ligament material is creep, which becomes apparent under quasistatic loading conditions. Creep is effectively a slow-flow process, within the ligament material, which tends to relieve the structure of load or stress. It may, however, cause the structure to elongate to such an extent that diminution of the ligaments' cross-section leads to rupture. This phenomenon was first shown by Smith (1954), for the rabbit anterior cruciate ligament. He found a full elastic recovery of length after applying a load equal to the body weight for 5 min. Application of a load approaching the rupture strength caused creep, leading either to a long-term rupture, or to only partial length recovery when the load was removed. The similar findings by LaBan (1962), for tendon material, are shown in Fig. 1.4(a): creep causes a slow elongation under load, which is not recovered when the load is

9

Ligament Injuries and their Treatment

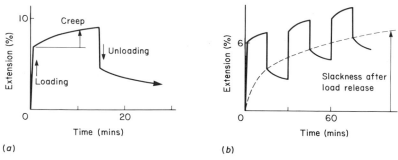

Fig. 1.4 (*a*) Load application causes an immediate elongation, which is followed by a slow creep elongation while the load is sustained; load removal leaves a residual elongation, which recovers slowly (from La Ban, 1962, loading to two-thirds of failure stress). (*b*) The cumulative effect of irreversible changes when loading is repeated.

removed. Part of this deformation is then taken up slowly by an elastic after-effect. The cumulative effect of load repetitions is shown in Fig. 1.4(b): insufficient time for full recovery of the initial length between load applications means that each load cycle causes an increment of elongation. It has been shown that these effects do apply to human knee ligaments *in vivo*. Pope *et al.* (1976) applied a lateral force of 32 N to the ankle, with the femur clamped in a test machine, and the knee flexed 30°. The ankle moved 11 mm immediately, then a further 5 mm, due to creep, in the next 2½ min (Fig. 5). The foot did not return to the starting position when the load was removed: 4 mm displacement remained even after 10 min relaxation.

The practical implication of these experiments is that the ligaments will be slightly slack during use. It is a general property of viscoelastic biological materials that stress induced by a permanent elongation will diminish with time – the material slowly relaxing, although it remains extended. This effect was shown, for the rabbit anterior cruciate ligament,

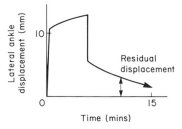

Fig. 1.5 Lateral deflection of the ankle, showing creep of medial collateral ligament under load, *in vivo* (from Pope *et al.*, 1976).

10

by Viidik (1966), who stretched the ligament until the tension reached 100 N, then kept the ligament at that extension. The load fell to 84 N after 2 min. Cyclic stress relaxation was demonstrated by Woo, Gomez and Akeson (1981) in the canine knee medial collateral ligament. After cycling the structure between 1.6 and 2.4% extension ten times in 160 sec, the peak stress had relaxed from 7.8 to 6.5 MPa. These results imply that tight ligaments will relax given time.

The literature of mechanical testing of the time-dependent properties of ligaments thus suggests that joints will not be stabilized by opposing sets of tensed ligamentous structures but, rather, that the ligaments will act progressively after allowing some small mobility. The progressive increase in resistance is caused by the increasing ligament stiffness with extension. Examination of cadaveric joints normally shows greater mobility than is apparent *in vivo*: the cadaver knee has 20° freedom for rotation of the tibia on the femur, compared with the 9° apparent when walking (Trent, Walker and Wolf, 1976). Similarly, the normal elbow does not appear to have a range of varus/valgus motion when examined clinically, yet the cadaveric joint allows the carrying angle to vary 9° at any angle of flexion (Amis *et al*, 1977). One must therefore conclude that it is the muscles which provide the initial joint stability in use, and that the ligaments act only after these active stabilizing actions have been overcome. Furthermore, attempts at prosthetic ligament replacement should allow sufficient free motion of joints, so that the stabilizing actions of the muscles and the joint geometry can be used to relieve the duty of the implant (Trent, Walker and Wolf, 1976).

1.3.3 THE EFFECT OF AGE ON MECHANICAL PROPERTIES

The morphological changes in ligament material associated with maturation were reviewed by Tkaczuk (1968), who found that the collagen fibres enlarge, and hence the water content (associated with the ground substance) diminishes. The effects of this are to increase the stiffness of the material and to cause it to rupture at a lower strain. This does not necessarily mean that mature ligaments rupture at a lower elongation than immature structures, because the changes in the ligament may be overshadowed by bony changes. This is shown by Fig. 1.6, the result of tensile tests on rabbit femur–anterior cruciate ligament–tibia specimens. The bone shafts were clamped into the test machine, in the posture shown in Fig. 1.6, then separated at a speed of 200 mm/min, after severing the joint capsule and other ligaments. The immature specimens failed by femoral epiphyseal separation. The mature specimens were stiffer, and failed by tibial or femoral bone avulsion, or ligament rupture, or a combination of these. Although this is an extreme example, it does

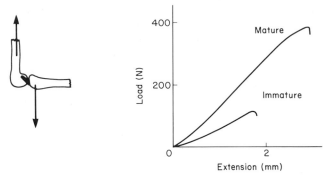

Fig. 1.6 Changing tensile behaviour with age, for rabbit anterior cruciate ligaments tested in the manner shown (from Amis, unpublished).

illustrate the clinical trend: juveniles presenting with epiphyseal traction lesions and their elders, who may have undergone similar injury mechanisms, presenting with ligament ruptures.

Further ageing of the material leads to degeneration, which gives easily demonstrable changes in mechanical behaviour. These are shown by Fig. 1.7, derived from the results of Noyes and Grood (1976), when testing the human femur–anterior cruciate ligament–tibia specimens from two age groups. Those from the age group 16–26 years had tensile strength, stiffness, and energy absorbtion properties averaging 2.4 times those in the age group 48–83 years. Not all of these large changes should be attributed to ligamentous material degeneration, though, because the ageing process also involves progressive weakening of the bones, and hence of the ligament anchorages. The anchorage zones normally have a

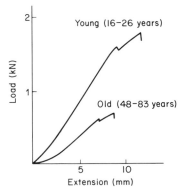

Fig. 1.7 The effect of degenerative changes with age on the tensile strength of the human anterior cruciate ligament (from Noyes and Grood, 1976).

12

thin cortical shell overlaying cancellous bone. Osteoporosity causes the cortical material to weaken, which is associated with reduced bone thickness, especially in females (Martin and Atkinson, 1977), so that bones fail under smaller loads, at lower deformations (Vose, Stover and Mack, 1961; Burstein, Reilly and Martens, 1976). Cancellous bone is affected dramatically by ageing: Weaver and Chalmers (1966) found that its strength dropped by nearly an order of magnitude with age. It is not surprising, then, that bone changes overshadow the ligament changes with age, leading to the mechanism of failure altering from ligamentous rupture to bone avulsion fractures (Noyes and Grood, 1976).

The most important factor shown by this section is that surgical repair processes which may be quite adequate for an elderly person, whose anterior cruciate will fail at 700 N load, will probably be totally inadequate for a younger subject with a ligament strength of 1700 N.

1.3.4 THE EFFECTS OF EXERCISE OR IMMOBILIZATION ON LIGAMENT STRENGTH

The immobilization of a limb creates effects similar to those seen during ageing. It has been noted that joint ligaments are among the most static in the body, with respect to metabolism, so their collagen turnover is low (Viidik, 1966). One would therefore expect only small changes to the ligaments, but greater changes in their bony anchorages. A difficulty which arises in experimental work on this subject is that caged laboratory animals probably suffer from disuse effects prior to any training or immobilization experiment (Noyes, DeLucas and Torvik, 1974), which explains the prevalence of bone avulsions seen in experiments, rather than ligament ruptures seen in life. This was shown by Laros, Tipton and Cooper (1971) for the collateral ligaments of the canine knee. The medial ligament had a strength of 3.3 × body weight in active animals, which was reduced 15% after 9 weeks in a cage, or 39% after 9 weeks in a plaster cast. These changes were principally due to subperiosteal bone resorption, leaving the collateral ligaments only a vascular fibrous tissue anchorage. Muscle weight returned to normal 12–18 weeks after activity recommenced but bone remineralization was only apparent after 12 weeks, and was not complete at 24 weeks. The ligaments had not regained full strength at 30 weeks, a fact which should be borne in mind when deciding when a sportsman can return to activity after injury, for example. Very similar results were shown by Noyes et al. (1974) for the anterior cruciate ligament in monkeys, the stiffness changes being summarized by Fig. 1.8.

The animals were immobilized for 8 weeks, some returning towards normal for a further 20 weeks. There was no significant effect on

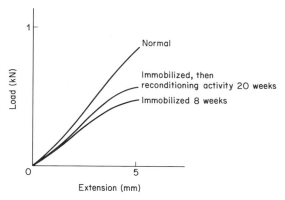

Fig. 1.8 The reduction in stiffness of the anterior cruciate ligament caused by 8 weeks' immobilization, showing that normal behaviour is not recovered after a further 20 weeks of reconditioning activity. Extension curves arbitrarily cut-off at 5 mm (from Noyes *et al.*, 1974).

elongation to failure, but the strength fell 39% after immobilization, and was still diminished 21% after 20 weeks of reconditioning activity. The stiffness changes must reflect a diminution of the ligaments themselves, although the strength change was caused largely by bone failures.

As might be expected, exercise leads to the opposite effects: a study of the rat anterior cruciate ligament (Cabaud *et al.*, 1980) showing significant increases in strength and stiffness of the ligaments after training.

1.4 The actions of ligaments at joints

1.4.1 GENERAL MECHANICAL PRINCIPLES

Having examined the properties of ligaments as isolated specimens, we are now able to use that data in its correct context – as part of a joint mechanism. The purpose of this section is to look at joints in their entirety, to elucidate some general principles relating to the functional reasons for joint architecture being what it normally is. This discussion will, of course, concentrate on the way in which ligaments act to stabilize joints and control movements.

(a) Lateral stability of joints

Many joints act in a hinge-like manner, in which one bone may move in an arc of flexion-extension in relation to the other (stationary) bone. The movement is not necessarily in a truly circular arc about a fixed axis, nor need it be confined to occur in a single plane, but, roughly speaking, even

14

the complexities of the knee joint lead to a hinge-like action. If motion is confined to this arc, then ligaments are needed to provide control over other movements, often in conjunction with the articular geometry. This is normally done by collateral ligaments situated on the sides of the joint, originating close to the joint axis, about which motion occurs, and passing to the other bone (Fig. 1.9(a)). It is immediately obvious that these are able to resist distraction of the joint (that is, a tension tending to separate the bones in a lengthwise direction). It is this property which allows them to resist moments tending to produce valgus or varus angulations, in combination with a compressive force within the joint. The bones of hinge-type joints are normally widened, in a direction along the flexion axis, to aid stability, often being adapted into a bicondylar form. The externally applied moment seen in Fig. 1.9(b) will cause the bones to rotate about the centre of rotation marked within one condyle. The other condyle will lift from the opposing bone until restrained by a ligament tension. Consideration of the leverage which the ligament tension produces, about the centre of rotation, shows that joint width aids stability. This, in other words, means that a small ligament tension will stabilize a wide joint.

One side-effect of this is that the design of a joint replacement may affect the ligament tensions required for stability, as shown in Fig. 1.10(a) and (b), where it can be seen that two prostheses with the same overall width may have very different stabilities. Thus the narrow intercondylar types tend to require larger ligament tensions than normal for stability.

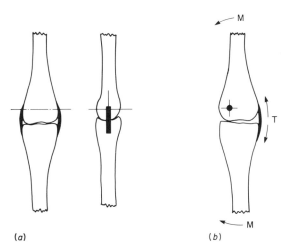

(a)   (b)

Fig. 1.9 (a) Collateral ligaments normally originate close to the flexion axis, on a wide bone end. (b) The externally applied moment M causes a collateral ligament tension T as the bones start to rotate about the condylar axis +.

Ligament Injuries and their Treatment

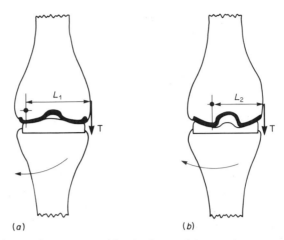

(a)   (b)

Fig. 1.10 Joint replacements with similar width may have different stability, depending on the location of the condylar centre of rotation, about which tilting occurs. Joint (b) is less stable, hence requiring greater ligament tensions for equilibrium, as L_2 is less than L_1.

(b) Limitation of motion

If a joint allows a large arc of motion, then various parts of the capsule surrounding it will have to accommodate large relative movements of the bones. Since the capsule will not normally be stretched, it follows that movement away from one extreme will lead to slackness. Capsular ligaments tend, therefore, to be very thin structures, to allow flexibility. They are normally found at the front and back of hinge joints, and all around spherical joints. The capsular structures tend to be broad sheets of tissue, thus remaining strong despite being thin. They are often augmented by an intimate relationship with overlying muscle tissues, for example, gastrocnemius over the femoral condyles, or brachialis over the humeral trochlea.

It can be seen in Fig. 1.11, that the taut capsular ligament has been deflected from a straight path by the intervening bulk of the articulation. This feature is typical of many joints. It causes the ligament tension to act at a greater distance from the joint axis. Since the restraining moment is the product of tension and moment arm, it follows that this geometry decreases the necessary capsular tensions.

(c) Progressive control of motion

This section concerns effects which constrain motion to occur within certain boundaries, rather than the limitation which arrests motion. This type of restraint normally depends on the ligaments' tension or degree of

16

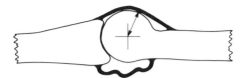

Fig. 1.11 The bulk of the articulation maintains the moment arm of the taut capsule from the joint axis, thus decreasing the tension required for equilibrium.

slackness varying with the posture of the joint. The variation of tension arises because the ligament origin does not coincide with the axis of the joint. At the metacarpophalangeal (mcp) joints, the collateral ligaments originate from tuberosities on the metacarpal bones (Wise, 1974) which are both proximal and dorsal to the flexion axis (Hagert, 1981). It has been reported that the eccentric location of their origin means that the collateral ligaments are slack when the metacarpophalangeal joint is extended, and tighten progressively as the joint flexes. This mechanism, in combination with the changing contour of the metacarpal head, allows a range of abduction–adduction of the finger, about the metacarpal head, when the metacarpophalangeal joint is extended, but causes it to diminish during flexion until there is no laxity at full flexion (Smith and Kaplan, 1967; Schultz, 1982).

A similar aspect is demonstrated at the knee, where the range of axial rotation of the tibia with respect to the femur gradually diminishes as the joint extends, culminating in the 'screw home' movement – an external rotation of the tibia, of approximately 9° when walking (Kapandji, 1970; Levens, Inman and Blosser 1948), after which there is no rotational laxity between the bones. This effect is caused by the ligaments tightening, the external rotation being due primarily to tension in the anterior cruciate ligament at full extension (Wang, Walker and Wolf, 1973; Kennedy, Weinberg and Wilson, 1974).

(d) Torque transmission

It was mentioned earlier that the lateral enlargement of bones, from the diaphysis towards the joint line, increases stability of the joint against laterally acting moments which tend to tilt one bone relative to the other. A byproduct of this form is that the joint is better adapted to transmit torque loads (that is, couples tending to produce rotation about the long axis) from bone to bone. The structure becomes analogous to the flanged coupling design of joints in transmission shafts (Fig. 1.12 (a)). Each of the shafts may be highly stressed by the torque load that it carries, but the shearing forces acting on the bolts (which transmit the torque across the joint between the flanges) are diminished by placing them at a large

17

Ligament Injuries and their Treatment

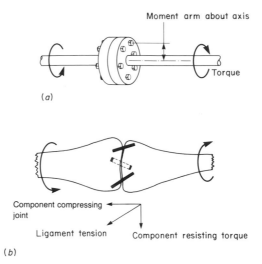

Moment arm about axis

Torque

(a)

Component compressing joint

Ligament tension

Component resisting torque

(b)

Fig. 1.12 (a) The large radius of the flanged joint diminishes the forces on the coupling bolts when transmitting a torque. (b) The spiral path of ligaments on wide bone ends transmits torque, the tensions also causing joint compression.

radius from the axis, because radius from the axis is analogous to 'leverage' about the axis. Some joints, of course, have their articular surfaces shaped in such a manner that the joint itself may transmit some torque, but the ligamentous and capsular structures usually augment this, as increasing torsion causes the bone ends to 'climb uphill' out of a close-packed arrangement. The relative movement of the bones causes the ligaments to tighten into a spiralling arrangement compared with their unloaded positions. Furthermore, many joints include spiralling components in their structures (for example, on the posterior aspect of the knee or the metacarpophalangeal collaterals). The slanting direction of the ligamentous or capsular tensions leads to an axial joint compression force, which augments the stabilizing effect of the joint surfaces, as well as the transverse component directly opposing torsion (Fig. 1.12 (b)).

1.4.2 DIFFERENTIAL ACTIONS WITHIN LIGAMENTS

The purpose of this section is to highlight the fact that ligaments are usually broad ribbons of collagenous material linking areas on adjacent bones, rather than thin string-like structures going from point to point. The result of this difference is that the function of the structures is more complex than might be imagined at first, a tendency which increases the problems of those who wish to design or implant artificial ligaments for example.

18

(a)   Tension differentials within ligaments

One direct consequence of the fact that ligaments originate from *areas* of bone surface is that only one point in a ligament origin can be coincident with the axis of rotation of a joint at any time. Thus a flexion motion will cause some fibres to tighten and others to slacken, as shown in Fig. 1.13. This phenomenon has been measured on the medial collateral ligament of the knee by Arms *et al.* (1982), although they did not seem to realize its cause, giving a result similar to that shown in Fig. 1.13.

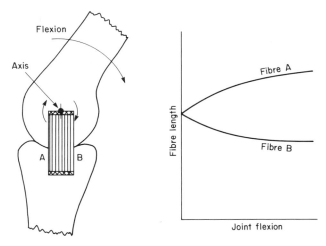

Fig. 1.13   The ligament origin is on both sides of the flexion axis, so flexion will tighten some fibres and slacken others.

The differential tightening behaviour is seen in an exaggerated form at other sites, where a separation of ligament fibres into discernible bundles has occurred. The anterior and posterior bands of the medial collateral ligament of the elbow are a good example. Their fibres originate from an area around the base of the medial humeral epicondyle. The anterior band passes distally, to the ulnar coronoid process, parallel to the forearm. Extension of the elbow joint causes this structure to tighten, as shown in Fig. 1.14(a), causing it to be the major passive stabilizer of the extended elbow against valgus actions. In normal conditions it is assisted by those muscles which originate from the common flexor origin, predominantly flexor digitorum superficialis. The posterior band tightens when the elbow is flexed, partly because the fibres have to pass around the posterior corner of the epicondyle (Fig. 1.14(b)). This band helps to stabilize the ulna against 'rolling' into pronation, the humero-ulnar

19

Ligament Injuries and their Treatment

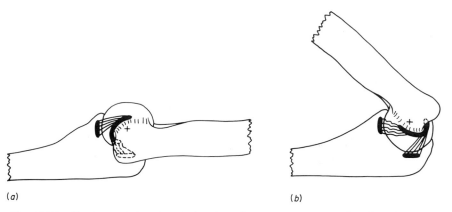

(a)   (b)

Fig. 1.14 Reciprocal tension behaviour between separate bands of medial collateral ligament of elbow: (*a*) elbow extension tightens anterior band; (*b*) flexion tightens posterior band.

articulation being much less stable in flexion, and valgus actions being diminished along with the carrying angle.

The anterior cruciate ligament is a more complex example of differential tightening phenomena, there being considerable controversy about its function, and hence its response to trauma. The more recent publications (such as Norwood and Cross, 1979; Welsh, 1980) have emphasized the differing roles of bundles of fibres within the ligament, the functions of which are made more difficult to discern by their spiralling path between origin and insertion. The situation has been confused by the publication of measurements of fibre lengths and tensions, which have neglected to allow for the complexity of the structure (Wang, Walker and Wolf, 1973; Trent, Walker and Wolf, 1976; Tremblay, Laurin and Drovin, 1980; Jasty, Lew and Lewis, 1982). A realistic summary seems to be that the wide areas of origin and insertion, allied to a 90° twist in the structure, allow some part of the ligament to be taut at any angle of knee flexion, while other parts are slack (Lam, 1968; Girgis, Marshall and Monajem, 1975). It has been reported that all the fibres have a uniform low tension, or even slackness, at 45° flexion (Kennedy, Weinberg and Wilson, 1974; Noyes, DeLucas and Torvik, 1974). This is in line with the finding that the anteromedial fibres are taut in extension, and the posterolateral fibres taut in flexion, as shown in Fig. 1.15 (Cowan, 1965; Smillie, 1970).

(b) *Strain differentials within ligaments*

Just as tensions in various parts of a ligament structure can vary because of the size of the areas of anchorage to bone, so too can the strains induced by the relative movements of the anchorages, even if all the fibres have

20

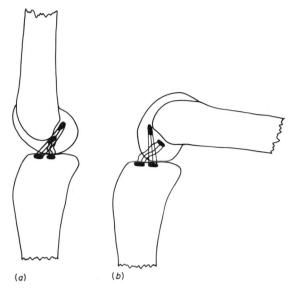

(a)   (b)

Fig. 1.15 (a) The anteromedial bundle of the anterior cruciate ligament is tight in extension, and (b) the posterolateral band is tight in flexion.

equal initial tension. This phenomenon is detailed in Fig. 1.16, which shows that when the bone anchorages move apart the shorter fibres undergo a greater strain (extension as a proportion of original length) than do the longer fibres. If this particular ligamentous material ruptures at 30% strain, say, then it means that the longer fibres will remain intact

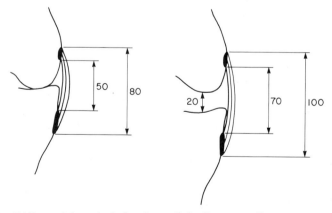

Fig. 1.16 Differential strain behaviour: if the ligament fibres rupture at 30–35% extension, the deep fibres will be ruptured and the superficial fibres intact when the bones move apart as shown, giving a deep fibre strain of 40% and a superficial fibre strain of 25%.

after the shorter fibres have failed. This mechanism is sometimes demonstrated at the medial collateral ligament of the knee, in which deep and superficial layers are discernible. The deep layer inserts into the tibia close to the joint line, while the superficial layer is mobile at this level and inserts distally (Mains, Andrews and Stonecipher, 1977). A valgus stress may rupture the deep layer of the ligament, while the superficial structure is intact, because of the differential strain phenomenon.

1.4.3 LIGAMENT LOADS AND STRAINS IN USE

Although, for a ligament, the imposition of a certain load will lead to a particular strain, ligament loads or strains in use have normally been studied as though they were unrelated phenomena.

The tensions in various ligaments have been estimated by biomechanical analyses of varying complexity. Such analyses normally commence by measuring an external force (for example, between foot and floor, or fingers on a lever), then model the internal structures in a form which allows mathematical analysis. This always involves assumptions regarding the sharing of muscle actions and the geometry of the system. If the forces thus calculated do not lead to equilibrium, then ligament tensions are invoked, to provide joint stability. This sort of exercise has normally aimed to provide data about joint forces (for prosthesis designers, for example), and perturbations in the muscle force sharing tend to have less effect on the predicted joint forces than on the marginal ligament forces which complete the picture. One should be aware, therefore, that published values of ligament forces may depend greatly on arbitrary choices (as far as the ligaments are concerned) made during a mathematical procedure deriving joint forces. Furthermore, since the ligamentous forces are often of secondary importance, when compared with muscle and joint forces, their structures and load-sharing characteristics may have been modelled in a manner which is oversimplified for the purpose of studying the ligaments.

One of the better-known analyses of joint forces examined the knee joint when subjects walked on level ground, steps, or ramps (Morrison, 1968, 1969). This work remains a classic for those interested in joint forces, but was completed prior to other work examining the manner in which the ligamentous and capsular structures share forces imposed across the knee joint. For example, Grood et al. (1981) showed that the collateral ligaments contribute only about 55% of the passive resistance of valgus or varus loadings at 5° flexion, the remainder being shared by the cruciate ligaments and joint capsule. Similarly, Piziali et al. (1980 a and b) and Butler et al. (1981) found that the cruciates may contribute only approximately 80% of the passive resistance to anterior-posterior shearing of the knee and are also the major stabilizers against lateral shearing actions. The incorporation of this sort of data into Morrison's analysis would change the predicted ligament tensions, but scarcely affect the joint force predictions.

Morrison predicted a maximal anterior cruciate ligament force of 445 N, when descending stairs, for example. This is similar to the predictions of Grood and Noyes (1976), who suggested a working load of 400 N, being 20% of the breaking load, or 360 N, being the force required to produce a 10% elongation. This latter suggestion was based on an analysis of strains in use (Wang, Walker and Wolf, 1973), which implies that stretching of the ligaments occurs because of relative movements between origin and insertion during normal flexion/extension of the joint, causing considerable ligament tensions in some joint postures, and hence also joint forces. A similar result was found by Tremblay, Laurin and Drovin (1980), who inserted a catheter along the anterior cruciate ligament, filled it with radiopaque dye and measured 14% strain during flexion/extension. If these results are correct, the ligament extensions must cause tensions even during passive joint movements, which will be in addition to the tensions needed to resist externally applied forces. The implication is that ligament reconstructions or replacements will have to accommodate to considerable elongations caused by the shapes of the bone ends, as well as by elastic stretching following external loading. This may be exacerbated by malpositioning of the bony attachments, which is sometimes done intentionally in order to take up ligamentous laxity. If this is to be done, then the geometrical implications must be examined so that the most efficacious site may be chosen, and excessive elongations avoided (Bartel et al., 1977).

1.4.4 POSTURAL EFFECTS ON LIGAMENT STRENGTH

Having read above that there are often tension and/or strain differentials between the fibres of a ligament, which depend on the geometry and relative movements of the bony anchorages, the reader may well have anticipated postural effects on the failure strength of ligaments. These have been well documented for the anterior cruciate ligament which, it was noted, has a changing pattern of fibre tensions with joint flexion. Two studies of canine knees, by Figgie et al. (1982) and Hurley, Cannon and Haynes (1982) found similar results: that when the ligament was stretched to failure by moving the tibia distally, the bone–ligament–bone specimen was strongest with the joint in full extension, when the failure was normally by avulsion of part of the tibial plateau, and had only 40% of this strength when the joint was flexed 90%, when the ligaments themselves failed. Thus both the ease with which a ligament may be

Ligament Injuries and their Treatment

damaged and the form which the damage takes both appear to be affected by the posture at the time of injury. A lower strength may be caused by differential tensions across the width of a ligament, so that tearing commences from the fibres which are initially tight. The failure mode may be affected by the direction in which tension is applied because this may load one side of an anchorage more than the other, causing a bone fragment to be lifted out.

The directional sensitivity, for a fixed posture, has been examined in the author's laboratory, using rabbit anterior cruciate specimens. The femur and tibia were always flexed 90°, but the bones were pulled apart, at 1000 mm/min. in various directions, as shown in Fig. 1.17. The high strength of this ligament in the rabbit (approximately 400 N, or eight to ten times body weight) meant that bone fractures were more common than ligament ruptures, especially since the bones of the caged laboratory animals used will have been atrophic. When the bones were distracted along the tibial axis (Fig. 1.17 (a)), the most common failure was an avulsion of part of the tibial plateau. Tension along the femoral axis – Fig. 1.17 (c) – produced avulsions of femoral condyles or intercondylar bone. The intermediate position caused the load to pass along the ligament from anchorage to anchorage, rather than causing the ligament to 'swing' into line under tension. The ligament itself tended to rupture in this posture, rather than the bones fracturing. Since this tended to be at a slightly higher load than in the other positions, it seems that the bone anchorages had then failed prematurely, due to eccentric loading.

This data helps to explain the diversity of joint injuries, the nature of which have been shown to vary with joint posture, the direction in which the injurious force is applied and even, as noted above, on the speed with

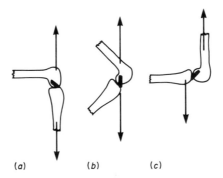

(a)   (b)   (c)

Fig. 1.17 Tensile tests of anterior cruciate ligament, with knee flexed 90°, in several directions: (a) load axis parallel to tibia causes tibial avulsion fracture; (b) ligament, bone, or combined failures occur in this test, at a higher force than in (a) or (c); (c) load axis parallel to femur leads to femoral fractures.

24

which the injury occurs. Thus it is not surprising that different research-ers have sometimes produced apparently contradictory results, and that clinicians often cannot agree about what has happened to a joint. It is the present author's hope that this chapter has brought together many aspects of the mechanical behaviour of ligaments, and discussed them in a manner which helps them to be seen in context and related to each other, thus explaining some of the clinical observations to be found later in the book.

Acknowledgements

The experimental work has been ably performed by Mr Derek Light, and was funded by the Arthritis and Rheumatism Council, to whom we are most grateful.

References

Amis, A. A., Dowson, D., Wright, V., Miller, J. H. and Unsworth, A. (1977), An examination of the elbow articulation, with particular reference to the variation of the carrying angle. *Eng. Med.*, **6**, 76–80.

Arms, S. W., Pope, M. H., Boyle, J. B., Davignon, P. J. and Johnson, R. J. (1982), Knee medial collateral ligament strain. *Proceedings 28th Annual ORS, New Orleans*, p. 47.

Bartel, D. L., Marshall, J. L., Schieck, R. A. and Wang, J. B. (1977), Surgical repositioning of the medial collateral ligament. An anatomical and mechanical analysis. *J. Bone Joint Surg.*, **59A**, 107–16.

Burstein, A. H., Reilly, D. T. and Martens, M. (1976), Ageing of bone tissue: mechanical properties. *J. Bone Joint Surg.*, **58A**, 82–6.

Butler, D. L., Noyes, F. R., Grood, E. S. and Miller, E. H. (1981), Ligamentous restraints in the human knee: anterior-posterior stability. *Proceedings 27th Annual ORS*, pp. 161–2.

Cabaud, H. E., Chatty, A., Gildengorin, V. and Feltman, R. J. (1980), Exercise effects on the strength of the rat anterior cruciate ligament. *Am. J. Sports Med.*, **8**, 79–86.

Cowan, D. J. (1965), Reconstruction of the anterior cruciate ligament by the method of Kenneth Jones. *Proceed. Roy. Soc. Med.*, **58**, 336–8.

Dorlot, J. M., Ait Ba Sidi, M., Tremblay, G. M. and Drouin, G. (1980), Load elongation behaviour of the canine anterior cruciate ligament. *J. Biomech. Eng.*, **102**, 190–3.

Figgie, H. E., Bahniuk, E. H., Heiple, K. G. and Davy, D. T. (1982), The effects of tibial-femoral angle on the failure mechanics of the canine anterior cruciate ligament. *Proceedings 28th Annual ORS, New Orleans*, p. 309.

Girgis, F. G., Marshall, J. L. and Monajem, A. R. S. (1975), The cruciate ligaments of the knee joint. *Clin. Orthop.*, **106**, 216–31.

Ligament Injuries and their Treatment

Grood, E. S. and Noyes, F. R. (1976), Cruciate ligament prosthesis: strength, creep, and fatigue properties. *J. Bone Joint Surg.*, **58A**, 1083–8.

Grood, E. S., Noyes, F. R., Butler, D. L. and Suntay, W. J. (1981), Ligamentous and capsular restraints preventing straight medial and lateral laxity in intact human cadaver knees. *J. Bone Joint Surg.*, **63A**, 1257–69.

Hagert, C. G. (1981), Anatomical aspects on the design of metacarpophalangeal implants. *Reconst. Surg. Traumatol.*, **18**, 92–110.

Ham, A. W. (1953), *Histology*. Lippincott, Philadelphia, p. 840.

Hurley, P. B., Cannon, H. C. and Haynes, D. W. (1982), The functional strength of the canine anterior cruciate ligament. *Proceedings 28th Annual ORS, New Orleans*, p. 357.

Jasty, M., Lew, W. D. and Lewis, J. L. (1982), *In vitro* ligament forces in the normal knee using buckle transducers. *Proceedings 28th Annual ORS, New Orleans*, p. 241.

Kapandji, I. A. (1970), *The Physiology of the Joints, Vol. 2: The Lower Limb*. Churchill Livingstone, Edinburgh, p. 134.

Kennedy, J. C., Weinberg, H. W. and Wilson, A. S. (1974), The anatomy and function of the anterior cruciate ligament, as determined by clinical and morphological studies. *J. Bone Joint Surg.*, **56 A**, 223–35.

Kennedy, J. C., Hawkins, R. J., Willis, R. B. and Danylchuk, K. D. (1976), Tension studies of human knee ligaments: yield point, ultimate failure, and disruption of the cruciate and tibial collateral ligaments. *J. Bone Joint Surg.*, **58A**, 350–5.

Kennedy, J. C., Roth, J. H., Mendenhall, H. V. and Sanford, J. B. (1980), Intraarticular replacement in the anterior cruciate ligament-deficient knee. *Am. J. Sports Med.*, **8**, 1–8.

LaBan, M. M. (1962), Collagen tissue: implications of its response to stress *in vitro*. *Arch. Physical Med. Rehabil.*, **43**, 461–6.

Lam, S. J. S. (1968), Reconstruction of the anterior cruciate ligament using the Jones procedure and its Guy's Hospital modification. *J. Bone Joint Surg.*, **50A**, 1213–24.

Laros, G. S., Tipton, C. M. and Cooper, R. R. (1971), Influence of physical activity on ligament insertions in the knees of dogs. *J. Bone Joint Surg.*, **53A**, 275–86.

Levens, A. S., Inman, V. T. and Blosser, J. A. (1948), Transverse rotations of the segments of the lower extremity in locomotion. *J. Bone Joint Surg.*, **30A**, 859–72.

Mains, D. B., Andrews, J. L. and Stonecipher, T. (1977), Medial and A–P ligamentous stability of the human knee measured with a stress apparatus. *Am. J. Sports Med.*, **5**, 144–53.

Martin, R. B. and Atkinson, P. J. (1977), Age and sex-related changes in the structure and strength of the human femoral shaft. *J. Biomech.*, **10**, 223–32.

Morrison, J. B. (1968), Bioengineering analysis of force actions transmitted by the knee joint. *Biomed. Eng.*, **3**, 164–70.

Morrison, J. B. (1969), Function of the knee joint in various activities. *Biomed. Eng.*, **4**, 573–80.

Norwood, L. A. and Cross, M. J. (1979), Anterior cruciate ligament: functional anatomy of its bundles in rotatory instabilities. *Am. J. Sports Med.*, **7**, 23–6.

Noyes, F. R. and Grood, E. S. (1976), The strength of the anterior cruciate ligament in humans and rhesus monkeys: age-related and species-related changes. *J. Bone Joint Surg.*, **58A**, 1074–82.

Noyes, F. R., DeLucas, J. L. and Torvik, P. J. (1974), Biomechanics of anterior cruciate ligament failure: an analysis of strain-rate sensitivity and mechanisms of failure in primates. *J. Bone Joint Surg.*, **56A**, 236–53.

Noyes, F. R., Torvik, P. J., Hyde, W. B. and DeLucas, J. L. (1974), Biomechanics of ligament failure II. An analysis of immobilisation, exercise, and reconditioning effects in primates. *J. Bone Joint Surg.*, **56A**, 1406–18.

Panjabi, M. M., White, A. A. and Southwick, W. O. (1973), Mechanical properties of bone as a function of rate of deformation. *J. Bone and Joint Surg.*, **53A**, 322–30.

Piziali, R. L., Seering, W. P., Nagel, D. A. and Schurman, D. J. (1980(a)), The function of the primary ligaments of the knee in anterior posterior and medial-lateral motions. *J. Biomech.*, **13**, 777–84.

Piziali, R. L., Rastegar, J., Nagel, D. A. and Schurman, D. J. (1980(b)), The contribution of the cruciate ligaments to the load-displacement characteristics of the human knee joint. *J. Biomech. Eng.*, **102**, 277–83.

Pope, M. H. and Outwater, J. O. (1974), Mechanical properties of bone as a function of position and orientation. *J. Biomech.*, **7**, 61–6.

Pope, M. H., Crowninshield, R., Miller, R. und Johnson, R. (1976), The static and dynamic behaviour of the human knee *in vivo*. *J. Biomech.*, **9**, 449–52.

Rigby, B. J., Hirai, N., Spikes, J. D. and Eyring, H. (1959), The mechanical properties of rat tail tendon. *J. Gen. Physiol.*, **43**, 265–83.

Schultz, R. J. (1982), *Total Metacarpophalangeal Joint Arthroplasty with Limited Metacarpal Head Resection. Total Joint Replacement of the Upper Extremity.* C. V. Mosby, St Louis, pp. 199–216.

Smillie, I. S. (1970), *Injuries of the Knee Joint.* Livingstone, London, pp. 130–50.

Smith, J. W. (1954), The elastic properties of the anterior cruciate ligament of the rabbit. *J. Anat.*, **88**, 369–81.

Smith, R. J. and Kaplan, E. B. (1967), Rheumatoid deformities at the meta-carpophalangeal joints of the fingers. A correlative study of anatomy and pathology. *J. Bone Joint Surg.*, **49A**, 31–47.

Tkaczuk, H. (1968), Tensile properties of human lumbar longitudinal ligaments. *Acta Orthop. Scand.*, Suppl. 115.

Tremblay, G. R., Laurin, C. A. and Drovin, G. (1980), The challenge of prosthetic cruciate ligament replacement. *Clin. Orthop.*, **147**, 88–92.

Trent, P. S., Walker, P. S. and Wolf, B. (1976), Ligament length patterns, strength, and rotational axes of the knee joint. *Clin. Orthop. Rel. Res.*, **117**, 263–70.

Viidik, A. (1966), Biomechanics and functional adaption of tendons and joint ligaments in *Studies on the Anatomy and Function of Bone and Joints* (ed. F. G. Evans), Springer, Berlin, pp. 17–39.

Vose, G. P., Stover, B. J. and Mack, P. B. (1961), Quantitative bone strength measurements in senile osteoporosis. *J. Gerontol.*, **16**, 120–24.

Wang, C. J., Walker, P. S. and Wolf, B. (1973), The effects of flexion and rotation on the length patterns of the ligaments of the knee. *J. Biomech.*, **6**, 587–96.

Weaver, J. K. and Chalmers, J. (1966), Cancellous bone: its strength and changes with ageing and an evaluation of some methods for measuring its mineral content. Part 1: Age changes in cancellous bone. Part 2: Osteoporosis. *J. Bone Joint Surg.*, **48A**, 289–308.

Welsh, R. P. (1980), Knee joint structure and function. *Clin. Orthop.*, **147**, 7–14.

Wise, K. S. (1974), The anatomy of the metacarpo-phalangeal joints with observations of the aetiology of ulnar drift. *J. Bone Joint Surg.*, **57B**, 485–90.

Woo, S. L. Y., Gomez, M. A. and Akeson, W. H. (1981), The time and history-dependent viscoelastic properties of the canine medial collateral ligament. *J. Biomech. Eng.*, **103**, 293–8.

Wright, T. M. and Hayes, W. C. (1976), Tensile testing of bone over a wide range of strain rates: effects of strain rate, microstructure and density. *Med Biol. Eng.*, **14**, 671–9.

2 Biomechanics of knee function and the ligaments of the knee

R. A. DENHAM

2.1 Introduction

It is important to remember that the knee joints are part of the complex musculoskeletal system which enables man to walk upright. Biomechanical factors should not be considered in isolation, for small changes in body posture greatly affect force transmission within all joints. The patient is balanced during standing so that the centre of gravity of the body is above and within the area covered by the margins of one or both feet. When the feet are wide apart the area is large, but balancing on tiptoe requires extremely accurate coordination (Fig. 2.1). An understanding of the mechanism by which forces are transmitted through the knee is necessary to any surgeon who operates upon that joint. It helps to appreciate the size and direction of these forces, their relationship to the line of action of the centre of gravity of the body, the shape of the joint surfaces, the position of the patella within the extensor mechanism and the thickness of the articular cartilage within the joint.

The forces transmitted by the knee are large, even under static conditions and when body weight and speed of action in the athlete are considered, it is remarkable how well the joint surfaces and the menisci stand up to sporting activity. Ligament injuries are frequent during contact games but damage is usually caused by external violence. Osgood–Schlatter's disease, patellofemoral pain, and other lesions of the extensor mechanism are also relevant. Before the transmitted forces are discussed, an important point related to the plane of movement and stress must be considered. This is, that small variations in posture, which move the position of the centre of gravity of the body in relation to the knee, may cause large differences in force transmission. In the sagittal plane, these changes are under voluntary control while in the coronal plane they are not; voluntary changes of posture can do little to diminish the destructive increase in force transmission which is caused by varus or valgus deformity (Fig. 2.2).

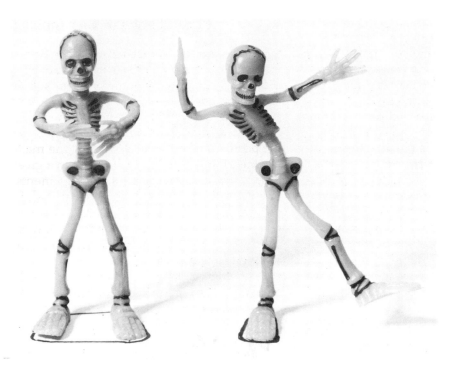

Fig. 2.1 When standing, the line of action of the centre of gravity of the whole body must be above the area bordered by the margins of the feet (or foot), if the line passes outside this area the model will fall.

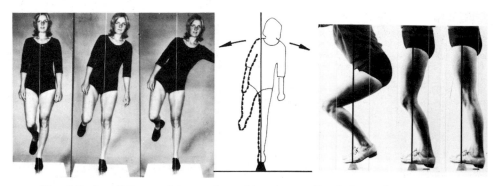

Fig. 2.2 In all these pictures, the subject is standing balanced upon a narrow wedge; a plumbline which intersects the centre of the wedge is shown. The centre of gravity of the body must be situated somewhere along this line for it must be directly above the supporting surface. The rotational effect of the parts of the body on the right of the line must equal exactly the rotational effect of those on the left. In the coronal plane changes in posture do not greatly affect the relationship between the line and the knee. In the sagittal plane, large variations do occur with alterations in the position of the trunk and limbs; force transmission in the knee changes dramatically with changes in posture.

Forces may be studied by measuring the distance between the line of body weight and the knee. This line can be located by asking a subject to balance on a narrow surface. The centre of gravity of the body must then be directly above this support and the line of action can be visualized and recorded on a radiograph by the use of a radiopaque plumbline which intersects the narrow surface. From the radiographs and the body weight, it is possible to determine the position, direction and value of the major forces which pass through the knee joint. Maintaining balance in a given position determines the need for muscle action and tension in ligaments.

In the *sagittal plane*, leaning backwards or forwards changes the distance between the line of body weight and the knee. If the line is moved away from the joint, muscle activity must be increased to maintain position and force transmission is greater. Conversely, the nearer the line is placed to the knee, the smaller is the active component, and the less the force passing through the different parts of the joint. These variations are not dependent upon the degree of flexion of the knee, but upon the posture of the body as a whole.

In the *coronal plane*, it can be seen (Fig. 2.3) that leaning to one side, by changing the posture of the trunk and upper limbs and abducting the hip of the supporting leg, causes only minor changes in the relationship between the centre of gravity of the body and the knee. The shape and

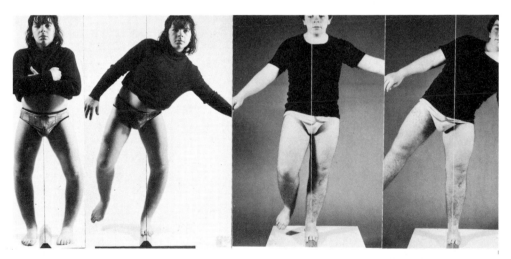

Fig. 2.3 This patient suffered from severe bilateral genu varum. When he stood upon one leg, his line of body weight passed well to the medial side of the left knee; leaning in either direction did not restore the line to its normal position; the medial condyle transmitted a greater force than the lateral condyle. Tibial osteotomy to restore normal leg alignment was performed. Postoperative pictures show that the centre of gravity of the body is now within the margins of the joint.

31

weight of the limbs and trunk are such, that significant additional varus or valgus forces are not put upon the normal knee. The *tibia remains almost vertical* and force transmission remains nearly perpendicular to the joint surface; the collateral ligaments are not stretched, and no additional closing action is required from the thigh muscles to protect the joint. But once a varus or valgus defomity has developed in the adult knee it will progress, for the increased force is transmitted through a fraction of the tibiofemoral joint surface. If the normal tibiofemoral angle is not restored accurately by operation, the ligaments and the joint surfaces will fail rapidly.

2.2 The forces involved

The work of Bishop (1977) and Denham and Bishop (1978) on static force transmission in the knee provides a key to an understanding of knee function, since the shape of the joint surfaces, the strength of the ligaments and muscles and the control of the position of the centre of gravity of the body are accurately related to the size and direction of the forces to which the knee will be subjected. These calculations are based upon the engineering analysis of line of body weight radiographs in the sagittal plane, and the practical application of line of leg alignment radiographs taken to show position in the coronal plane (Fig. 2.4).

Bishop has shown that axial force transmission in the femur, in the

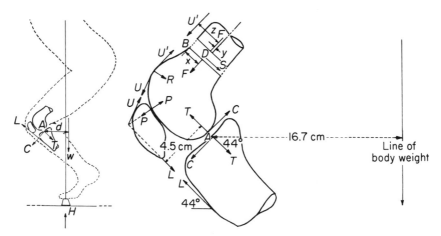

Fig. 2.4 Bishop's analysis of force transmission in the knee has been made from tracings of lateral radiographs which show the outline of the bones and the position of the line of body weight. From a series of these tracings the forces acting about the knee in different postures has been calculated.

patellofemoral joint and in the quadriceps expansion above the knee all rise to as much as six to eight times half body weight in each knee (each leg bearing half of the body weight) as the subject crouched to the ground. Tension in the patellar ligament and compression in the tibiofemoral joint also rise to high levels, but the shearing force at the tibiofemoral joint remains small, rising to a maximum of half body weight. The forces tending to produce anteroposterior glide are much smaller than the tibiofemoral compressive force (Fig. 2.5). During normal activity, tension in the cruciate ligaments will never be greater than about one-quarter of the force transmitted by the tibiofemoral joint. These large compressive forces across the joint surfaces are spread and transmitted through the large area of the articular surfaces and menisci and the especially thick articular cartilage of the patella and of the femoral and tibial surfaces. Any deformity at the knee can cause a great increase in force transmitted during activity since muscles and ligaments must exert a protective action to support the joint and these forces are added to the 'normal' forces acting on the knee (Fig. 2.6).

Normal anatomy in the coronal plane can be shown by radiographs taken of the whole leg, in a vertical, weight-bearing situation. A line drawn from the centre of the head of the femur to the centre of the talus should pass through the medial tibial spine in the normal patient

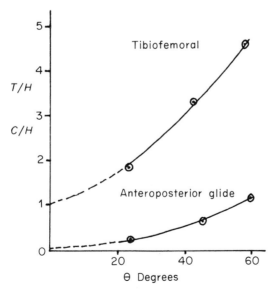

Fig. 2.5 As the subject crouches to the ground, the force pressing the tibia and the femur together is nearly four and a half times as great as the force at right angles to it which tends to sublux the knee (H is half body weight).

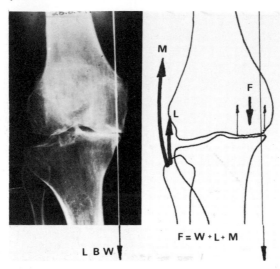

Fig. 2.6 With varus deformity, the line of action of body weight passes through the medial margin of the joint. Force is concentrated in a small area. Muscles and lateral ligaments act to preserve the joint; in this way joint pressure is increased and degenerative arthritis in the medial compartment is progressive. Meanwhile the load transmitted by the lateral tibiofemoral compartment is much reduced and disuse atrophy occurs.

LBW: line of body weight; F: tibiofemoral force transmission; M: muscle action; L: ligament tension.

(Maquet, 1972) (Fig. 2.7). A long film taken with the patient standing provides much greater accuracy than that obtained from a smaller radiograph, but it is important to be aware that rotation, in the presence of fixed flexion, can cause errors. Every effort must be made to obtain a truly anteroposterior view of the knee and to record radiologically (by a fully extended lateral view) the presence of any fixed flexion. When leg alignment is normal, normal force transmission occurs; with varus or valgus deformity, the forces passing through the joint are exaggerated. Increased force transmission associated with flexion or extension of the knee in the sagittal plane can easily be compensated by leaning the trunk forwards or backwards; but only very small errors in leg alignment in the coronal plane can be corrected. When varus or valgus deformity at the knee is more than 3° from normal, leaning to one side or the other does little to restore force transmission to normal. When deformity is more than 10°, the line of leg alignment is beyond the limits of the knee. Ligaments are strained, joint pressure rises steeply and deterioration is likely to occur.

34

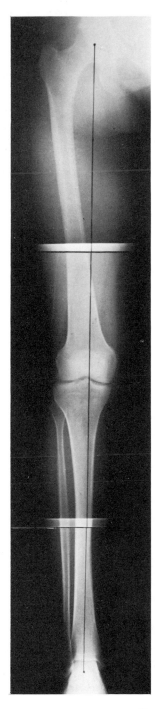

Fig. 2.7 In the normal leg alignment radiograph, a line which joins the centre of the femoral head to the centre of the body of the talus should pass through the medial tibial spine. The picture should be taken with one exposure using a 105.5 by 35.5 cm. Cronex 4 film in a 109.5 by 38 cm cassette with a Dupont Cronex screen at 180 cm from the knee using 100 mA for 0.05 sec at 105 kV, −5 to +10 according to the thickness of the leg.

2.3   The function of ligaments

Movement at the knee is mainly in one plane, with very little abduction or adduction, and limited rotation. Unwanted movements are restricted by the shape of the joint surfaces which are protected by strong sensitive ligaments. Muscles can thereby concentrate their effect upon the important movements of flexion and extension. This economy reduces the weight of the lower limb.

Ligaments act as strong sensitive check reins which ensure that the surfaces of a joint articulate correctly and function properly. These thickenings in the capsule help restrict the joint to its normal range of movement and are probably not stressed under gentle activity. During movement, they help to guide the surfaces. It can be demonstrated on a cadaver knee that the joint surfaces connected only by the cruciate and collateral ligaments will move passively with all the characteristics of a normal knee, including the screw home of full extension.

Excessive loads on the ligaments initiate protective muscle action through a neuromuscular reflex arc tending to close the joint and to minimize damage to soft tissues. When full muscle power is not sufficient to maintain the joint, or when the muscles are caught off guard or at a disadvantageous position, the capsule and one of more ligaments may be torn or avulsed from bone. Without the protective action of muscles and reflexes, ligaments are relatively weak, and as the femur and tibia are long compared with the width of the knee, the ligaments can easily be damaged. Ligaments which are deprived of their nerve supply become stretched and joint surfaces will be damaged by movement past their normal range. Failure of normal muscle action allows an increasing abnormality to develop and traumatic arthritis evolves as the range of abnormal movement increases.

Ligaments which have contracted after injury and inadequate treatment may cause painful limitation of movement. Recovery is sometimes prevented by reflex inhibition of muscle action and treatment by manipulation, with or without anaesthesia, followed by well-directed physiotherapy may be needed. The protection afforded to a joint by its ligaments is only part of the complex mechanism which guards it from abnormal movements. In the normal patient the relation between the line of body weight and the knee is constantly monitored by the sensory mechanisms of the body so that during static or dynamic conditions, muscle activity is varied to produce the correct posture. The importance of vision to normal action is illustrated by the difficulty of a jump from a window in the dark. It is probable that, at the point of landing, the centre of gravity of the body will be incorrectly placed, and an awkward fall may damage ligaments. From experience, a footballer has learned to rotate his leg so that a damaging force in the coronal plane of the knee is absorbed by harmless flexion. The ability to turn away from a hyperextending force can reduce the danger of ligament injury. Most injuries to the knee occur when the subject is not prepared for external violence or when the foot is temporarily immobilized.

The tension in the tendons above and below the patella are different during activity (Figs. 2.8 and 2.9). Furthermore, the direction of the compressive force at the patellofemoral joint is not midway between the tendons above and below the patella. The assumption that the forces above and below the patella are equal invalidates further calculations of force transmission. Tension in the extensor mechanism can be considerable in the normal patient, rising to between four and six times half body weight in each knee, even in a static crouching position. If surgical repair of the extensor mechanism is needed, it should be done very carefully and exercises started gently, so that suture lines are not strained.

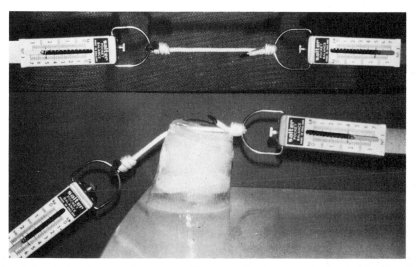

Fig. 2.8 A simple experiment can illustrate force transmission in the patello-femoral joint. An ice cube is placed at the edge of a smooth surface. A piece of string with a small spring balance at each end is stretched over the ice cube which is held near the edge of the table. One spring balance is pulled horizontally and the other is pulled in the opposite direction, but also 45° downwards over the end of the table. The friction between the ice and the table is very low. When the tension in each string is gently increased so that the ice cube does not move upon the table, it will be noted that the readings in the two spring balances are different. Some of the force exerted by the oblique pull is expended pressing the ice against the table top. A parallelogram of forces shows that the horizontal component exerted by both balances is the same.

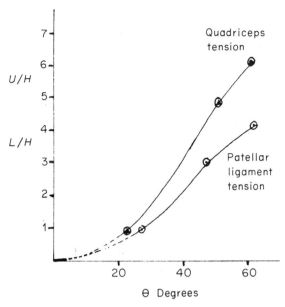

Fig. 2.9 Tension in the quadriceps tendon and in the patellar ligament is not the same during function of the knee. (Where U is the tension in the quadriceps tendon, L the tension in the patella ligament and H half the body weight).

The restoration of good extensor function is an important factor in all operations upon the knee joint. This is difficult because of the complexity of the patellofemoral pathway and the large forces which are transmitted. Analysis shows that at 25° of weight-bearing flexion, forces at the patellofemoral joint are equal to those passing through the tibiofemoral articulation (Fig. 2.10). Approaching full flexion, before the patient's buttocks touch the heels, this value can rise to almost twice the force passing through the tibiofemoral joints. This explains the large area of very thick articular cartilage of the patella and the femoral condyle. These surfaces must be able to adapt to changes in contour during movement. The irregular patellar pathway seems to ensure that forces about the knee are resolved to give axial stress in the femur and tibia and minimal shearing in the tibiofemoral joint. The broad deep areas of articular cartilage at the patellofemoral joint help to spread the load just as the menisci enlarge the area of contact at the tibiofemoral joint.

Cruciate ligaments are essential for full athletic activity but limited function is possible in a patient who has sustained a complete rupture of both ligaments and in whom treatment has restored good muscle function. Results (see Fig. 2.5) show that the forces producing anteroposterior glide during static force transmission in the knee are only one-quarter of

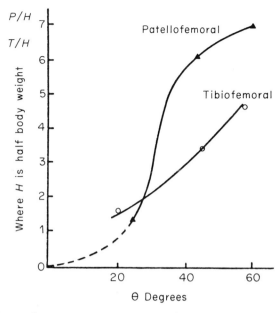

Fig. 2.10 This graph compares compressive force at patellofemoral and tibio-femoral joints in a subject who crouches to the ground. After 25° the force exerted by the patella is greater than that sustained by the tibiofemoral joint.

the compressive tibiofemoral force. Limited function can be expected without additional constraints to movement in the sagittal plane but the knee is unlikely to feel very stable.

The posterior capsular ligament has three parts, two overlie the posterior femoral condyles and a shorter section passes between them. These three parts can limit extension and maintain lateral stability in extension if the joint surfaces are normal. Stability in full extension is fundamental to the success of any operation upon the knee. If a permanent degree of fixed flexion is present muscle effort is wasted. If too much hyperextension is allowed, the knee feels unstable, and flexor and extensor muscles must act together to maintain a normal standing position.

2.4 Applications to knee replacement

If degenerative arthritis is associated with severe varus or valgus deformity in the knee joint, the collateral ligament on the convex side is stretched whilst fibrosis occurs on the overrelaxed concave side and that collateral ligament contracts as the tibiofemoral angle increases. When operative reduction of the deformity is attempted during some knee replacement operations, the tight ligament on the concave side may cause translocation or even persistent angulation of one component of the prosthesis upon the other. To obtain correct tension in all parts of the posterior capsular ligament with the knee in full extension it is often necessary to divide a contracted collateral ligament at operation. Provided the tibial component of a knee replacement is convex (thus ensuring some limitation of anteroposterior glide during healing) there will be no ill-effects from cutting this ligament. Indeed, failure to release a tight collateral ligament may result in a painful unstable knee. Reflex inhibition from a tight ligament may actually prevent correct reduction of the joint surfaces. In the Portsmouth series of knee replacements (Laskin, Denham and Apley, 1983) the collateral ligament on the concave side was divided in 25% of all knee arthroplasties. The lateral expansions of the extensor mechanism overlying the collateral ligament protected the knee during early recovery, and healing with stability in flexion as well as in extension occurred within 6 months. The posterior capsular ligament is most important during arthroplasty. All parts of this ligament must be tight in full extension, holding the wide congruous artificial joint surfaces together so that the normal tibiofemoral angle of 7° is maintained.

2.5 Conclusion

In a normal patient the ligaments of the knee guard the joint against abnormal movement by their passive action as strong fibrous structures and also by initiating the reflex protective action of muscles. Ligaments guide joint surfaces during movement in a way which permits the physiological range of movement within the limits of the articular cartilage. During normal activity, tension in ligaments is never more than one-quarter of the force transmitted between joint surfaces. Indeed, it would be wasteful use of muscle force to increase tension in ligaments. The shape of the joint surfaces, the line of action of muscles and the position and direction of the force of gravity upon the subject all interact, so that during activity ligaments are protected from the considerable forces generated by muscles and transmitted by joints.

References

Bishop, R. E. D. (1977), On the mechanics of the human knee. *Eng. Med.*, **6**, 46–52.
Denham, R. A. and Bishop, R. E. D. (1978), Mechanics of the knee and problems in reconstructive surgery. *J. Bone Joint Surg.*, **60B**, 345–52.

Laskin, R., Denham, R. A. and Apley, A. G. (1983), *Total Knee Replacement.* Springer–Verlag, Berlin.

Maquet, P. (1972), Biomechanique de la gonarthrose. *Acta Orthop. Belg.*, **38**, Suppl. 33, 54.

Cellular and biochemical composition of .ling tendon

ISABEL F. WILLIAMS

3.1 The structure of normal tendon

In this section it is proposed to cover the most important aspects of the structure of normal tendon with particular reference to its major component, collagen. Limitations of space necessarily restrict the scope of this discussion, however more comprehensive information may be obtained from several recent reviews (Bailey and Etherington, 1980; Bornstein and Sage, 1980).

The extracellular matrix of the normal tendon is composed of the fibrous protein collagen, which forms 86% of the dry weight, associated with proteoglycans, glycoproteins, elastin and mucopolysaccharides. Developing tendon contains more tenocytes than tendon taken from older animals. In mature tendon completely acellular areas are common.

To achieve the high tensile strength necessary to efficently transmit muscular force the collagen is organized into parallel arrays of fibre bundles oriented along the stress axis. The hierarchical structure of the tendon has as its smallest unit the collagen fibril. These are grouped into bundles or fascicles which themselves are grouped to form the tendon (Kastelic, Galeski and Baez, 1978). The fibrils consist of type I collagen, one of several genetically distinct collagens now recognized (Table 3.1), with an ordered surface coating of proteoglycan (Scott, 1979). The fibre bundles are enclosed by a membranous network, the endotendineum and peritendineum. These have been shown to contain types III, IV and V collagen (Duance *et al.*, 1977), and also hyaluronic acid (Reid and Flint, 1974). The nature of the fibre changes during the maturation of the animal (Cetta *et al.*, 1982). The diameter of the fibrils increases with age and the resultant increase in collagen content and decrease in accompanying proteoglycan is associated with an enhancement of the tensile strength of the tissue. It has been proposed that the larger the fibril diameter the greater the ultimate tensile strength of a tissue because of the increased

43

we have mentioned, large fibre bundles are arranged parallel to the axis and as such will not be deformed by the applied stress. On the hand, in the skin the fibres are found in a crisscross network throu the dermis which allows the tissue some flexibility and elasticity, but with some sacrifice of tensile strength. In the cornea the same collagen is found in small regularly sized bundles in sheets of parallel fibres. The fibre axis of one sheet is almost perpendicular to the fibre axis of the sheets above and below. In this well-structured form the tissue maintains its transparency and any disruption, as in wound-healing, leads to opacity.

3.3 Disruption of normal tendon

When the tendon is extended beyond its point of elasticity, which is at approximately 8% extension of total length, overstretching and rupture of some collagen fibres occurs, accompanied by cell damage. Healing is initiated by the invasion of the area by cells which remove debris and synthesize a new connective tissue matrix. The resultant granulation tissue is well vascularized, highly cellular and poorly organized but undergoes substantial remodelling during the maturation of the scar. The electron microscope shows that the major non-inflammatory cell type present in early granulation tissue is the myofibroblast, which is the source of the new collagenous matrix.

The myofibroblast can be distinguished morphologically from normal tendon fibroblasts. It contains a well-developed endoplasmic reticulum, indented nucleus and pronounced bundles of microfilaments parallel to the long axis of the cell (Nakanishi et al., 1981). It may therefore be considered to have contractile ability, although there is no direct evidence to this effect.

The source of the myofibroblasts is not known. It has been suggested by Williams, Heaton and McCullagh (1980) that they are derived from the peripheral smooth muscle cells of invading small blood vessels, which may then transform to a fibroblastlike cell, or that they arise from a partially differentiated cell already present in the damaged area by completion of the differentiation process (Nakanishi et al., 1981).

Inflammatory cells are thought to be the main cell type involved in the clearing of debris and haemorrhage. However, recent evidence has shown that cultured fibroblasts applied to an artificial matrix of collagen and proteoglycan can have a degradative capacity ten times that of activated macrophages (Laub et al., 1982). It is therefore possible that the myofibroblasts contribute to both synthesis and degradation during wound healing.

During the maturation of the scar the myofibroblasts become more scarce and are replaced by cells which are more like normal tendon fibroblasts in appearance. These are orientated, in parallel with the collagenous matrix, in the plane of stress of the tendon. The period of time over which this occurs appears to be somewhat different in various species. Postacchini and de Martino (1980) have stated that the calcaneal tendon of the rabbit reaches full morphological and biochemical normality within 4 months after partial section. This conclusion was based primarily on the fact that the diameter of collagen fibrils in the healed scar was similar to that of fibrils from uninjured tendon.

Studies of the injured equine tendon in our laboratories have indicated that such rapid recovery may not occur in all species. After acute injury to the superficial digital flexor tendon, collagen fibril diameter was found to be much smaller than normal (Silver *et al.*, 1983 (Williams *et al.* 1985)), and this was the case for the whole period under study, 14 months after injury. The biochemical composition of the healing tendon, described below, was also found to be abnormal during this period (Williams, McCullagh and Silver, 1984).

3.3.1 THE SYNTHESIS OF NEW PROTEIN FOLLOWING TENDON INJURY

Studies have been carried out on new protein synthesis in the healing tendon using *in vivo* labelling techniques. Protein synthesis was shown by Banes *et al.* (1981) to be maximal in the healing avian flexor profundis tendon 10 days after section and suturing while partial devascularization of the cut tendon resulted in a lesser increase in protein synthesis.

Vailas *et al.* (1981) have shown that levels of both collagen and non-collagen protein synthesis are elevated above normal in the healing medial collateral ligament of the rat 8 weeks after complete section. However, studies were not carried out during later stages of scar maturation. Synthesis of collagenous and non-collagenous proteins remained high in injured tendon compared with that in the opposite or contralateral tendon in the horse at 3 months after acute injury (Silver *et al.*, 1983; Williams, McCullagh and Silver, 1984). Also the concentration of crosslinks found mainly in newly synthesized collagen was substantial at this time. Normal adult equine tendon contains only trace amounts of these crosslinks (Silver *et al.*, 1983; Williams, McCullagh and Silver, 1984a).

3.3.2 THE BIOCHEMICAL COMPOSITION OF NEW GRANULATION TISSUE AND SUBSEQUENT CHANGES DUE TO SCAR REMODELLING

Electronmicrographs of tissue from healing skin wounds (Gabbiani, Majno and Ryan, 1973) and from patients suffering from a variety of

Ligament Injuries and their Treatment

pathological syndromes, such as fibrosarcoma (Nakanishi *et al.*, 1981) and Dupuytrens contracture (Salamon and Hamori, 1980) show that the myofibroblast is surrounded by abundant collagen fibrils and amorphous electron-dense material. The staining of sections of healing tissue with silver reveals a reticulin network shown recently to have several biochemical components (Unsworth *et al.*, 1982). These include type III collagen, fibronectin or LETS protein (large external transformation sensitive protein), and at least one other glycoprotein of a non-collagenous nature. Recent studies have shown that the healing equine tendon shows similar characteristics (Williams, McCullagh and Silver, 1984). Fibronectin and type III collagen are found throughout the matrix in the early stages of healing in high concentration by comparison with normal tissue in which both molecules are confined to the endotendineum (Fig. 3.1). Type I collagen is also present at this stage, and throughout the entire period of healing. It has been demonstrated that a fibroblast is capable of simultaneous synthesis of both types I and III collagen (Gay *et al.*, 1976). It therefore seems likely that the myofibroblasts are the source of both types of collagen.

The glycoprotein fibronectin found in the early wound is probably derived from several sources. It is possible that the fibronectin in the healing tendon has a myofibroblastic origin, although it may also be synthesized by endothelial cells (Clark *et al.*, 1982). Fibronectin may also derive from plasma which has leaked from damaged vessels (Oh, Pierschbacher and Ruoslahti, 1981). The fibronectin forms a complex with fibrin present at the site of haemorrhage and forms a network which is then further complexed with type III collagen, a molecule which is synthesized at an abnormally high level in the early wound as early as 10 hours after injury (Clore, Cohen and Diegelmann, 1979). It seems likely that other molecules also participate in this complex, but these have not so far been elucidated. Other molecules present in the matrix in addition to the reticulin complex include chondroitin sulphate-rich proteoglycans, also present at abnormally high levels.

During later stages of healing, up to 14 months after acute injury to the equine tendon, type III collagen is still present throughout the matrix (Fig. 3.2). The persistence of type III may have reflected the continuation of a low level of chronic inflammation and this is discussed in the section below in relation to factors which may predispose towards tendon injury.

3.3.3 FACTORS WHICH CONTRIBUTE TO THE POSSIBILITY OF TENDON RUPTURE OR SPRAIN

The normal tendon is capable of bearing a load of approximately 50–100 N/m^2 (Viidik, 1969). If this is exceeded as a result of misapplied load during normal use, sprain or rupture occurs. However, this does not explain why some areas of the tendon fibrillar population remain unaffected, some fibrils are only stretched to just above their elastic limit while some are ruptured completely. The possibility that areas of microtrauma may be found in an apparently clinically normal tendon has been raised by several workers. Webbon (1977) noted the presence of small acellular necrotic areas in equine digital flexor tendons which constituted part of a study of normal tendon structure, and Pool, Wheat and Ferraro (1980) found that microscopic lesions involving the absence of tenocyte nuclei and the hyalinization of adjacent tendon fibres were not uncommon in the digital flexor tendons of clinically normal adult racehorses.

It is likely that this apparent morphological degeneration is accompanied by a local cellular response to the microtrauma, including an increased synthesis of type III collagen, as occurs in healing tendons after more radical injury. It is not known if type III collagen fibrils are less capable than type I of maintaining tensile strain, but discontinuity created by the presence of an area of different biochemical composition could contribute to a predisposition to partial sprain or rupture.

A substantial amount of type III collagen has been found in human Achilles tendon excised within 24 hours after acute rupture (Coombs, 1981). Normal Achilles tendon has been shown, by similar biochemical techniques, to contain no detectable type III collagen (Hanson and Bentley, 1983) and it is tempting to speculate that the presence of an abnormal concentration of type III collagen accumulated as a result of repeated minor injury was at least partially responsible for the final rupture.

One piece of evidence which would support this conclusion is the observation that type III collagen levels are raised in the tendon contralateral to the affected equine tendon after acute injury (Williams, McCullagh and Silver, 1984). The opposite or contralateral tendon is often found to be more prone to damage during a period of recovery following tendon injury. This may be due to the presence of areas made weaker by the accumulation of type III collagen as a result of extra stress experienced during healing of the opposite leg.

Type III collagen is known to be present in high concentration in tissues which are exposed to a high degree of mechanical stress, for example, periodontium, subjected to the process of mastication, and this would also apply to the chronically injured tendon. Another tissue which might also be included in this group is the palmar fascia taken from human patients who are suffering from Dupuytrens syndrome. This disease is frequently associated with repeated mechanical stimulation of the palm and involves the growth of a band of tissue connecting the palm with the base of one of the fingers, usually the ring or little finger. The morphological and

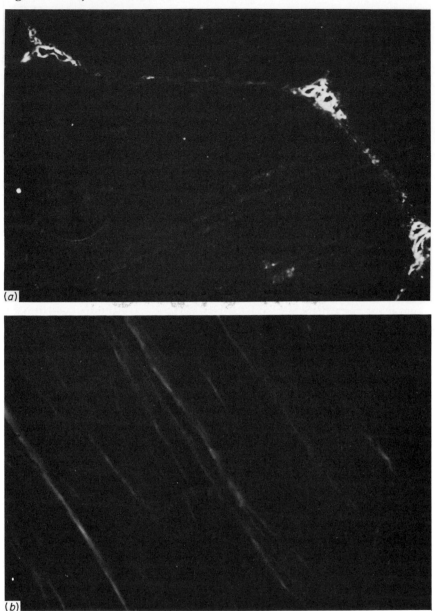

Fig. 3.1 Immunofluorescent localization of type III collagen and fibronectin in normal and healing tendon. (*a*) Frozen section (transverse) of normal tendon incubated with anti-fibronectin serum. (× 197). (*b*) Frozen section (longitudinal) of normal tendon incubated with antitype III collagen serum. (× 385). (*c*) Frozen section (longitudinal) of injured tendon incubated with antifibronectin serum (× 197). 1 week after injury. (*d*) Frozen section (longitudinal) of injured tendon

50

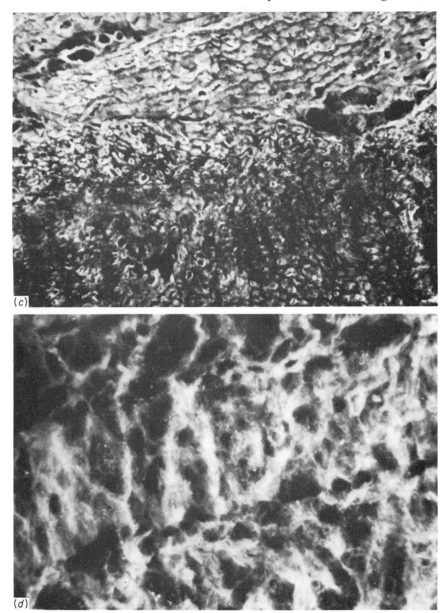

incubated with anti-type III collagen serum (× 500). 1 week after injury. Frozen sections were cut on a Slee cryostat and incubated in specific antiserum to either collagen or fibronectin. The immunoglobulins which had bound to the section were then localized by incubation in anti-immunoglobulin serum which had been labelled with fluorescein. This compound was visualized by viewing under ultraviolet light which causes the fluorescein to fluoresce.

51

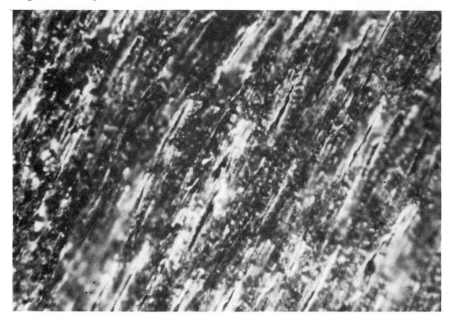

Fig. 3.2 Immunofluorescent localization of type III collagen in healing equine tendon at 14 months after injury. (× 500).

biochemical characteristics of this tissue are well described in the current literature (Bazin *et al.*, 1980; Brickley-Parsons *et al.*, 1981) and are very similar to those of healing tendon (Williams, McCullagh and Silver, 1984) and healing palmar fascia (Brickley-Parsons *et al.*, 1981). This would also seem to suggest that a similar response occurs in the tendon when it is subjected to repeated stress.

If cells are removed from the palmar fascia of Dupuytrens patients into tissue culture, their synthetic characteristics become indistinguishable from those of normal fascia fibroblasts (Slack, Flint and Thompson, 1982), indicating that local environmental conditions are important in determining the synthetic expression of the cells.

The reaction of rabbit cranial fibroblasts to tensile strain *in vivo* by synthesizing large amounts of type III collagen (Meikle *et al.*, 1982) is another indication that a small local change in the biomechanical environment of a fibroblastic cell within a tendon might cause a metabolic response which could subsequently result in further adverse effects on tissue structure and function.

3.4 The treatment of tendon injury

To some extent preventive measures may be taken which decrease the possibility of tendon sprain or rupture. The normal tendon can be induced to hypertrophy in the same way as a muscle by means of concentrated exercise regimes (Woo et al., 1980) although this does not appear to be as effective in older as younger animals (Viidik, 1969). The insertion of the tendon is not strengthened by this approach. The use of exercise regimes in the treatment of tendon injury has been explored by several groups. Gelberman et al. (1980) have found an increase in the rate at which the network of small blood vessels and capillaries in the injured dog flexor tendon is replaced by fewer and larger vessels, orientated in the longitudinal axis of the tendon, as a result of a gradually increasing range of passive motion initiated 3 weeks after injury. Vailas et al. (1981) showed that if treadmill exercise was initiated within 2 weeks after section of the rat medial collateral ligament and continued for 6 weeks, dry weight, collagen content and the force required to separate the ligament were all significantly greater than control values at the end of this time.

The transplantation of tendon grafts has also been considered as a possible treatment for tendon injury (Fackleman, 1973). Klein and Lewis (1972) compared the rate of destruction of isograft, allograft and xenograft of young rat tendon, and isograft of old tendon, by radiolabelling the grafts before implantation into the Achilles tendons of rats or guinea-pigs. Scar formation in tendon isografts or allografts was minimal, although 50–64% of the grafted tendon turned over within 3 months of implantation. The xenograft showed an almost complete loss of pre-existing tendon within a period of 1 month. Although successful transplantations of autologous tendon have been carried out in horses (Fackleman, 1973) the surgery involves considerable trauma to the tendon and paratenon, which may cause adhesion formation at a later stage.

The implantation of artificial prostheses as a support for healing tendons or as complete replacements for particular tendons or ligaments has been applied in both human and veterinary medicine, following the use of filamentous carbon fibre to replace ligaments and tendons in experimental animals (Jenkins et al., 1977, Jenkins, 1978). In human patients ruptured cruciate ligaments have been replaced with carbon fibre twists (see Chapters 14–15), while carbon fibre plaits have been implanted in the superficial digital flexor tendons of horses after tendon breakdown on the racetrack or hunting field (Goodship et al., 1980). A fuller discussion of the clinical aspects of this subject may be found elsewhere in this publication. There is little information in the literature about the biochemical nature of the connective tissue produced within and around an inorganic implant, carbon or other material. Coombs *et al.* (1981) have stated that tissue formed around a carbon fibre replacement for rat Achilles tendons was biochemically and morphologically normal within 4 months after implantation. This may have reflected a species difference, as it is well known that rodents do not become skeletally mature and have a very high metabolic rate. There is, therefore, a strong possibility that the turnover rate of connective tissue molecules is proportionally faster and that comparison between the rat and larger mammals may not be reliable.

3.5 Conclusion

On the basis of the biochemical and clinical evidence available, it seems unlikely that a tendon, once injured, will return to complete normality of structure and function in the adult animal. It can, however, be strengthened by the means of exercise regimes or by the implantation of inorganic prostheses. Studies are currently proceeding in our laboratory in order to develop new biochemically based treatments of tendon injury.

ACKNOWLEDGEMENTS

Some of the work described in this chapter was carried out as part of a recent study of 'line firing', used in the treatment of equine tendon injury. This study was initiated by Professor I. A. Silver, Department of Pathology, University of Bristol and funded by the Horserace Betting Levy Board.

References

Bailey, A. J. and Etherington, D. G. (1980), Metabolism of collagen and elastin in *Comprehensive Biochemistry 19B* (eds M. Florkin, E. Stotz) Part I, Elsevier, Amsterdam, pp. 299–460.

Banes, A., Enterline, D., Bevin, A. and Salisbury, R. (1981), Effects of trauma and desvascularization on protein synthesis in the avian flexor profundis tendon. *J. Trauma*, **21(7)**, 505–12.

Bazin, S., LeLous, M., Duance, V. C., Sims, T. J., Bailey, A. J., Gabbiani, G., D'Andiran, G., Pizzolato, G., Browski, A., Nicoletis, C. and Delauney, A. (1980), Biochemistry and histology of the connective tissue of Dupuytren's disease lesions. *Eur. J. Clin. Invest.*, **10**, 9–16.

Brickley-Parsons, D., Glimcher, M. H., Smith, R. J., Albin, R. and Adams, J. P. (1981), Biochemical changes in the collagen of the palmar fascia in patients with Dupuytren's disease. *J. Bone Joint Surg.*, **63A**, 787–97.

Bornstein, P. and Sage, H. (1980), Structurally distinct collagen types. *Ann. Rev. Biochem.*, **49**, 957–1003

ıca, G., Ippolito, E., De Martino, C. and
ıl and morphological modifications in
on and ageing. *Biochem. J.*, **204**, 61–7.
[., Dellepe, P. and Colvin, R. B. (1982),
s in response to injury. *J. Exp. Med.*, **156**,

n, R. F. (1979), Quantitation of collagen
ı rat skin. *Proc. Soc. Exp. Biol. Med.*, **161**,

D., Narcissi, P., Nichols, A. and Pope,
ı-fibre-induced tendon. *J. Bone and Joint*

ıture. Thesis submitted for the degree of

., Bourne, F. J. and Bailey, A. J. (1977),
ıkeletal muscle. *FEBS Lett.*, **79**, 248–52.
he nature, structure and function of the
ınical Interactions at the Endothelium* (ed.
sterdam, pp. 41–78.
, Structure of the trophoblast basement
membrane in *Biology of Trophoblast* (eds Y. W. Loke and A. Whyte) Elsevier/
North-Holland, Amsterdam, pp. 597–625.

Fackelman, G. E. (1973), The nature of tendon damage and its repair. *Equine Vet. J.*, **5**, 141–9.

Gabbiani, G., Majno, G. and Ryan, G. B. (1973), in *Biology of the Fibroblast* (eds E. Kulonen and J. Pikkarainen) Academic Press, London, pp. 39–154.

Gay, S., Martin, G. R., Muller, P. K., Timpl, R. and Kuhn, K. (1976), Simultaneous synthesis of types I and III collagen by fibroblasts in culture. *Proc. National Academy Science* **73**, 4037–40.

Gay, S., Gay, R. and Miller, E. J. (1980), The collagens of the joint. *Arth. Rheum.*, **23**, 937–41.

Gelberman, R. H., Menon, J., Gonsalves, M. and Akeson, W. H. (1980), The effects of mobilization on the vascularization of healing flexor tendon in dogs. *Clin. Orthop.*, **153**, 283–9.

Goodship, A. E., Brown, P. N., Yeats, J. J., Jenkins, D. H. R. and Silver, I. A. (1980), An assessment of filamentous carbon fibre for the treatment of tendon injury in the horse. *Vet. Rec.*, **106**, 217–21.

Jenkins, D. H. R. (1978), The repair of cruciate ligaments with flexible carbon fibre. *J. Bone Joint Surg.*, **60B**, 520–2.

Hanson, A. N. and Bentley, J. P. (1983), Quantitation of type I to type III collagen ratios in small samples of human tendon, blood vessels and atherosclerotic plaque. *Anal. Biochem.*, **130**, 32–40.

Kastelic, J., Galeski, A. and Baer, E. (1978), The multicomposite structure of tendon. *Conn. Tiss. Res.*, **6**, 11–23.

Jenkins, D. H. R., Forster, I. W., McKibbin, B. and Ralis, Z. A. (1977), Induction of tendon and ligament formation by carbon implants. *J. Bone Joint Surg.*, **59B**, 53–7.

Ligament Injuries and their Treatment

Klein, L. and Lewis, J. (1972), Simultaneous quantification of ^{3}H-collagen loss and ^{1}H-collagen replacement during healing of rat tendon grafts. *J. Bone Joint Surg.* **54A(1)** 137–46.

Laub, R., Huybrech, G., Peeters, J. C. and Vaes, G. (1982), Degradation of collagen and proteoglycan by macrophages and fibroblasts – individual potentialities of each cell type and co-operative effects through the activation of fibroblasts by macrophages. *B.B.A.*, **721(4)**, 425–33.

Light, N. D. and Bailey, A. J. (1979), Covalent crosslinks in collagen: characterization and relationships to connective tissue disorders in *Fibrous Proteins: Scientific, Industrial and Medical Aspects*, Vol. I (eds D. A. D. Parry and L. K. Creamer), Academic Press, London, pp. 151–77.

Meikle, M. C., Heath, J. K., Hembry, R. M. and Reynolds, J. J. (1982), Rabbit cranial suture fibroblasts under tension express a different collagen phenotype. *Arch. Oral Biol.*, **27**, 609–13.

Nakanishi, I., Kajikawa, K., Okada, T. and Eguchi, K. (1981), Myofibroblasts in fibrous tumours and fibrosis in various organs. *Acta. Pathol. Jap.*, **31**, 423–37.

Oh, E., Pierschbacher, M. and Ruoslahti, E. (1981), Deposition of plasma fibronectin in tissues. *Proc. National Academy Science*, **78**, 3218–221.

Parry, D. A. D., Barnes, G. R. G. and Craig, A. S. (1978), A comparison of the size distribution of collagen fibrils in connective tissues as a function of age and a possible relation between fibril size distribution and mechanical properties. *Proc. Roy. Soc. Lond. B.*, **203**, 305–21.

Pool, R. R., Wheat, J. D. and Ferraro, G. L. (1980), Corticosteroid therapy in common joint and tendon injuries of the horse. Part II. Effects on tendons. *Proc. Am. Assoc. Equine Pract.*, **26**, 407–10.

Postacchini, F. and de Martino, C. (1980), Regeneration of rabbit calcaneal tendon. Maturation of collagen and elastic fibers following partial tenotomy. *Conn. Tissue Res.*, **8**, 41–7.

Reid, T. A. and Flint, M. H. (1974), Changes in glycosaminoglycan content of healing rabbit tendon. *J. Embryol. Exp. Morphol.*, **31**, 489–95.

Salamon, A. and Hamori, J. (1980), Possible role of myofibroblasts in the pathogenesis of Dupuytren's contracture. *Acta Morphol. Acad. Sci. Hung.*, **28**, 71–82.

Scott, J. E. (1979), Hierarchy in connective tissues. *Chem. Brit.*, **15**, 13–18.

Silver, I. A., Brown, P. N., Goodship, A. E., Lanyon, L. E., McCullagh, K. G., Perry, G. C. and Williams, I. F. (1983), A clinical and experimental study of tendon injury, healing and treatment in the horse. *Equine Vet. J.*, Suppl. 1, **July**, 1–43.

Slack, C., Flint, M. H. and Thompson, B. M. (1982), Glycosaminoglycan synthesis by Dupuytren's cells in culture. *Conn. Tiss. Res.*, **9**, 263–9.

Unsworth, D. J., Scott, D. L., Almond, T. J., Beard, H. K., Holborow, E. J. and Walton, K. W. (1982), Studies on reticulin. I. Serological and immunohistological investigation of the occurrence of collagen type III, fibronectin and the non-collagenous glycoprotein of Pras and Glynn in reticulin. *Br. J. Exp. Pathol.*, **63**, 154–66.

Vailas, A. C., Tipton, C. M., Matthes, R. D. and Gart, M. (1981), Physical activity and its influence on the repair process of medial collateral ligaments. *Conn. Tiss. Res.*, **9**, 25–31.

Viidik, A. (1969), Tensile strength: Properties of Achilles tendon systems in trained and untrained rabbits. *Acta. Orthop. Scand.*, **40**, 261–72.

Webbon, P. M. (1977), A post mortem study of equine digital flexor tendons. *Equine Vet. J.*, **9**, 61–7.

Williams, I. F., Craig, A. S., Parry, D. A. D., Goodship, A. E. Shah, J. and Silver, I. A. (1985), The development of collagen fibril organisation and collagen crimp patterns during tendon healing. *Int. J. Biol. Macromolecules* (in press).

Williams, I. F., Heaton, A. and McCullagh, K. G. (1980), Cell morphology and collagen types in equine tendon scar. *Res. Vet. Sci.*, **28**, 302–10.

Williams, I. F., McCullagh, K. G. and Silver, I. A. (1984), The distribution of types I and III collagen and fibronectin in the healing equine tendon. *Conn. Tiss. Res.* **12,** 211–27.

Williams, I. F., McCullagh, K. G. and Silver, I. A. (1984a), The synthesis of collagenous and noncollagenous proteins following tendon injury (in preparation).

Woo, S.L-Y., Ritter, A., Amiel, D., Sanders, T. M., Gomez, M. A., Kuei, S. C., Garfin, S. R. and Akeson, W. H. (1980), The biomechanical and biochemical properties of swine tendons – long term effects of exercise on the digital extensors. *Conn. Tiss. Res.*, **7**, 177–83.

PART TWO
Treatment

4 *Elbow lesions*

J. H. MILLER

4.1 Collateral ligaments

Even with the additional stability supplied by the capsule, the incomplete middle range stability demands the addition of the collateral ligaments. The more important of these is the medial one. The carrying angle and its potential medial instability demands the presence of resilient medial soft tissue structures strong on tensile loading. This is achieved by an equilateral triangle of three bands, the anterior and posterior limbs of which originate from the inferior surface of the medial epicondyle close to the junction with the medial face of the trochlea; indeed the deep fibres originate from the proximal aspect of the medial face of the trochlea at this junction. The anterior band passes anteromedially and is attached to the sublime tubercle of the coronoid process; the posterior band passes to the edge of the articular margin of the olecranon process and the oblique band joins the bases of these two bands (Fig. 4.1(a))

The lateral collateral ligament arises from the lateral epicondyle and is isosceles in shape, passing distally to mingle intimately with the transverse fibres of the annular ligament (Fig. 4.1(b)). Muscles stabilize the soft tissue. The arrangement is such that the humeral muscles are attached to the coronoid and olecranon processes distally whereas the hand and forearm muscles are attached to the humerus proximally; similarly with the pronator and supinator muscles which originate in the humerus and are inserted into the forearm. The common extensor origin greatly strengthens the lateral collateral ligament. Biomechanical implications of these arrangements are shown below (Fig. 4.2).

There are three main peripheral nerves which, like the brachial artery, are closely related to the joint. Damage can occur to these in situations of gross ligamentous laxity, or because of post-traumatic or postoperative fibrosis in the natural repair of ligamentous damage.

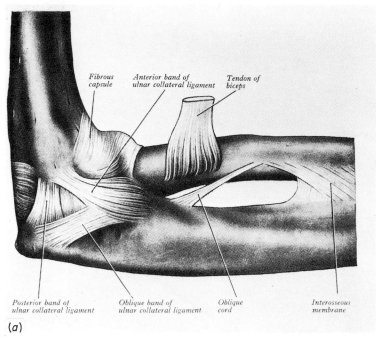

Fibrous capsule   Anterior band of ulnar collateral ligament   Tendon of biceps

Posterior band of ulnar collateral ligament   Oblique band of ulnar collateral ligament   Oblique cord   Interosseous membrane

(a)

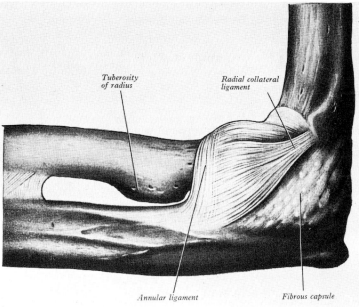

Tuberosity of radius   Radial collateral ligament

Annular ligament   Fibrous capsule

(b)

Fig. 4.1 (a) Equilateral triangular arrangement of the bands of the medial ligament. (b) Isosceles triangular arrangement of the structure of the lateral ligament blending with the annular ligament. (Reproduced from Gray's Anatomy, published by Churchill Livingstone.)

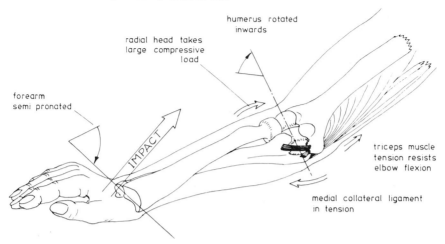

Fig. 4.2 Normal forces exaggerated as shown in biomechanical analysis in falls on the outstretched hand. (Amis *et al.*, 1984.)

4.2 Cadaveric and radiographic studies

The following equations show the stabilizing features of the normal elbow:

(1) Stability = intact ligaments + intact bones
(2) Intact ligaments = medial + lateral + annular + capsule
(3) Intact bones = (coronoid + trochlea) + (radial head + capitellum)

In my own research involving extensive cadaveric studies I have been able to analyse the harmony of action between ligaments and bones forming the joint. Further by the systematic creation of selected lesions it has been possible to observe the patterns of instability and to apply manual force to the limb in three directions, that is, valgus/varus, anteroposterior and rotation. The sequences of disruption were recorded photographically and radiologically.

From the lesions simulated and the forces applied many interesting facts have emerged.

(1) The initial lesion created was division of the proximal end of the anterior band of the medial collateral ligament. The joint was then subjected to forces and the only significant instability resulted from those

63

forces in a valgus/varus and hyperpronation direction producing widening of the medial side of the joint.

(2) Anterior band rupture plus increasing rupture of the medial capsule increases the degree of medial instability with an increasing tendency to posterior subluxation by applying manual forces in a valgus/varus and a hyperpronation direction.

(3) Division of the anterior band alone will not allow an anteroposterior force to produce posterior displacement of the ulna. The intact lateral ligament will prevent this. However, if its attachment to the lateral epicondyle is divided a manual force applied in an anteroposterior direction will produce a posterior shift of the ulna and radial head. This will only proceed posteriorly until the intact capsule becomes taut and stops further movement resulting in the coronoid process being locked directly below the surface of the humerus, its point being impinged against the trochlear groove. This is usually an unstable position because of the guarding spasm in the extensor and flexor muscles, and the fact that the latter are stronger results in reduction of the latent or occult subluxation.

(4) The application of a manual force in a varus direction causes lateral instability, in other words, widening of the lateral side of the joint where the attachment of the lateral ligament to the lateral epicondyle has been divided; the radial head will displace anteriorly or posteriorly where there is the application of an additional force in a pronated or supinated direction.

(5) Increasing lateral instability is produced by increasing the division of the lateral capsule.

(6) The division of both collateral ligaments has been stated to produce posterior displacement with an anteroposterior force; where the anterior capsule has been divided this force results in complete posterior displacement of the ulna and radial head the coronoid passing to the posterior surface of the humerus. As stripping of the anterior capsule increases, posterior dislocation becomes more pronounced.

(7) Stripping up of the posterior capsule and the posterior band of the medial ligament occurs with the continued application of the manual force in an anteroposterior direction; the result is complete posterior dislocation.

(8) Division of the coronoid process diminishes the bony protection afforded to the collateral ligaments and the application of a manual force to the forearm increases the tension of the collateral ligaments. Division of their attachments will still be necessary for the posterior subluxation to occur. Similarly, osteotomy of the anterior third of the radial head will transfer the anteroposterior manual force directly to the ligaments and only then will the radial head and forearm pass posteriorly. Division of both processes will further increase the joint laxity and the ability to

sublux the joint posteriorly on the application of the anteroposterior force.

(9) The division of the medial epicondyle produces medial instability and lessens the protection of the medial capsule afforded by the intact epicondyle and medial ligament.

(10) The lateral capsule is similarly exposed by dividing the lateral epicondyle and its rupture causes widening of this joint space.

Any loss of bony integrity results in exposure of the soft tissues to forces applied to the limb particularly in an axial or angulatory direction. This applies to all intracapsular components of the joint in addition to the ones mentioned, that is, the capitellum, lateral condyle, trochlea and olecranon.

In summary, therefore, a compressive force applied along the longitudinal axis of the limb loaded either in a valgus or a varus direction with or without rotation may produce each of these fractures. Should the force continue then displacement will be restrained by tension in the collateral ligaments, usually the anterom medial band. Should the damage be restricted to a simple strain or partial rupture, stability will be maintained. However, forces in excess of those producing such lesions will result in total rupture allowing displacement. One can therefore say that stable fractures are those in which the force has at the most produced a strain or partial rupture of the ligament or ligaments concerned; an unstable fracture is one where the force has produced a total rupture of the ligament or ligaments concerned. If the anterior capsule remains intact then the instability remains latent or occult; should the anterior capsule be totally ruptured a complete dislocation results.

A *stable fracture* is a fracture with no more than a partial rupture of a collateral ligament or ligaments, for example, crack or minimally displaced fractures. An *unstable fracture* is a fracture plus total rupture of ligament or ligaments, for example, fracture subluxation or dislocation of the radial head or neck or medial epicondyle.

4.2.1 ARTHRITIS

The tension in the ligaments is due to a normal depth of cartilage and bone stock. Where this diminishes due to degenerative changes in the articular cartilage in osteoarthritis or erosive disease as in rheumatoid arthritis, laxity of the collateral ligaments results. This is more obvious in rheumatoid arthritis where chondrolysis is associated with subsequent erosion of bone with loss of bone stock. That such changes are responsible for the laxity rather than disease of the ligaments can be demonstrated experimentally in the cadaver by incising the capsule longitudinally allowing access to the joint. Bone nibblers can then be used to remove the articular cartilage and bone. Clinical testing of joint stability will show increasing degrees of instability with the diminution of cartilage and bone.

4.3 Clinical patterns of instability in acute injuries and disease

4.3.1 SIGNIFICANT POINTS IN EXAMINATION OF THE ELBOW

(1) *Inspection of arm.* Medial bruising will be missed if the arm is not elevated from the chest wall and externally rotated.

(2) *Medial bruising signifies serious soft tissue damage.* This is confirmed by aspiration of a haemoarthrosis and by detection of medial instability on examination under anaesthesia.

(3) *Ligamentous rupture.* If the elbow is examined in full extension, this lesion could be overlooked, because in this position the olecranon is contained in the olecranon fossa. The examiner must therefore test for instability with the elbow in 30–40° flexion.

(4) *Occult posterior subluxation.* This instability will also be missed unless the anteroposterior force is applied with the elbow in the same degree of flexion.

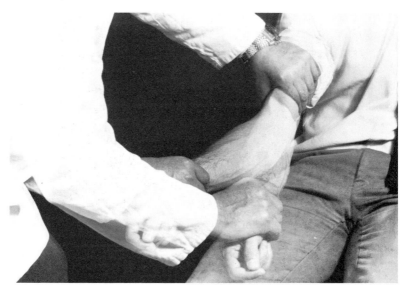

Fig. 4.3 Method of clinical testing of integrity of the collateral ligaments.

4.3.2 ASSESSMENT OF JOINT STABILITY

This is best carried out with the humerus at the side of the chest when both medial and lateral ligaments can be subjected to valgus and varus strains; the examiner restrains the elbow with one hand while the forearm is manipulated with the other (Fig. 4.3). This often proves difficult, however, in the assessment of lateral ligament stability as shoulder rotation causes the limb to move. Where the shoulder is unaffected therefore, the arm should be elevated to 90° and the upper arm firmly supported while the forearm is depressed to determine ligamentous integrity (Fig. 4.4). Where rheumatoid disease affects the shoulder, examination should be carried out with the arm by the chest and the ligaments tested with the elbow in 30–40° flexion.

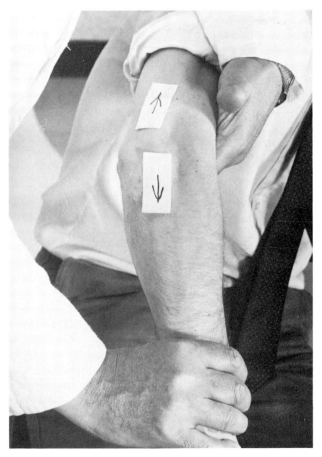

Fig. 4.4 Specific method of clinical testing of integrity of lateral ligament.

Ligament Injuries and their Treatment

4.3.3 RADIOGRAPHY

Stress views of the ligaments can be taken either with or without anaesthesia but care must be taken to maintain 30–40° flexion of the elbow when taking the anteroposterior views. The position of the X-ray plate is demonstrated in Fig. 4.5. The medial collateral ligament can also be tested by hyperpronation. For the right arm two fingers of the left hand can be applied to the medial epicondyle and the olecranon while the right hand hyperpronates. Instability will be indicated by the widening of the gap between the two left-hand fingers. Hyperpronation also tests the stability of the annular ligament; here the two fingers of the left hand are applied to the lateral epicondyle and the head of the radius. Instability of the radial head will be demonstrated by its anterior movement (Fig. 4.6).

Instability of the anterior band of the medial collateral ligament can be demonstrated by longitudinal compression the long axis of the limb combined with hyperpronation (Fig. 4.7). Latent instability involving laxity of both collateral ligaments will be revealed by a thrust in the long axis of the limb without rotation. Where the anterior capsule is intact, subluxation occurs but when ruptured, then posterior dislocation will be clearly demonstrated (Fig. 4.8).

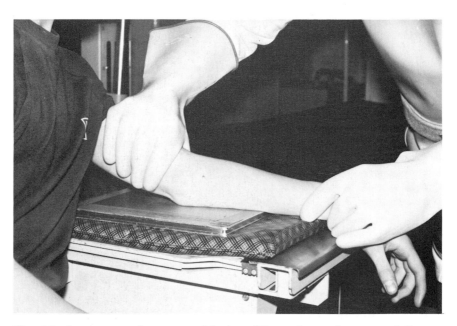

Fig. 4.5 Importance of correct positioning of X-ray plate and posture of elbow to get accurate stress views in diagnosis of ligamentous instability.

On inspecting the medial side of the elbow a swelling with, in some cases, early bruising medially will be noted. It is important to look for tenderness localized to the region of the medial epicondyle and along the line of the anterior band of the medial ligament down to its attachment to the coronoid to enable one to diagnose from simple strains to total rupture. This along with a restricted range of motion indicates the necessity for aspiration of the joint to confirm the presence of a haemarthrosis, followed by an examination under anaesthesia to test for medial instability with stress X-ray views where necessary.

The clinical picture of the injured elbow following falls on the outstretched hand or the point of the elbow varies. A contusion is the mildest injury of the joint and presents as a painful limitation of the range of motion with slight lateral swelling increasing the girth of the joint no

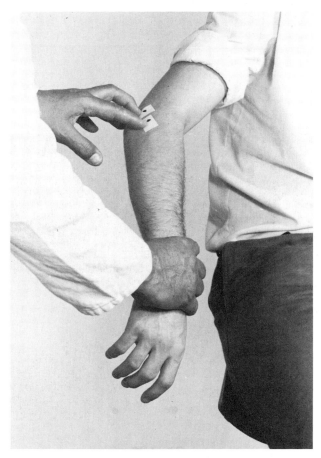

Fig. 4.6 Clinical testing of the stability of the radial head.

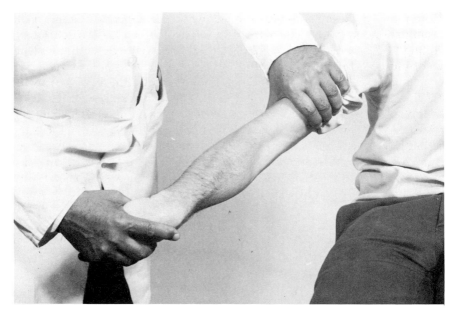

Fig. 4.7 Specific clinical examination to test integrity of anterior band of medial ligament.

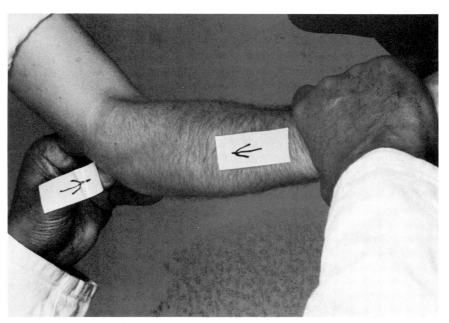

Fig. 4.8 Clinical 'thrust' method to produce subluxation or dislocation which will be confirmed radiographically.

more than 1 cm, and in which the ligaments are shown to be intact on examination under anaesthesia. The more severe injuries of which we are talking show generalized swelling of the joint with or without some deformity and bruising increasing the girth by at least 2–3 cm. There is very painful limitation of motion and the patient supports his arm by holding the wrist with the opposite hand. Medial bruising should always be looked for as it indicates rupture of the medial collateral ligament or fracture of the medial epicondyle. Examination of the joint includes aspiration; a copious haemarthrosis indicates a contusion or stable fracture. A minimal one suggests total rupture of ligaments and capsule. Examination under anaesthesia will allow testing of the stability of the joint. There are five types of acute instability:

(1) Medial
(2) Lateral
(3) Posterior
(4) Anterior
(5) Rotational

4.3.4 MEDIAL INSTABILITY

By this is meant a loss of control of the stability of the medial side of the joint. The causes are two-fold: (a) soft tissue, or (b) bony damage. Falls on the outstretched hand in a forwards or lateral direction increase the carrying angle by strong tensile/rotational forces rupturing the ligament or its attachments in pronation or avulsing the epicondyle in supination; compression loading of the joint with the arm in an adducted position is rarer and decreases the carrying angle by fracturing the coronoid or trochlea with tearing of the anterior and posterior capsules.

Usually fractures of the medial epicondyle have the medial ligament as well as the common flexor origin attached to the fragment. It is for this reason that I strongly favour reattachment of the epicondyle by internal screw or pin fixation so re-establishing the joint stability. Distal reattachment with fibrous union may lead to slight ligamentous laxity where compression loading in the longitudinal axis occurs. If gross disability is to be avoided, early recognition of an entrapped epicondyle where capsular tearing has allowed this, is important. Cubitus valgus with painful restriction of range of motion and danger of tardy ulnar palsy results.

In mature adults isolated rupture of the medial collateral ligament is more commonly seen as a result of a rotational force such as hyperpronation applied to the joint. This lesion is often produced as a result of the method of apprehension exerted by the forces of the law in which a

71

detainee's forearm is grasped in one hand while the other holds the shoulder vigorously internally rotating it with the elbow flexed to beyond 90° and the forearm twisted strenuously into hyperpronation (Fig. 4.9). This stretches the medial collateral ligament to the full, straining it and at the worst totally rupturing it; either its proximal or distal attachment may be avulsed or its substance disrupted. If the force continues tearing of the capsule ensues and rotational dislocation of the elbow occurs. Surgical exploration has shown this lesion to be rupture of one, or more, bands of the medial collateral ligament with capsular tearing (Fig. 4.10).

Ruptures of the medial collateral ligament, however, are more often seen as combined lesions with the lateral collateral ligament, capsule and fracture of the coronoid process, radial head or neck due to falls on the outstretched hand.

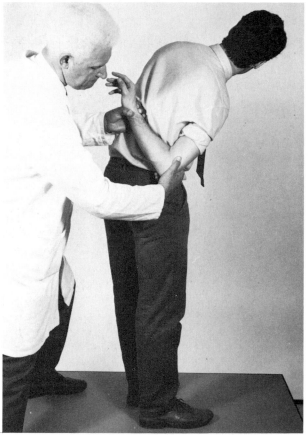

Fig. 4.9 A common mechanism of rupture of medial collateral ligament.

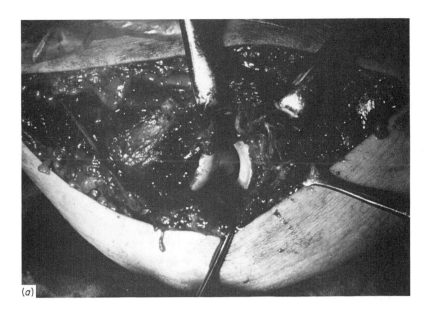

(a)

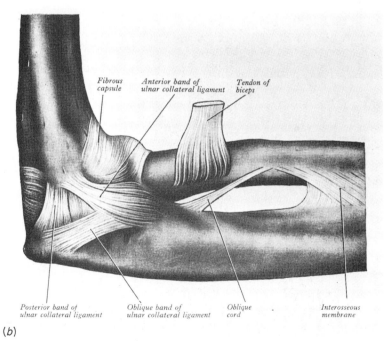

| Fibrous capsule | Anterior band of ulnar collateral ligament | Tendon of biceps |

| Posterior band of ulnar collateral ligament | Oblique band of ulnar collateral ligament | Oblique cord | Interosseous membrane |

(b)

Fig. 4.10 (a) Lesion of medial collateral ligament – rupture of all three bands. (b) Diagram inset showing sites of lesion. (Reproduced from Gray's Anatomy, published by Churchill Livingstone.)

73

Ligament Injuries and their Treatment

The clues leading to the detection of these injuries clinically are marked swelling, points of tenderness over known sites of bone and soft tissue damage and painful restriction of elbow motion. X-ray examination will reveal the type of bony damage and aspiration and examination under anaesthesia the extent of the soft tissue damage.

4.3.5 LATERAL INSTABILITY

Because of the carrying angle, lateral instability is not commonly seen. A fall on the oustretched hand has to be with the shoulder adducted and the arm internally rotated to put the lateral collateral ligament on the stretch resulting in avulsion of the lateral epicondyle. This may be seen as an isolated lesion or in combination with the medial ligament and bony lesions already stated. In general this lesion does not require reduction and fixation. However, slackening of the pull on the annular ligament can consequently give the radial head more freedom to displace.

(a) Annular ligament lesions

Isolated lesions of the annular ligament are likely to occur in children in falls on the outstretched hand resulting in hyperpronation to the flexed elbow. Where the medial ligament remains intact tension builds up in the annular ligament resulting in avulsion of the ligament from its attachment to the ulna with or without a fragment of bone. This can be seen to lie anteriorly in the antecubital fossa, a prominent feature of the lateral radiograph. Rupture of the interosseous membrane also occurs, the radius becoming mobile and slipping anteriorly with the radial head (Fig. 4.11). Rupture of the annular ligament may occur in combination with fractures of the ulna in Monteggia fracture dislocation. Axial forces exerted on the pronated forearm and extended elbow result in annular ligament rupture probably with the avulsion of the lateral ligament from the epicondyle, and radial head dislocation occurs anteriorly. Where the impact force on a flexed elbow produces a Monteggia fracture dislocation the annular ligament ruptures posteriorly to allow posterior dislocation of the radial head.

Rupture of the annular ligament can also occur in displaced fractures of the radial head, neck or epiphysis. Where the interosseous membrane also ruptures displacement of the radial shaft occurs with the radial head.

The clinical detection of these lesions depends on relating the clinical features of lateral swelling, bruising and hypermobility of the radius to an accurate lateral radiograph of the elbow enabling one to decide whether or not the relationship of the radial head to the capitellum is normal (Fig. 4.12).

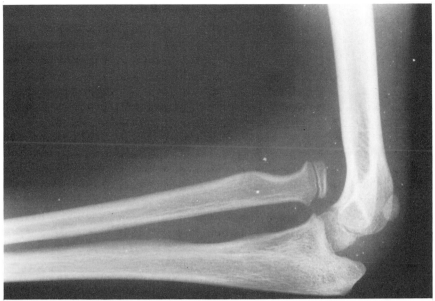

Fig. 4.11 Lateral X-ray showing dislocation of radial head due to rupture of annular ligament.

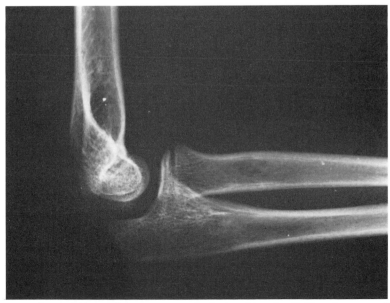

Fig. 4.12 Lateral X-ray showing normal relationship of radial head to capitellum.

Ligament Injuries and their Treatment

4.3.6 POSTERIOR INSTABILITY

The mechanism and pathology responsible for posterior, posterolateral and posteromedial displacements of the elbow joint have been fully discussed in appropriate sections. The clinical entities that result are latent or occult subluxation with or without associated fractures particularly of the radial head or coronoid process and also posterior dislocation which is more often posterolateral but can be posteromedial in displacement.

Whereas the swan neck deformity and swollen bruised elbow in posterior dislocation is well known, it is important to remember the clinical picture of latent subluxation is less well appreciated. Swelling should be looked for, with or without bruising medially, that is, in excess of localized lateral swelling seen with the simple contusion. Stronger evidence is that of medial bruising; deep palpation showing tenderness along the attachments of the collateral ligaments strengthens this suspicion. Provisional diagnosis can be strengthened by aspiration of a haemarthrosis under anaesthesia. This enables one to test the ligament for stability establishing the diagnosis. A lateral radiograph shows the displaced 'pointing' coronoid process (Fig. 4.13). The diagnosis should not be based on radiography alone, for instance, fracture of head of radius or fractured coronoid, as it does not take account of the soft tissue lesion which may exist. It is still important to decide on the stability of the fracture. A simple crack or minimally displaced fracture of the radial

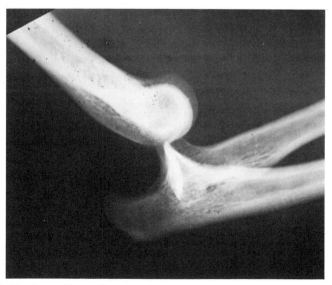

Fig. 4.13   Later X-ray showing displaced 'pointing' coronoid process.

head, neck or epiphysis, the coronoid process, lateral condyle or trochlea may each be associated with occult or latent instability resultant on the ligamentous damage. This will only be revealed on early examination under anaesthesia; it becomes more difficult to demonstrate on the day following fracture.

4.3.7 ANTERIOR INSTABILITY

Forward displacement of the forearm bones can occur where there is a severe or comminuted fracture of the upper end of the ulna, the quarter-staff injury (Hendry). Forward displacement occurs due to the rupture of the collateral ligaments but the anterior capsule may not be torn because in the flexed position there is a laxity of the capsule. This laxity allows forward displacement of the forearm bones until the capsule becomes taut and if the force continues rupture will occur with wider displacement. An ugly deformity with gross swelling and bruising results, and there is a danger of neurovascular problems. Again one must beware of the seemingly innocuous olecranon fracture moderately displaced (Fig. 4.14(a)) but with potential displacement due to occult instability (Fig. 4.14(b)). Aspiration will of course show a haemarthrosis and this lesion can be inferred from the facts or stability tested under anaesthesia.

4.3.8 ROTATIONAL INSTABILITY

The mechanism and pathology behind this lesion have been discussed in the appropriate sections. The clinical picture is again of a grossly swollen elbow with very severe and widespread medial bruising associated with the limitation of motion. The radiograph is striking in that there is less posterior displacement than one would expect normally associated with the lateral shift; this varies in degree according to the capsular tearing and stripping of the lateral ligaments from the humerus (Fig. 4.15). It is important to remember in severe cases of medial instability showing an apparently normal X-ray, or with fractures of the lateral epicondyle, that examination under anaesthesia for occult or latent instability should be made.

4.3.9 CHRONIC INSTABILITY

(a) Disease

That loss of cartilage alone or with increasing amounts of bone stock can lead to laxity of the collateral ligaments has been shown in earlier sections of this chapter. This is seen in both osteoarthritis and rheumatoid

Ligament Injuries and their Treatment

arthritis. Both primary and secondary osteoarthritis show this feature.

Following the initial synovitis, rheumatoid arthritis has two patterns of disease both of which pass through an early stage of chondrolysis. Either increasing erosion of bone with progressive loss of bone stock follows or, as a result of cartilage loss, progressive joint stiffness and indeed ankylosis occurs.

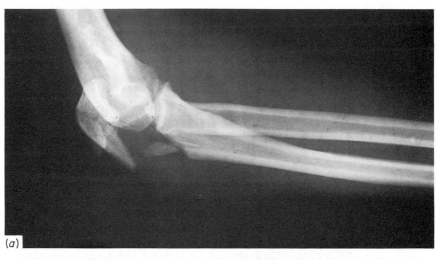

(a)

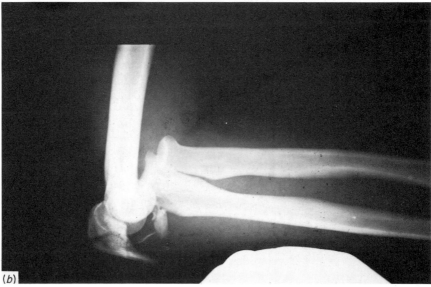

(b)

Fig. 4.14 (a) Fracture of olecranon with apparent moderate displacement. (b) Testing of same fracture under anaesthesia showing 'occult' instability.

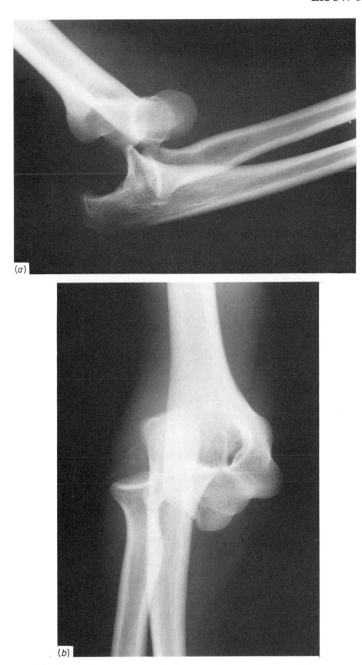

Fig. 4.15 (*a*) Limited posterior displacement on lateral X-ray in rotational dislocation. (*b*) Antero-posterior X-ray showing limited lateral shift in rotational dislocation.

Ligament Injuries and their Treatment

The former is associated with increasing degrees of joint instability, medial, lateral, posterior and rotational all occurring with steady progression in the worst cases. Initially the laxity is due to relative lengthening of the ligaments because of loss of solid tissue but later there is destruction of the ligaments which on exploration can be hard to find. This is particularly true of the annular ligament. In late pictures of the disease it is not uncommon to see grossly deformed upper limbs with wasted soft tissues, posterior subluxation of the elbows, a carrying angle varying from gross valgus to gross varus and all degrees of rotational instability. X-ray examination shows gross loss of bone stock and classical patterns of disease. Initially, in the earlier stages where pain has settled, it is possible to test for ligamentous instability without anaesthesia. Where, however, there is severe pain this is impractical and general anaesthesia will be required; it is usually done once the patient is anaesthetized prior to surgery on the elbow.

(b)   Trauma

This is usually occupational. Various occupations throw an undue load on the arms and elbows in particular. In some types of labouring, for instance where a heavy hammer has to be used, degenerative arthritis may occur in the elbow with increasing laxity of the lateral collateral ligament. Gymnastics can throw excessive loads on the elbow joint in young enthusiasts. Osteochondritis dissecans may occur with degenerative change. In both these instances discomfort in the elbow is associated with a loss of confidence in its use. Clinical signs are few; there is no evidence of deformity or swelling. One must look for the slight loss of extension or hyperextension and also for the slight but definite degree of ligamentous laxity present. It may be more obvious where the other elbow is normal.

4.3.10   RECURRENT INSTABILITY

Recurrent dislocation of the elbow joint is uncommon. Most surgeons see no more than three or four cases throughout their career. However, with the advent of total elbow arthroplasty, all the forms of instability including recurrent dislocation are likely to be seen more often. It is therefore worthwhile looking at this entity in more detail than its occurrence might justify. The work of Osborne and Cotterill (1966) goes a long way towards clarifying this ill-understood condition and, further, suggesting a logical method of treatment.

Recurrent instability occurs in both children and adults. The initiating cause is an acute dislocation which subsequently becomes recurrent. This instability may be a patent dislocation but some merely subluxate. These cases may have their origin in 'latent instability' which has healed incompletely, although the majority of cases of latent instability on follow-up are usually seen to have regained full stability. It is suggested that the lesion is similar to that of the Bankhart lesion described for recurrent dislocation of the shoulder. The transmission of the impact force to the elbow joint causes the coronoid process to abut against the trochlear groove and the radial head against the capitellum. The coronoid guides the forearm bones out posteriorly, laterally and into lateral rotation. The radial head impact damages the capitellum posteriorly and strips up the posterolateral capsule off the bone taking with it an osteochondral fragment. The coronoid process may be fractured as well. It is a non-union of the osteochondral fragment which leads to posterior capsular laxity and, together with the 'shovel-like' bony defect on the radial head, leads to instability.

The medial ligament may also have a laxity which contributes to the instability of the joint. Osborne and Cotterill (1966) say further that the displacement is initiated by transmission of the impact force through the ulna to the coronoid process causing it to pass posteriorly and rotate posterolaterally in its passage through the trochlear groove. In my opinion falls on the outstretched hand undoubtedly produce medial loading of the joint causing one of the lesions producing diminution of the carrying angle, for example, fracture of the coronoid or trochlea with subluxation or dislocation. The majority of cases, however, result in an increase in the compression loading of the humeroradial side of the joint, for example, fractures of the radial head or capitellum combined with a tensile force on the medial side leading to strain or rupture of the medial collateral ligament increasing the carrying angle. There would therefore appear to be an underemphasis of the role of, and damage to, the medial ligament in the production of this lesion. Even in cases where there is a coronoid fracture, the carrying angle still leads to resolution of the forces with tensile loading in the medial side of the joint. Not all cases of recurrent dislocation show the lesion of Osborne and Cotterill, and it is important to note that some may be produced by other mechanisms, for instance that of rotational dislocation described earlier. In the surgical repair of this lesion, therefore, it is as imperative to explore the medial side of the joint as it is the lateral.

Clinically, recurrent subluxation of the elbow joint should always be considered where there is a vague history of discomfort and 'locking' as this may be an expression of underlying instability. The frequency of dislocation varies from one or two incidents a year to monthly or weekly. There may be little evidence of abnormality, even the absence of swelling and bruising, although bruising should be looked for medially immediately after an acute incident. Tenderness may be elicited along the lines of

Ligament Injuries and their Treatment

the medial and lateral ligaments. It may be possible clinically to reproduce instability with subluxation if the joint does not present as a patent dislocation. The radiological picture may be unremarkable or there may be evidence of past bony damage, such as 'loose body' formation along the lines of the collateral ligaments; of course the joint may present as a dislocation.

4.4 Flexion deformities of the elbow

In the knee, angulatory forces rupture the collateral ligaments and collateral capsule, but even in the most severe anteroposterior force injuries, rupturing of the anterior cruciate ligament seldom involves the capsule. In the elbow these forces, in the less severe degree, produce isolated ligamentous rupture and, in the more severe degrees, varying extents of anterior capsular and brachialis tears (Fig. 4.16). In the knee, weight-bearing stretches the fibrous repair tissue resulting in laxity and

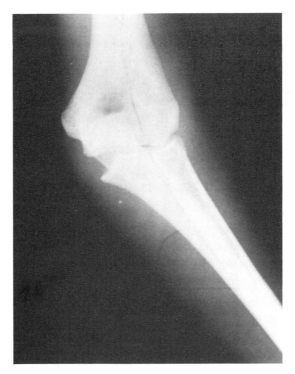

Fig. 4.16 Widening of joint space due to collateral ligament and capsular rupture.

82

instability. Absence of weight forces in the elbow allows fibrosis to progress to contracture especially if injudicious stretching by manipulation or exercising activity occurs. Indeed heterotopic bone formation may occur anteromedially in the substance of the ruptured capsule or brachialis.

Severe functional disability results; for example, there is difficulty in reaching forward for objects at a distance, and carrying heavy weights is uncomfortable and can aggravate the range restriction. Some patients also show gross restriction of flexion and indeed the elbow may be practically ankylosed in the extension/flexion range. Fibrous contracture occurs in arthritis too, due to scarring in the fibrous layer of the synovium and capsule.

Rotation too can be affected, either pronation or supination being grossly restricted by contracture in the supinator or pronator muscles. A pronation deformity is well tolerated where the shoulder remains mobile. Inability to supinate is a most severe disability poorly compensated for even by strenuously adducting the upper arm across the chest.

It is common to think of valgus deformity as being the main reason for the development of a tardy ulnar palsy. However, prolonged flexion deformity is also associated with this lesion in a significant proportion of cases; presumably the immobility of the nerve leads to its being bound down by adhesions. The loss of the gliding potential of the nerve in its groove causes traction damage on movements of the hand, forearm and elbow. Conduction studies by the neurophysiologist confirm the presence of this lesion.

4.4.1 CHRONIC LIGAMENTOUS LAXITY

This results where the damaging force is dissipated early and ruptures the ligaments only, the capsular integrity being retained; flexion contracture in these cases is minimal. Instability may not be gross so the lesion must be looked for carefully as it is easily missed. Gross laxity in severe rheumatoid arthritis will be obvious clinically.

4.5 Treatment

Ligamentous lesions should ideally heal by a process of regrowth of the damaged collagen fibres reproducing the normal ligament. Hypothetically, this would require absence of a haematoma, the type of lesion encountered in 'sprain' injuries. Tears, partial or complete, heal by the process of repair with fibrosis. This results in (a) normal healing, (b) contracture with loss of motion, or (c) lengthening and instability. The

Ligament Injuries and their Treatment

elbow is particularly prone to developing fibrous contracture rather than instability. Concern lest the patient, often a child, develops a 'stiff elbow' determines the plan of conservative or operative regimes of management. prolonged immobilization in a collar and cuff sling or plaster in 90° flexion and varying positions of rotation together with dependency may doom this elbow to permanent stiffness just as much as injudicious manipulation, ill-planned surgical approaches or late surgery. Post-traumatic or postoperative oedema aggravates the degree of fibrosis. It is important to treat severe lesions in elevation in order to get early resolution of swelling (Fig. 4.17). The avoidance of these errors will go a long way to diminishing the number of stiff elbows following treatment.

The lesions themselves resultant on injury must bear the major blame for the post-traumatic stiff elbow; for example, there can be fewer likelier causes of stiffness than either the notorious comminuted fracture of the radial head with posterolateral dislocation of the joint or the displaced intercondylar fracture with capsular disruption. The fact that a recently injured or operated elbow may spend considerable periods of time in a flexed position in the presence of a steadily organizing pannus of fibrous scar tissue results in the development of a tight knot of scar in the antecubital fossa; conversely it may be stretched too early and too much by unwisely ignoring immobilization altogether thus producing an abundance of fibrous tissue by overstretching and tearing of the fine

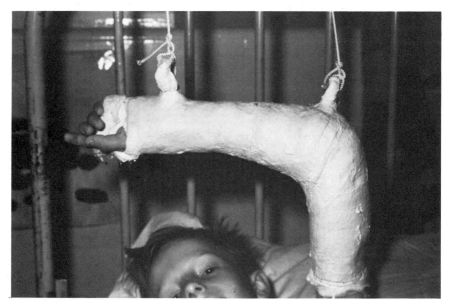

Fig. 4.17 Elevation method of treatment in severe injuries of the elbow.

vascularized scar. Immobilization limited to 1 week followed by graduated actions of daily living for up to 3 weeks provides the basis from which
physiotherapy can rehabilitate the arm over the next 6–8 weeks. It is the
management of this phase, whether conservative or operative that makes
or mars the elbow. Where surgery is decided on it should be carried out
immediately. Delay even for 36 or 48 hours predisposes to significant
postoperative stiffness particularly where the brachialis has been damaged. In these cases it is generally wiser to accept that the opportunity for
surgery has been missed. The patient should be treated conservatively
and the subsequent orthopaedic problems dealt with at a later date,
usually some 6–9 months later; flexion deformity will be less.

4.5.1 MEDIAL INSTABILITY

Avulsion fractures of the medial epicondyle have not only the common
flexor origin attached to the bone fragment but also the fibres of the
medial ligament. Accurate reattachment of the fragment by manipulation
or operation will lead to complete restitution of the function of the
ligament. Where the displacement is minimal a simple collar and cuff
sling with the elbow in as much flexion as the circulation will allow will
often reduce the fracture completely. The danger is that where it is more
distally displaced, it may heal in this position with chronic medial
instability of varying degrees. It is likely that the displacement will be
wider in those cases with increasing capsular rupture. Also inclusion of
the epicondyle in the joint is more likely in this situation.

It is because of these facts and because early stabilization allows one to
mould the fibrous pannus at the right stages of healing that I prefer to
stabilize all but the most minimally displaced fractures of the medial
epicondyle by open reduction and internal screw or pin fixation. It is
important to do the operation with the patient in the prone position
where possible. A much better view of the fracture will be obtained. The
ulnar nerve is usually left in its bed but if at risk then or in the future,
transposition can be carried out readily after the method of Osborne
(1970).

(a) The place of surgery for the medial ligament in trauma

Is there a place for it? It has been said that, as there is a natural tendency
for fibrous organization of the ruptured ligament and capsular areas to
occur, the joint is stable thus eliminating the necessity for surgical repair.
It can of course be excessive leading to flexion contraction. Surgery can be
useful in the following conditions.

(1) In the hyperpronation injuries, rupture of the ligament may be

Ligament Injuries and their Treatment

isolated or combined with increasing degrees of capsular damage. Surgical repair of these lesions can be most rewarding, full joint function being obtainable. The rupture may be found either at the proximal or distal attachments of the anterior or even the posterior band. Repair of the avulsed ligament necessitates its reattachment to the bone; this is achieved using synthetic absorbable sutures anchored through drill holes in the bone. The aim is to diminish the degree of fibrous tissue produced and so lessen the chance of flexion contracture.

(2) In rupture of the medial collateral ligament in association with fracture of the head of the radius and/or dislocation of the elbow. In severe fracture dislocation of the elbow the worst results as far as mobility is concerned are in cases where there is a fracture of the head of the radius. It has been our practice therefore to reduce the problems of bony instability by radial head replacement on the one hand and where a large coronoid fracture exists stabilizing it by screw fixation, although one appreciates that many cases show severe comminution and internal fixation is not always possible. This regime has resulted in stability and an excellent range of motion.

However, in some cases serious medial instability persists even with the elbow immobilized in flexion just above a right angle as far as the circulation and swelling will allow. In these cases repair of the medial collateral ligament where some of the ligamentous tissue persists, however tenuously, is advocated; this should be carried out using synthetic absorbable sutures.

Where the ligament is deficient, present work supports the case for using a polyester synthetic fibre replacement (Amis *et al.*, 1984). In rheumatoid arthritis, total arthroplasty is being used increasingly. Should there be ligamentous laxity, particularly involving the anterior band of the medial collateral ligament, perhaps synthetic fibre implantation to stimulate neoligament formation may provide stability.

4.5.2 LATERAL INSTABILITY

Repair of the lateral epicondylar fracture by suturing the epicondyle back in position or the proximal attachment of the lateral ligament by means of a suture through a drill hole in the bone may be necessary where instability of the radial head associated with laxity of the annular ligament is present. Otherwise lateral instability seldom proves troublesome.

(a) Rupture of the annular ligament

Where hyperpronation has led to disruption and dislocation of the head of the radius in the child it is essential to reduce this displacement as soon as possible allowing the replaced radial head to act as a mould for the healing annular ligament. In the adult this would apply to radial head dislocation in Monteggia fractures. Stabilization of the ulnar fracture with supination of the forearm will generally replace the head and allow such remoulding. In the childhood injury where the annular ligament has avulsed a fragment of bone this can be replaced accurately giving an excellent chance of success. In late cases stabilization of the head may be carried out by the method of Bucknill (1977) using a strip of triceps aponeurosis to fashion a fresh annular ligament or effect repair of the damaged one.

4.5.3 POSTERIOR INSTABILITY

Latent instability will generally heal by conservative measures although associated lesions may need surgical treatment, such as internal fixation or excision and replacement of the radial head. Fracture of the radial head in association with a dislocation is a positive indication of radial head replacement using either a silastic or a metallic head (MacKay, Fitzgerald and Miller, 1970).

4.5.4 ANTERIOR INSTABILITY

Despite the risk of late stiffness, comminuted fractures of the olecranon should be treated by stabilizing the fragments with a bone plate rather than by excision which leads to dislocation.

4.5.5 ROTATIONAL INSTABILITY

In severe injuries of the elbow joint rupture of the medial collateral ligament may predispose to stripping up of the lateral ligament resulting in lateral dislocation; this requires manipulative reduction. If undue medial instability persists repair of the medial ligament is necessary.

4.5.6 RECURRENT INSTABILITY

The method of Osborne and Cotterill (1966) is aimed at the obliteration of the pocket in which the radial head is situated posterolateral to the lateral condyle. A lateral approach exposes the ballooned capsule which is divided and opened allowing access to the condyle to freshen up the bony surface and encourage subsequent readhesion of the capsule. This is ensured by suturing the capsule down to the bone using sutures which pass through both the capsule and drill holes in the bone. The author's preference is for a bilateral approach through the medial method of Molesworth and Campbell (1980) to expose the medial side of the joint. It

Ligament Injuries and their Treatment

may be that the medial collateral ligament is virtually non-existent or else lengthened. Reconstitution or tightening of the ligament can be carried out by using synthetic polyester fibre sutures passed through drill holes in the base of the medial epicondyle. Some cases may be better suited to the use of the method of Schwab *et al.* (1980) who modify Molesworth and Campbell's approach by transferring the osteotomized medial epicondyle proximally. It may be that a similar tightening after osteotomy of the lateral epicondyle could be used and combined with polyester sutures through the capsule. It is likely that a flexion deformity of 30° will have to be accepted if stability is to be regained. It is imperative that antero-posterior, valgus/varus and rotational stability should be tested after the procedure has been completed. Immobilization in this instance would be necessary for a period of 3 weeks prior to commencing the graduated actions of daily living and the physiotherapeutic programme mentioned above.

4.5.7 FLEXION DEFORMITY

Correction of flexion deformity should be reserved for cases of 45–60° or more and should not be attempted earlier than 1 year from the time of injury. Although complete resolution of the flexion contracture is unlikely, correction to 20–30°, in other words minimal deformity, would certainly be worthwhile. The results of arthrolysis are debatable (Bhattacharya, 1974). Because of the hazards involved in the surgical approach and the likelihood of wound contractures subsequently, collateral and posterior surgical approaches are preferred to anterior ones even though they offer more limited access to the desired site. Limited access inhibits the confident division of soft tissue by the surgeon lest damage is inflicted on nerves and blood vessels particularly where there is a lack of familiarity with the area. Peroperative electromyography (EMG) monitoring of neural conduction may lessen this hazard. Using the principles of plastic surgery in the plan of approach to prevent scar contraction over a flexure, together with careful handling of the tissues and meticulous attention to haemostasis, it should be possible to expose the brachialis and anterior capsule directly; thus lengthening of these structures where bony and cartilagenous articular problems are non-existent or minimal can be carried out. More severe bony damage especially of the humeral condyles may necessitate surface arthroplasty, in addition.

The postoperative regime must be carefully planned and will entail control of postoperative haematoma. Suction drains must be used, and swelling must be avoided by elevation of the arm. Prolonged immobilization is undesirable therefore a bulky compression bandage should be applied which affords comfortable splintage but allows minimal voluntary movement. About 1 week later an elasticated support is substituted thus maintaining compression but at the same time permitting gentle activities of daily living. For this reason a long collar and cuff sling is essential replacing the more commonly adopted right angled position of the elbow (Fig. 4.18). The patient commences rehabilitation by the gentler activities of daily living which merge into a planned programme of more active physiotherapy; once maximum function is achieved maintenance exercises retain this range of movement. Vigorous movements or manipulation only increase the chance of recurrence of the flexion deformity, which is a high risk in any case. Following arthroplasty for the treatment of post-traumatic osteoarthritis or rheumatoid arthritis, an undesirable degree of flexion deformity may develop. This can be minimized if one adopts the routine practice of measuring the range of

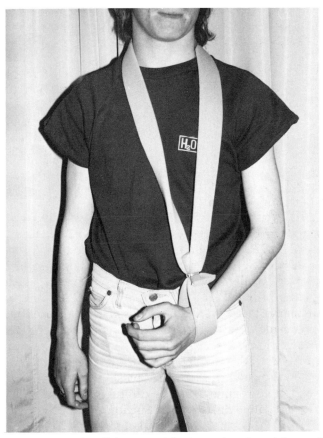

Fig. 4.18 Long collar and cuff sling in 30° flexion rather than right-angled sling to allow freer activity in extension as well as flexion.

Ligament Injuries and their Treatment

joint movements, extension in particular, at the stage of insertion of the trial prosthesis enabling one to make any adjustments necessary; this should guarantee the final ranges of movement once the definitive prosthesis has been inserted.

4.5.8 JOINT STABILITY AND ARTHROPLASTY

In the field of joint replacement strict adherence to the principles ennunciated in this chapter is essential. Biomechanics of the implant design and its surgical insertion must not break any of the rules, otherwise complications occur just as in trauma and disease (Miller *et al.*, 1981). Damage to the medial ligament or to the medial epicondyle will lead to medial instability. If this is excessive then posterior subluxation occurs. Indeed if

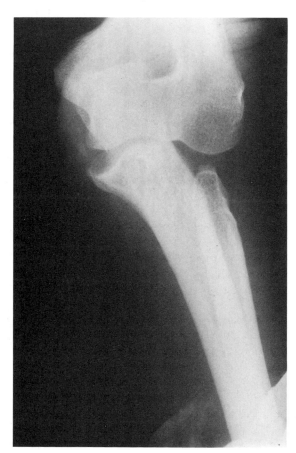

Fig. 4.19 Antero-posterior X-ray of elbow showing cubitus valgus deformity following excison of radial head.

the capsule has been divided full dislocation follows. Should the coronoid implant be malaligned or deficient in its design then posterior displacement will result. Again where the radial head has been excised without replacement the lack of this spacer will increase the tendency to valgus and posterior instability of the joint (Rymaszewski *et al.*, 1984) (Fig. 4.19). If the radial head has been replaced. but the soft tissue attachments of the lateral ligament to the epicondyle have been slackened, instability of the radial head will occur (Fig. 4.20). When the rheumatoid process has severely damaged the annular ligament, control of the radial head after operation may be difficult. Posterior instability may occur where the surgical exposure has divided the attachment of the triceps to the olecranon.

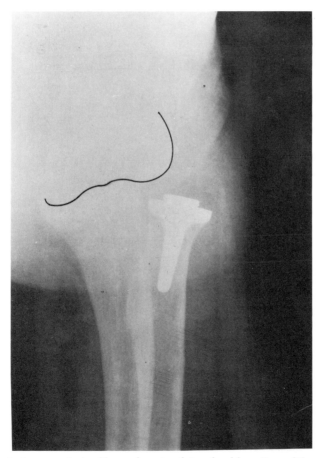

Fig. 4.20 Antero-posterior X-ray showing lateral subluxation of the radial head due to incomplete soft tissue repair.

Ligament Injuries and their Treatment

It is therefore important to repair all ligaments, muscular insertions, or origins divided in the course of the surgical approach or subsequent surgery in order to retain the integrity of the capsule where possible. The radial head must be replaced. A period of immobilization following operation will allow a plaque of scar tissue to form round the implants, immobilizing them.

4.6 Conclusion

Studies of stiff or unstable elbows provide one of the greatest challenges in orthopaedic and accident surgery. Advances have been made but much more remains to be done. In the field of trauma, knowledge that the occult soft tissue lesions are an important complement to the patent bony damage is of vital importance in the analysis and detection of the soft tissue lesion. Its severity cannot be stressed enough. Early treatment of the joint injury within the first 8–24 hours will determine the subsequent fate of this elbow joint. Post-traumatic and postoperative fibrosis will destroy the results of the most meticulous operation. Should the injury fall outside this time-scale then it is wiser in most cases to follow conservative treatment and only tackle the subsequent orthopaedic problems at a much later date, around 6–9 months from the time of the injury. In the field of rheumatoid surgery much remains to be done. There may be some place for the use of synthetic fibre ligaments as an adjuvant to arthroplasty in some cases. To patients with late stage IV rheumatoid disease and gross instability, late synovectomy is often all that can be offered. Some measure of pain relief may be attained but there remains the problem of instability. While recognizing that many surgeons favour the modern non-constrained hinge replacement, an alternative, to conserve bone stock, would be the use of a stemned surface hemi-arthroplasty combined with synthetic polyester fibre ligamentous replacement.

Had man been quadruped, the elbow could have claimed equal status with the knee. Had there been as many elbow surgeons as knee surgeons, greater progress might have been made in this field; but the recent interest in the elbow joint created by the challenge of designing a suitable arthroplasty is fortunately altering this situation.

References

Amis, A. A., Campbell, J. R., Kempson, S. A. and Miller, J. H. (1984), Comparison of the structure of neotendon induced by implantation of carbon or polyester fibre. *J. Bone Joint Surg.*, **66B,** 138.

Bhattacharya, S. (1974), Arthrolysis: a new approach to surgery of post-traumatic stiff elbow. *J. Bone Joint Surg.*, **66B,** 567.

Bucknill, T. M. (1977), Anterior dislocation of the radial head in children. *Proc. Roy. Soc. Med.*, **70,** 622.

MacKay, I., Fitzgerald, B. and Miller, J. H. (1979), Silastic replacement of the radial head in trauma. *J. Bone Joint Surg.*, **61B,** 497.

Miller, J. H., Amis, A. A., Wright, V. and Dowson, D. (1981). Anatomical study of the factors responsible for failure in 'total' elbow arthroplasty. *Proceedings of XV World Congress of SICOT*, p. 407.

Molesworth, W. H. L. and Campbell, W. C. (1980), Medial approach to the elbow with ostoeotomy of the medial epicondyle. *Campbell's Operative Orthopaedics*, Vol. 1, p. 96.

Osborne, G. V. (1970), Compression neuritis of the ulnar nerve at the elbow. *Hand*, **2,** 13.

Osborne, G. and Cotterill, V. (1966), Recurrent dislocation of the elbow. *J. Bone Joint Surg.*, **48B,** 341.

Rymaszewski, L. A., MacKay, I., Amis, A. A. and Miller, J. H. (1984), Long-term effects of excision of the radial head in rheumatoid arthritis. *J. Bone Joint Surg.*, **66B,** 112.

Schwab, G. H., Bennett, J. B., Woods, G. W. and Tullos, H. S. Biomechanics of elbow instability: the role of the medial collateral ligament. *Clin. Ortho. Rel. Res.*, **146,** 50.

5 ⏞

P. A.

5.1 Iɪ

Ligam   e distinct groups;
simple   ty of these injuries
in clir   tears. Unlike the
compl   stability or dislocation o   objective physical
signs.   nisdiagnosed and
poorly managed. Only too often the patient is told that there is no underlying fracture but is offered nothing in the way of specific treatment for the soft tissue injury. In order to appreciate the general principles governing the treatment of ligament injuries, it is first useful to have an understanding of the process of ligament repair.

5.2 Ligament healing

The main ideals of the repair process are for the damaged ligament to heal as rapidly as possible with no elongation of the ligament tissue, no loss in tensile strength, and minimal adhesion formation. Failure to achieve these objectives may result in instability of the neighbouring joint or prolonged discomfort for the patient.

Much of the experimental work on ligament healing has been carried out on the collateral and cruciate ligaments of animal knee joints. As with other connective tissue structures, ligaments have a distinct blood supply derived from the surrounding soft tissues and osseous attachments (Arnoczky, Rubin and Marshall, 1979). Following a ligament rupture the two ends retract and the surrounding elastic areolar tissue grips the divided fibrils of the ligament stumps, thereby preventing apposition of the ligament ends when the rupturing force is discontinued (Jack, 1950). In oblique tears the ligament ends recoil but tend to remain in reasonable apposition, whereas in transverse tears a wide gap develops between the divided ligament ends. During the first week following injury there is a diffuse infiltration of the deficit by polymorpholeucocytes, immature fibroblasts and undifferentiated round cells. This is followed by a progressive infiltration of mature fibroblasts and the deposition of collagen, so that by 6 weeks following injury heavy collagenization has often occurred.

Experimental evidence suggests that ligament injuries are often associated with pathological changes in the neighbouring joint (Miltner, Hu and Fang, 1937). It has been shown that simple sprains are frequently associated with a traumatic synovitis, with inflammation and small haemorrhagic foci seen in the synovial membrane. These acute inflammatory changes may persist for up to 3 weeks following injury. More severe trauma resulting in partial or complete ligament tears, may produce a fibrillar degeneration of the surface layer of cartilage on the same side as the ligament rupture, with cell damage and fissuring of the intermediate cell layer on the opposite side. It is possible that this cartilage damage at the time of injury might be a contributory factor in the development of late onset traumatic osteoarthritis following a previous ligament injury.

Although histochemical studies have demonstrated that the rate of healing of ligament ruptures is unaffected by surgical repair (Wray, Dillon and Harper, 1971), experimental evidence suggests that the quality of the repair process is influenced by adequate immobilization and accurate apposition of the ligament ends (O'Donaghue *et al.*, 1961). Complete tears treated conservatively without adequate immobilization heal with a large amount of undifferentiated scar tissue with no real deposition of collagen. The healed ligament is elongated and lax, and the overall tensile strength of the repaired ligament is markedly reduced, failing at the site of the previous repair. When complete tears are treated conservatively with adequate immobilization, the repair process is more advanced with a significant increase in collagenization of the scar tissue. In the case of the collateral ligaments of the knee joint, surgical repair of complete tears with adequate immobilization produces the optimum results. The torn ligament ends are accurately apposed, and 4 weeks following injury heavy collagenization is seen at the site of repair. The degree of ligament elongation and laxity is greatly reduced, and on testing for tensile strength the ligament fails at the ligament–osseous junction rather than at the site of previous repair.

As a result of the experimental work to date, three important factors should be borne in mind when considering the treatment of ligament injuries:

(1) Following a ligament injury there is often associated damage to the neighbouring joint; there is frequently an associated traumatic synovitis with or without damage to the articular cartilage of the joint surface.

(2) The amount of scar tissue laid down in partial and complete ligament tears is inversely proportional to the degree of immobilization of the affected ligament.

(3) Accurate apposition of the divided ligament fibrils plays a significant role in the quality of the repair process; the greater the gap between the ligament ends, the greater the amount of scar tissue laid down, with ensuing laxity and impaired tensile strength in the healed ligament.

5.3 Treatment of ligament injuries in general

As a general rule the majority of ligament injuries heal adequately with conservative treatment, and it is only a small percentage of complete ligament ruptures which benefit from surgical repair. Complete ruptures of the collateral ligaments of the knee joint undoubtedly benefit from surgical apposition of the ligament ends, but operative repair of complete ruptures of the ankle ligaments is very much open to debate. It must, however, be remembered that surgical apposition of completely torn ligaments improves the quality of the repair process, thereby reducing the disability of instability of the neighbouring joint, and this in itself might be an important factor when considering whether or not a complete tear should be repaired surgically. Adequate immobilization of complete and partial ligament tears is of great importance in reducing the amount of scar tissue and ensuing ligament laxity, and failure to adequately immobilize a complete rupture will undoubtedly lead to an unsatisfactory end result.

The majority of ligament injuries are simple sprains. By definition the ligament fibres are stretched but the ligament as a whole remains in continuity. Instability of the neighbouring joint is not a feature. The objective physical signs are of local tenderness overlying the damaged ligament, swelling and often an associated joint effusion. In the initial stages the damage sustained may appear trivial, and as a result these injuries are frequently poorly managed resulting in prolonged disability and discomfort for the patient.

The objectives of treatment are threefold; the relief of pain, the minimization of soft tissue swelling and the associated joint effusion, and the prevention of adhesion formation.

Ligament Injuries and their Treatment

5.3.1. REST

In the acute phase following injury resting of the affected ligament plays an important role in promoting the healing process. In simple sprained ligaments affecting the limbs, a correctly applied support crêpe bandage or elastoplast strapping helps alleviate pain and reduces local swelling, or in the case of a whiplash injury to the cervical spine a cervical support collar has a markedly beneficial effect. Following more severe trauma resulting in partial or complete ligament injuries, plaster of paris casts should be used to rest the affected part, thereby reducing the amount of scar tissue laid down in the repair process.

5.3.2 ANTI-INFLAMMATORY AGENTS

A short course of anti-inflammatory non-steroidal drugs (NSAID), to dampen down the inflammatory reaction in the neighbouring joint, helps to reduce pain and decrease the associated joint effusion.

5.3.3 COLD

The application of cold in the form of icepacks or cold water is of great value in the early treatment of many ligament sprains. It has two main effects. First, it produces a sensory effect numbing the affected part thereby acting as a counter-irritant and analgesic, and second, it produces a vasoconstriction of the local blood vessels reducing bleeding into the damaged area and decreasing local swelling and inflammation of the neighbouring joint. Evenly applied compression following cooling prevents the danger of a reactive flush and further bleeding into the affected area. In the initial phase following injury cooling of the affected part may be of great therapeutic value.

5.3.4 HEAT

The application of deep heat in the form of short wave diathermy is often beneficial once the danger of bleeding into the affected region has passed. Like the application of cold in the initial stages of treatment it promotes a feeling of comfort and pain relief via a sensory feedback mechanism, and has the added effect of promoting local blood flow.

5.3.5 ULTRASOUND

The use of high frequency mechanical vibrations in the form of ultrasound plays an important role in the early management of ligament sprains and partial ligament tears. It has the effect of dispersing haematoma formation and stimulating local blood flow to the affected parts, and alleviates pain by a micromassage effect.

5.3.6 MOBILIZATION OF THE AFFECTED NEIGHBOURING JOINT

One of the most difficult decisions in the treatment of ligament sprains and partial tears is when best to commence active physiotherapy of the affected joint. As a general rule following simple sprains gentle mobilization of the neighbouring joints should be encouraged as soon as swelling has subsided and pain relief allows, in order to reduce the risk of adhesion formation and joint stiffness. In more severe injuries when adequate immobilization is required to reduce scar formation in the repair process, mobilization of the affected joint should be commenced as soon as the plaster cast is removed. It must, however, be stressed that in the acute phase following injury, active mobilization of acutely inflamed and swollen joints will only aggravate the condition and retard recovery.

In summary the following points are guidelines in the general treatment of ligament injuries.

(1) Complete ligament tears should be adequately immobilized for a minimum of 6 weeks following injury, and in the case of certain ligaments (such as the collateral ligament of the knee joint and the collateral ligaments of the metacarpophalangeal (MCP) joint of the thumb) may benefit from surgical repair with adequate immobilization; this should be followed up by active physiotherapy to reduce joint stiffness and promote strength in the supportive muscles.

(2) In the acute stage following injury the combination of cold, compression and elevation helps to alleviate pain and reduces local swelling and the associated joint effusion.

(3) The use of short wave diathermy and ultrasound in the early phase following injury has a therapeutic sensory effect and promotes local blood flow to the injured part thereby reducing swelling; in the case of ultrasound local haematoma formation is dispersed, thereby reducing the development of adhesion formation.

5.3.7 CHRONIC LIGAMENT STRAIN

The phenomenon of 'strain pain' may be encountered following a ligament sprain or partial tear and is only too frequently seen in injuries treated inadequately in the early stages following injury. The lateral ligament of the ankle is particularly susceptible, but it can also be encountered in injuries to the shoulder joint and cervical spine. In these cases the local injection of hydrocortisone acetate and manipulation under general anaesthetic often has a beneficial effect.

5.4   The ankle joint

5.4.1   SURGICAL ANATOMY

Although the ankle joint is commonly described as a form of hinged joint, the axis of rotation of the ankle changes between the extremes of plantar flexion and dorsiflexion. The stability of the ankle is in part dependent on the strong deltoid ligament on the medial side and the lateral ligament complex on the lateral side (Figs. 5.1. and 5.2).

The lateral ligament (see Fig. 5.1) is made up of three distinct bands radiating out from the lateral malleolus. The *anterior talofibular ligament* runs forwards and almost horizontally between the anterior border of the lateral malleolus and the neck of the talus as a flat band; the *calcaneofibular ligament* which is a cord-like structure runs from the front of the tip of the lateral malleolus posteriorly and downwards to the lateral aspect of the os calcis; and the *posterior talofibular ligament* lies as a horizontal band between the lateral malleolar fossa and the posterior tubercle of the talus. These three ligaments, the anterior talofibular, the calcaneofibular and posterior talofibular ligaments, make up the lateral ligament complex.

The medial aspect of the ankle is supported by the strong *deltoid ligament*. The ligament fans downwards from its attachments to the

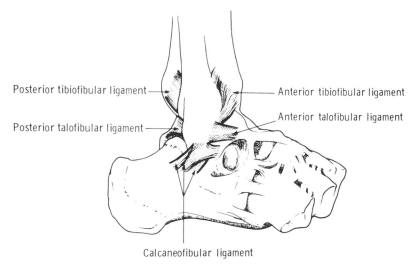

Posterior tibiofibular ligament —

Posterior talofibular ligament —

Anterior tibiofibular ligament

Anterior talofibular ligament

Calcaneofibular ligament

Fig. 5.1   The lateral ligament complex.

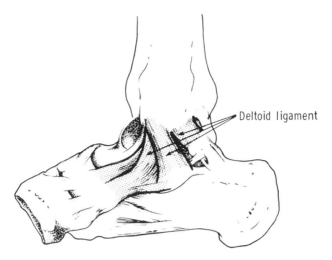

Fig. 5.2 The medial ligament.

medial malleolus and is attached in a triangular-shaped fashion to the medial tubercle and inferior border of the talus, the sustentaculum tali, the spring ligament, neck of the talus and base of the navicular tuberosity (see Fig. 5.2). It is strongest in its middle portion where it is fused with the capsule of the ankle joint.

The syndesmosis of the distal tibiofibular articulation is strengthened by two ligaments and the interosseus membrane. The *anterior tibiofibular ligament* runs as a triangular band extending obliquely downwards and laterally between the tibia and fibula on the anterior aspect of the syndesmosis, while the *posterior tibiofibular ligament* is smaller and runs as a triangular band obliquely downwards between the posterior aspect of the tibia and the lateral malleolus on the posterior aspect of the syndesmosis (Fig. 5.3). The *interosseus ligament* is continuous above with the interosseus membrane, and constitutes the main bond between the distal tibia and fibula.

It must be remembered that although ligament injuries can occur in isolation about the ankle, they may frequently be associated with ankle fractures.

5.4.2 INJURIES TO THE LATERAL LIGAMENT

Of all the ligaments in the body the lateral ligament of the ankle is perhaps the most commonly injured ligament seen in clinical practice. When the body is in the erect position the foot lies in the neutral position at right angles to the leg. The two malleolar processes firmly embrace the talus so

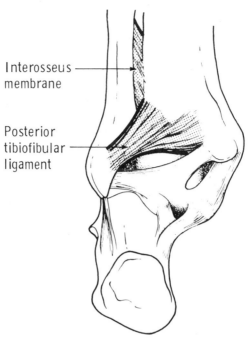

Fig. 5.3 Posterior view of the ankle mortice showing the posterior tibiofibular ligament.

that any side-to-side movement of the talus in the ankle mortice is only permitted by stretching of the ligaments of the distal tibiofibular joint. The strong middle portion of the deltoid ligament together with the calcaneofibular ligament bind the bones of the foot to the leg resisting displacement in all directions. The anterior talofibular ligament prevents displacement of the foot forwards from the ankle mortice, and the calcaneofibular ligament assisted by the talofibular ligament resists backward displacement of the foot relative to the ankle. Plantar flexion of the ankle joint is in part limited by the anterior fibres of the deltoid ligament medially and the anterior talofibular ligament laterally, whilst dorsiflexion of the ankle is limited by the posterior fibres of the deltoid ligament medially, and the calcaneofibular ligament laterally.

Forcible adduction of the talus relative to the ankle mortice places the lateral ligament complex on stretch, and depending on the magnitude of the deforming force a simple sprain, partial or complete disruption of the lateral ligament will ensue. The most common sequence of events resulting in injuries to the lateral ligament complex is seen as a result of a forced adduction or inversion injury with the ankle joint fully plantar-flexed (Coltart, 1951; Ruth, 1961; Broström, 1964). With the ankle plantar flexed the anterior talofibular ligament is under tension and assuming the adduction force is minor a simple sprain or partial tear of this ligament will result. This isolated injury is the so-called 'sprained ankle'. If the adduction force is increased a complete tear of the anterior talofibular ligament will develop, and as the disrupting force continues will extend both posteriorly to involve the calcanofibular ligament and medially across the anterior capsule towards the anterior fibres of the deltoid ligament. The resulting ruptures of the anterior talofibular ligament, calcaneofibular ligament and anterior fibres of the deltoid ligament allows for the talus to sublux forwards, medially rotate and tilt into varus.

Although most commonly encountered as a result of the sequence following a forced adduction of the talus in the plantar-flexed ankle joint, isolated injuries of the calcaneofibular ligament may occur when the plantigrade foot is forcibly adducted. Depending on the magnitude of the disrupting force this may take the form of a simple sprain, partial or complete tear of the calcaneofibular ligament.

(a) Sprained lateral ligament

It has already been mentioned that the most common ligament injury about the ankle is a sprain of the anterior talofibular ligament. The mechanism of injury is that of an adduction or inversion force in the plantar-flexed ankle and clinically there is definite tenderness and swelling distal to and in front of the lateral malleolus overlying the fibres of the anterior talofibular ligament. By definition the ligament is structurally intact and as a result the ankle joint remains quite stable. The diagnosis can be confirmed by gently stressing the inverted heel with the ankle joint fully plantar-flexed causing discomfort at a site anterior to the lateral malleolus.

Although less frequently seen, an isolated sprain of the calcaneofibular ligament can occur following an inversion injury in the plantigrade ankle. When this injury occurs the swelling and tenderness is maximal immediately below and just posterior to the tip of the lateral malleolus overlying the affected ligament. In this form of injury the heel inversion test evokes pain at this site when the plantigrade ankle is inverted. Following a sprain of the anterior talofibular ligament or the calcaneofibular ligament the ankle joint remains quite stable and the only abnormal radiological features are of a soft tissue swelling overlying the site of injury.

(b) Treatment of lateral ligament sprains

Treatment of acute sprains of the lateral ligament should be along the lines previously outlined in the general treatment of ligament injuries. In the immediate stages following injury a combination of cold compresses, elevation and support bandaging helps to minimize soft tissue swelling and oedema, thereby reducing the risk of adhesion formation. Early active movements of the ankle joint should be encouraged. The support bandage may take the form of an elastic adhesive strapping or a crêpe bandage. It is important that this support should be applied in such a way as to control inversion of the heel. Ultrasound and short wave diathermy administered by a trained physiotherapist may result in a more rapid period of recovery.

(c)   Partial and complete tears of the lateral ligament

As with a simple sprain the most common mechanism of injury in a partial or complete tear of the lateral ligament complex is a violent adduction force of the talus in the plantar-flexed ankle. This may result in a partial tear of the anterior talofibular ligament alone, a complete tear of the anterior talofibular ligament, a complete tear of the anterior talofibular ligament with an associated partial tear of the calcaneofibular ligament, or at the worst a complete tear of both the anterior talofibular and calcaneofibular ligaments. In the same manner, depending on the degree of the traumatizing force, a violent inversion injury of the plantigrade foot may result in an isolated partial or complete tear of the calcaneofibular ligament.

Severe swelling, ecchymosis and marked pain following a violent inversion injury to the ankle must raise the possibility of a partial or complete tear of the anterior talofibular and/or calcaneofibular ligaments. From a clinical standpoint, the importance in distinguishing between partial and complete tears revolves around instability of the neighbouring ankle joint, and at the time of initial presentation stress radiographs of the ankle joint in both an anteroposterior and lateral plane are mandatory.

Stress radiographs may be carried out under local or general anaesthesia, and comparable views should be taken of the uninjured ankle for comparison. The varus stress view is best obtained by forcibly inverting the heel with the foot plantar flexed and the leg medially rotated approximately 20° so that the radiograph is taken in an anteroposterior plane at right angles to the bimalleolar axis. To obtain an anterior stress view, the heel is rested on a sandbag at the end of the X-ray table and downward pressure exerted over the distal end of the tibia. A true lateral view of the talus in the ankle mortice is achieved with the leg medially rotated by approximately 20° (Glasgow, Jackson, and Jamieson, 1980). Significant varus instability may be diagnosed (Fig. 5.4) when the talar tilt is in excess of 5° compared to the uninjured side (Rubin and Witten, 1960); and for anterior subluxation (Fig. 5.5) a gap of more than 6 mm between the posterior lip of the tibia and the articular surface of the talus, or a difference of more than 3 mm in this measurement when compared to the

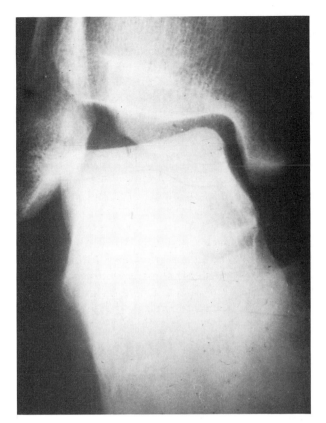

Fig. 5.4 Standard varus stress view demonstrating a marked talar tilt.

uninjured ankle is significant (Noesberger, Hachenbruch and Muller, 1977). The importance of the anterior stress view should not be over-looked. In their study of 56 unstable ankles, Glasgow, Jackson and Jamieson (1980) found that 48% of the ankles examined showed radio-logical evidence of anterior instability without any abnormal talar tilt demonstrated on the varus stress views.

Evans and Frenyo (1979) have advocated the use of stress-tenograms as an aid in the diagnosis of lateral ligament ruptures. The test comprises of a combination of the varus and anterior stress radiographs together with a peroneal tenogram. It can be carried out under local anaesthetic.

(d)   Treatment of partial tears of the lateral ligament

Having excluded instability of the neighbouring ankle joint on presen-tation, partial tears of the lateral ligament may in the initial phases be treated symptomatically. The soft tissue injury and accompanying joint

105

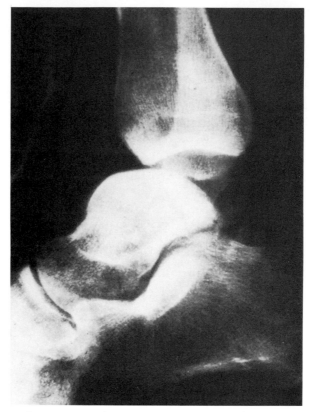

Fig. 5.5 Lateral stress view demonstrating marked anterior subluxation of the talus.

inflammation is more severe than that seen following a simple sprain, and as a result there is often marked swelling and pain around the injured ligament. If the partial tear of the ligament tissue is transverse a definite gap will develop between the torn ligament fibres, whereas if the torn portion is oblique the fibres remain in closer apposition. Clinically it is not possible to distinguish between the two types of tear.

For the sake of pain relief and quality of scar formation it is wise to treat partial tears in below-knee plasters for 2–3 weeks, although unlike complete tears this is not mandatory. Anti-inflammatory drugs afford pain relief and help to decrease inflammation in the neighbouring ankle joint. Following removal of the plaster cast, active movement of the ankle and subtalar joints should be encouraged to prevent or break down early adhesion formation, and this may be enhanced by the added use of ultrasound and short wave diathermy treatment. 'Wobble-board' exercises have been shown to be of definite value in increasing the sense of ankle stability, by re-educating the proprioceptive function of the healed ligament (Freeman, Dean and Hanham, 1965).

5.4.3 COMPLETE TEARS OF THE LATERAL LIGAMENT

Opinions differ over the acute treatment of ~~   · ̣e tears of the lateral
ligament A ̃ ̃ ̇   ınstrated improved
long-   ir (Anderson and
Lecoc   ers have suggested
that e   ple immobilization
of the   , 1965; Gross and
MacIn   ent healing have
demoı   f the torn ligament
ends o   ?t al., 1961), which
suppoı   ɔuld, however, be
empha   ılly demonstrate
instabil

It has   disruption of the
lateral l   te rupture of the
anterior   te rupture of the
anterior   ıd posterior talofibular li   ı isolated tear of
the ante   ɔluxation of the
talus, and   . ̣ ......ugıı a positive shift is demonstrated
on the anteroposterior stress views, the varus stress view is negative. A complete tear of both the anterior talofibular ligament and the calcaneofibular ligament results in a positive tilt on both varus and anteroposterior stress views (Anderson, Lecocq and Lecocq, 1952; Dietshi and Zollinger, 1977; Glasgow, Jackson and Jamieson, 1980).

Before deciding on the mode of treatment of a particular patient a number of factors should be considered. First, the age and physical activity of the patient must be taken into account. In young athletic patients who place high demands on their ankle joints, consideration should be given towards primary surgical repair of the ruptured complex, whereas in the older age group who place less demands on the ankle joint conservative treatment in a plaster cast will suffice. Second, consideration must be given to the extent of the damage sustained. In cases of complete rupture of both the anterior talofibular and calcaneofibular ligaments the argument in favour of primary surgical repair must be stronger than in the case of an isolated rupture of just the anterior talofibular ligament alone.

Whether treatment is by primary surgical repair or by immobilization alone, the ankle joint must be immobilized in a below-knee cast for a period of 6 weeks. Following removal of the plaster cast the ankle and subtalar joints should be mobilized with a course of physiotherapy, and 'wobble-board' type exercises encouraged to re-educate the propriocep-tive function of the muscles supporting the foot and ankle (Freeman, Dean and Hanham, 1965).

5.4.4 CHRONIC ANKLE INSTABILITY

Inadequate treatment of a complete rupture of the lateral ligament will often result in chronic instability of the ankle joint.

The patient presents with a history of having sustained a severe inversion injury in the past, and complains of the ankle feeling weak and giving way. There is often a history of repeated inversion injuries for no apparent reason. Although it is sometimes possible to clinically demonstrate ankle instability, the diagnosis is made after taking stress radiographs in both an anteroposterior and varus plane.

(a)   Treatment of chronic ankle instability

A small percentage of patients may be helped by a course of 'wobble-board'-type exercises combined with a laterally placed heel raise, but more often than not surgical intervention is indicated.

A number of procedures have been described to reconstruct the lateral ligament complex, ranging from tenodeses and tendon grafts to the insertion of artificial structures such as carbon fibre.

In the Watson–Jones procedure, the tendon of peroneus brevis is dissected from its muscle belly which is sutured to the peroneus longus tendon, and is then passed through drill holes in the fibula and neck of the talus to recreate the anterior and middle part of the lateral ligament complex, the new ligament being protected by the tenodesis between the base of the fifth metatarsal and the lateral malleolus. Evans (1953) has suggested that the technically easier procedure of passing the peroneus brevis tendon obliquely upwards from its insertion, through the lateral malleolus alone gives equally good results. In order to minimize restric-tion of movement at the subtalar joint, Sefton *et al.* (1979) have devised a procedure to recreate the anterior talofibular ligament with a free tendon graft of the plantaris tendon.

5.4.5 INJURIES TO THE DELTOID LIGAMENT

Although injuries to the deltoid ligament are much rarer than those of the lateral ligament complex, forced abduction of the talus in the ankle mortice may result in a simple sprain, partial or complete tear of the deltoid ligament. More often than not complete ruptures of the deltoid

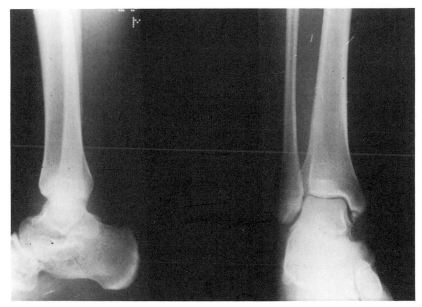

Fig. 5.6 Old avulsion fracture from the tip of the medial malleolus associated with an injury to the deltoid ligament.

ligament are associated with an avulsed fragment of bone from the tip of the medial malleolus (Fig. 5.6) or seen in combination with fracture dislocations of the ankle joint.

Simple sprains and partial tears of the medial ligament should be treated conservatively along the same lines outlined in the treatment of injuries to the lateral ligament complex. In cases of a complete rupture of the medial ligament, particularly when associated with an avulsed fragment of the medial malleolus, surgical repair is indicated.

5.4.6 INJURIES OF THE INFERIOR TALOFIBULAR JOINT

The syndesmosis of the distal talofibular joint is strengthened by two ligaments; the anterior and posterior talofibular ligaments. Although most commonly damaged in association with external rotation–pronation fractures around the ankle joint, resulting in a complete diastasis of the inferior talofibular joint, sprains and partial tears of the anterior talofibular ligament may occur in isolation. The mechanism of injury is that of an external rotation of the talus with the forefoot supinated.

Clinically there is tenderness to palpation over the anterior aspect of the syndesmosis (as distinct from tenderness over the insertion of the anterior talofibular ligament), and on gently externally rotating the foot pain is felt at this site.

It is not uncommon for this injury to give rise to chronic discomfort around the ankle joint. More often than not the symptoms subside following one or more local injections of hydrocortisone acetate and lignocaine around the tender site, but rarely screw fixation of the inferior talofibular joint is indicated for persistent disability (Mullins and Sallis, 1958).

References

Anderson, K. J., Lecocq, J. F. and Lecocq, E. A. (1952) Recurrent anterior subluxation of the ankle joint. *J. Bone Joint Surg.*, **34A**, 853–60.

Anderson, K. J. and Lecocq, J. F. (1954) Operative treatment of injuries to the fibular collateral ligament of the ankle. *J Bone Joint Surg.*, **36A**, 825–32.

Arnoczky, S. P., Rubin, R. M. and Marshall, J. L. (1979) Microvasculature of the cruciate ligaments and its response to injury – an experimental study in dogs. *J. Bone Joint Surg.*, **61A**, 1221–9.

Broström, L. (1964) Sprained ankles I: Anatomic lesions in recent sprains. *Acta Chirurg. Scand*, **128**, 483–95.

Coltart, W. D. (1951) Sprained ankle. *Br. Med. J.*, **2**, 957–61.

Dietschi, C. and Zollinger, H. (1977) Radiological diagnosis of lateral laxity of the ankle joint, *Injuries of the Ligaments and Their Repair* (ed. G. Chapchal), Georg Thieme, Stuttgart, pp. 181–2.

Evans, D. L. (1953) Recurrent instability of the ankle – a method of surgical treatment. *Proc. Roy. Soc. Med.*, **46**, 343–4.

Evans, G. A. and Frenyo, S. D. (1979) The stress-tenogram in the diagnosis of ruptures of the lateral ligament of the ankle. *J. Bone Joint Surg.*, **61B**, 347–51.

Freeman, M. A. R. (1964) Treatment of ruptures of the lateral ligament of the ankle. *J. Bone Joint Surg.*, **47B**, 661–8.

Freeman, M. A. R., Dean, M. R. E. and Hanham, I. W. F. (1965) The aetiology and prevention of function instability of the foot. *J. Bone Joint Surg.*, **47B**, 678–85.

Glasgow, M., Jackson, A. and Jamieson, A. M. (1980) Instability of the ankle after injury to the lateral ligament. *J. Bone Joint Surg.*, **62B**, 169–200.

Gross, A. E. and MacIntosh, D. L. (1973) Injury to the lateral ligament of the ankle; a clinical study. *Can. J. Surg.*, **16**, 155–7.

Jack, E. A. (1950) Experimental rupture of the medial collateral ligament of the knee. *J. Bone Joint Surg.*, **32B**, 396–403.

Miltner, L. J., Hu, M. D. and Fang, H. C. (1937) Experimental joint strain. *Arch. Surg.*, **35**, 232–41.

Mullins, J. F. P. and Sallis, J. G. (1958) Recurrent sprain of the ankle joint with diastasis. *J. Bone Joint Surg.*, **40B**, 270–3.

Noesberger, B., Hackenbruch, W., and Muller, M. E. (1977) Diagnosis of lateral ligament lesion in the ankle joint, in *Injuries of the Ligaments and Their Repair* (ed. G. Chapchal). Georg Thieme, Stuttgart, pp. 182–3.

O'Donaghue, D. H., Rockwood, C. A., Zariczny, B. and Kenyon, R. (1961) Repair of the knee ligaments in dogs. *J. Bone and Joint Surg.*, **43A**, 1167–78.

Rubin, G. and Witten, M. (1960) The talar-tilt angle and the fibular collateral ligaments. A method for determination of talar tilt. *J. Bone Joint Surg.*, **42A**, 311–00.

Ruth, C. J. (1961) The surgical treatment of injuries of the fibular collateral ligaments of the ankle. *J. Bone Joint Surg.*, **43A**, 229–39.

Sefton, G. K., George, J., Fitton, J. M. and McMullen, H. (1979) Reconstruction of the anterior talofibular ligament for the treatment of the unstable ankle. *J. Bone Joint Surg.*, **61B**, 352–4.

Staples, O. S. (1975) Ruptures of the fibular collateral ligaments of the ankle. Result study of immediate surgical treatment. *J. Bone Joint Surg.*, **57A**, 101–7.

Wray, J. B., Dillon, G. P. and Harper, G. E. (1971) Histochemical studies of ligament healing. *J. Bone Joint Surg.*, **53A**, p. 1029.

6   Knee lesions I

J. F. FETTO

6.1   Introduction

The knee is an anatomic region that contains four bones (the femur, tibia, fibula, patella) and their three articulations; femorotibial, patellofemoral, and tibiofibular. The geometry of these articulations would imply that they are inherently unstable. This is particularly so at the femorotibial articulation. The femur, a bicondylar surface, articulates with the relatively flat tibial plateau. As such it can accommodate multidirectional mobility between the distal femur and tibia: flexion–extension; internal–external rotation; anterior–posterior glide; and varus–valgus angulation. However for normal knee kinematics during both static loading as well as dynamic function, stability is critically necessary for this articulation. It has been demonstrated that excessive motion whether acquired post-injury or congenitally, in any or a combination of these degrees of freedom, will result in dysfunction and premature senescence of the knee. Protection against such excessive motion is afforded through a dual mechanism of restraints, some static and some dynamic. The primary static stabilizers are the ligaments; the dynamic stabilizers are the musculotendonous units. Hypothetically there exists through recruitment and training of muscle tendon units a potential means of compensation for static stabilizer dysfunction (that is, post-traumatic). It is the intention of the discussion below to address the following issues concerning knee ligament injuries:

(1) the anatomy and function of the static stabilizers of the knee;
(2) the pathomechanics of knee ligament injuries;
(3) the techniques of diagnosis of these injuries;
(4) the available means of compensation for static stabilizer dysfunction;
(5) the available treatment options for ligament injuries;
(6) the future directions of research and investigation.

Ligament Injuries and their Treatment

Although it is recognized that the knee is composed of many more than four static stabilizing structures, this discussion of knee ligament injuries, their diagnosis, treatment, and future directions of investigation will be primarily directed towards consideration of the superficial medial collateral (MCL), the lateral collateral (LCL), anterior cruciate (ACL), and posterior cruciate (PCL) ligaments. Other static stabilizers (such as capsular ligaments, arcuate ligament, etc.) will be discussed in conjunction with these four main categories as appropriateness and space allow.

6.2 Superficial medial collateral ligament (MCL)

6.2.1 ANATOMY

As well described by numerous authors, the medial collateral ligament presents as a distinct and robust structure. It is easily palpable as a vertical band with a well-demarcated anterior edge as it traverses the mid-medial joint line. It is a broad and flat structure lying between the superficial investing fascia of the extremity and the deep capsular tissues. The medial collateral ligament originates at the medial femoral epicondyle approximating the medial aspect of the knee flexion–extension axis. The ligament is divided such that one-quarter of its length lies proximal to the medial joint line; and its tibial insertion attaches beneath the pes anserine. Deep to the medial collateral ligament is the 'deep' medial collateral or capsular ligament. It originates just proximal to the medial femoral articular margin and extends distally to insert onto the medial side of the proximal tibia. As it does so it is attached to the medial meniscus. Hence the deep ligament may be considered as having two halves: the femoral–meniscal, and the meniscal–tibial. The deep medial collateral ligament is a much less robust structure than is the superficial medial collateral ligament. These structures are quite distinct at the mid-medial joint line but do coalesce into a single layer at the posteromedial corner of the knee.

6.2.2 FUNCTION

Functionally the superficial medial collateral ligament has two components: an anterior longitudinal component which tightens during flexion, and a posteromedial expansion which becomes taut in extension.

During single leg stance loading, the body's centre of gravity falls medial to the knee joint. As such there is a varus moment at the knee. This results in a *compressive* loading across the medial compartment of the knee joint. As such there is no significant longitudinal tensile loading of the medial collateral ligament under such conditions. The medial collateral is most often under tensile stress during dynamic loading (in other words 'push-off').

114

'Push-off' as the term implies, is the initiation of locomotor activity. At this time the driving lower extremity is positioned such that the foot and leg are externally rotated relative to the femur. The foot is planted and the ipsilateral knee is flexed in anticipation of forward acceleration of the body. In this posture a valgus stress is applied to the knee. The resultant tensile loading of the medial static stabilizers places them at risk of excessive strain (elongation) and failure. This failure may be classified into one of three grades: I, II, III, in proportion to the grade of anatomic and functional distortion created. A grade I sprain shows only microscopic collagen disruption in the face of painful but preserved gross anatomic and functional integrity. A grade III lesion is one in which total mechanical integrity is compromised (with or without apparent anatomic integrity). A grade II injury is therefore one in which both anatomic and mechanical integrity are affected but not totally compromised. (This classification will be similarly applied in the cases of other static stabilizers to be discussed below.) The medial collateral ligament therefore functions primarily to stabilize the knee against valgus loading particularly at the initiation of locomotion, or 'push-off'.

6.2.3 MECHANISM OF INJURY

Clinical and cadaveric investigation incorporating radiographic, arthrographic and surgical techniques have demonstrated that the superficial medial collateral ligament is the prime static stabilizer of the medial side of the knee joint. These studies attempted to reconstruct and reproduce the mechanism of medial collateral ligament injury. They conclusively demonstrated agreement with earlier investigators that a valgus stress to the knee will be resisted sequentially by first the superficial medial collateral ligament followed by the 'deep' medial collateral ligament capsular ligament, anterior cruciate ligament (ACL), and finally the posterior cruciate ligament (PCL).

6.2.4 DIAGNOSIS

Proper and accurate diagnosis of medial collateral ligament injuries (as in other ligament injuries) is predicated upon three fundamental medical principles: (1) the eliciting of a complete and thorough history; (2) the performance of a meticulous physical examination based upon the understanding of knee anatomy and function; and (3) accessibility and availability of ancillary testing capabilities (such as stress X-ray, arthrography, etc.)

Crucial to the diagnosis of medial collateral ligament injury is a reconstruction of the recent traumatic event and any previous such events. An analysis of the *mechanism of injury* (Fig. 6.1) will direct the examiner's attention towards the appropriate static stabilizer which would have been stressed during the insult. For example, a medially directed force applied against the lateral aspect of the knee will create a valgus stress upon the knee joint. The medial collateral ligament is the primary static stabilizer against such a stress. Therefore, injury occurring in this manner would raise a strong index of suspicion regarding medial collateral ligament injury and possible compromise. Also important is the patient's functional capability at the time of injury. A knee which is unable to bear weight due to exquisite medial pain may imply at least partial anatomic disruption of the medial collateral ligament. A medially unstable yet relatively painless knee may indicate complete disruption of the ligament. This relative absence of pain is due to the lack of an intact structure to resist tensile loading.

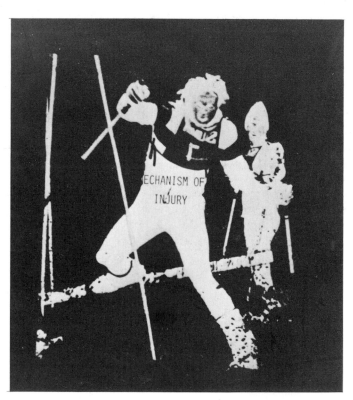

Fig. 6.1 Mechanism of injury: as observed in the figure, the mechanism of injury can be easily constructed by review of the patient's activity at the time of injury; the example seen here demonstrates flexion–valgus–external rotation of the injured right lower extremity.

At physical examination, the medial collateral ligament is normally palpable as a 1 cm band having a distinct anterior margin crossing the medial joint line. Area of maximal tenderness may be localized as the length of the ligament is traced from its origin at the medial femoral epicondyle to its disappearance beneath the pes anserine. Functional integrity of the medial collateral ligament may be clinically assessed by its ability to resist tensile loading under valgus stress. Classically medial collateral ligament injury is said to be proportional to the amount of the medial 'opening' observed during an applied valgus stress. However the exact interpretation of this opening has been a source of great controversy.

As the primary static stabilizer against valgus stress, it is reasonable to assume that a clinically applied valgus stress would be useful to assess medial collateral ligament integrity. The critical issues at hand are: (1) in which position should the knee be held at the time valgus stress is applied; (2) what is the anatomic significance of 'medial opening'; and (3) the observations made should always be compared against the unaffected contralateral knee.

Under controlled cadaveric and prospective clinical studies correlations were established between observed clinical findings and anatomic lesions. First, valgus stress of the medial collateral ligament is most accurate when the knee is held at 30° of flexion. In this position the anterior and posterior cruciate ligaments are relaxed. This is important because both the anterior and posterior cruciate ligaments are valgus stabilizers in the face of medial collateral ligament compromise at full and hyperextension positions of the knee. Second, it has been demonstrated that increased medial opening as compared to the unaffected knee is of importance but equally important is the quality of the terminal ('endpoint') resistance provided by the ligament to an applied stress. A functionally intact ligament will produce a firm, discrete endpoint at the termination of a medial opening (grade I). This is in contrast to the 'spongy' or 'soft' endpoint resistance of a compromised ligament (grade II or grade III). Comparison X-rays at 30° of flexion will assist in substantiating a clinical impression of medial 'opening'. Opening at 0° of flexion may indicate not only medial collateral ligament compromise but should also raise suspicion of anterior cruciate ligament insufficiency. Single contrast arthrography has been demonstrated to be an accurate tool for the assessment of the degree of ligamentous damage present. Specific radiographic patterns have been shown to hold significant correlation to specific degrees of injury. Containment of the dye within the knee implies integrity of the deep ligament, while diffusion of the dye into the periarticular soft tissues would suggest rupture of both the medial collateral ligament and capsular tissues. This technique is especially useful in assessing a knee too painful to allow other form of manual examination.

6.2.5 TREATMENT OPTIONS

Treatment of medial collateral ligament injuries may be divided into two categories: non-operative and operative; each of which may be further divided according to individual physician training, experience, and preference. The decision of whether or not to operate always includes consideration of a patient's age, goals, comprehension, level of function, compliance, and motivation. However two major factors have been identified through long-term analysis of medial collateral ligament injuries which have been demonstrated to significantly affect the prognosis of a given injury and therefore mitigate for or against specific treatment options. These factors are the grade of the lesion (as defined earlier) and the complexity of the lesion, that is, whether or not other static stabilizers have been compromised coincident with the medial collateral ligament. This is especially of concern when the anterior cruciate ligament is not functionally preserved. It has been demonstrated that the end result for *acute* (less than 2 weeks postinjury) comparable-grade isolated medial collateral ligament injuries is not affected by the alternative of either adequate closed or operative treatment chosen. Adequate closed treatment is defined as 2 weeks (in splint), 6, and 10 weeks (plaster) immobilization for grade I, II, and III lesions respectively. However the prognosis of *mixed* medial collateral ligament lesions (that is, ones with coincident anterior cruciate and/or posterior cruciate ligament compromise) regardless of the grade, was significantly diminished under closed treatment. Mixed medial collateral ligament injuries fared well only if primary surgical repair of all injured structures was performed.

Surgical repair of acute medial collateral ligament injuries may be performed by primary anastomosis with or without supplementation of the ligament by adjacent soft tissue structures. The anterior advancement of the posteromedial soft tissues (that is, capsule and semimembranosis tendon) is one such option. The second is incorporation of the semitendonosis tendon after anterior advancement and staple fixation of that tendon at the medial femoral epicondyle (Bosworth procedure). Immobilization postoperatively is accomplished by a Jones dressing for 5–7 days with the knee held at 30° of flexion. Weight-bearing status is slowly progressed from non-weight-bearing to full weight-bearing during the balance of 6 weeks' plaster immobilization. Following immobilization after operative and non-operative treatment, the knee is protected with a medial–lateral hinged elasticized brace (knee cage). Rehabilitation is directed initially at restoration of joint range of motion, followed by strength and endurance training. The former is accomplished through a combination of passive, active-assisted, and active range of motion exercises together with joint mobilization and electrical muscle stimulation therapy as indicated. The latter will be accomplished through a programme which includes isometric, isotonic, and isokinetic exercises. The patients may return to previous levels of sports participation when they have demonstrated recovery of at least 75% endurance and power as compared with the unaffected limb by isokinetic techniques (such as, Cybex).

6.2.6 SUMMARY

The medial collateral ligament is the prime static stabilizer of the knee against valgus stress. As an isolated lesion, injury of this ligament demonstrates full recovery regardless of the severity of the injury and treatment modality employed. However, when complicated by coincident ligament compromise, the prognosis is maximized only by simultaneous primary surgical repair of all injured structures.

6.3 Anterior cruciate ligament (ACL)

6.3.1 ANATOMY

The anterior cruciate ligament is a dense collagenous structure which lies intra-articular and extrasynovial to the knee joint (Fig. 6.2). Its average dimensions are approximately 10 mm in width × 40 mm in length. It is divided into a 'distinct anteromedial band and a main posterolateral part'. The ligament originates at the posteromedial intercondylar surface of the lateral femoral condyles, and inserts 15 mm posterior to the anterior edge of the tibial plateau articular surface *between* the tibial spines. Its overall direction is therefore posterosuperior to anteroinferior, coursing across and anterior to the posterior cruciate ligament. The blood supply of the ligament arises from: (1) its articular attachments; (2) posterior meniscal attachments; (3) ligamentum mucosum, infrapatellar fat pad attachment (Fig. 6.3).

6.3.2 FUNCTION

Following the paraphrased design principle, 'function follows structure' the anterior cruciate ligament is the primary static stabilizer of the knee against anterior displacement of the tibia on the femur. It is also a static stabilizer against hyperextension and internal rotation; and after the medial collateral ligament is a secondary restraint against valgus angula-

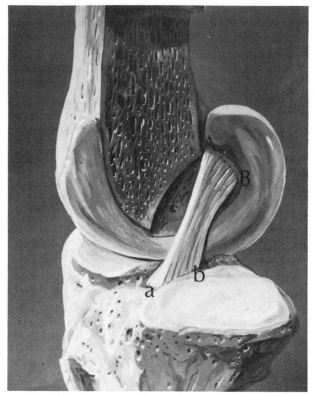

Fig. 6.2   Anatomy of anterior cruciate ligament.

tion. Within the ligament these functions are divided among the antero-medial band, posterolateral bulk, and anterior ligament respectively. Historically, although most authors express little expectation for spon-taneous healing of the anterior cruciate ligament postinjury, the func-tional consequences of anterior cruciate ligament insufficiency have been hotly contested. This difference of opinion arises primarily out of the duration of follow-up postinjury one chooses. Within the initial 6–10 weeks postinjury, although originally presenting as a significant injury, an anterior cruciate ligament insufficient knee will appear to have recovered full function. But anterior cruciate insufficiency does result in an instability. This instability may not initially appear to be clinically significant nor pose a compromise to function. However, it does place an increased burden upon secondary stabilizers against anterior displace-ment and internal rotation. These secondary stabilizers are: statically the posterior horn of the lateral meniscus; and dynamically the hamstring musculature. In spite of these secondary stabilizers episodes of clinical

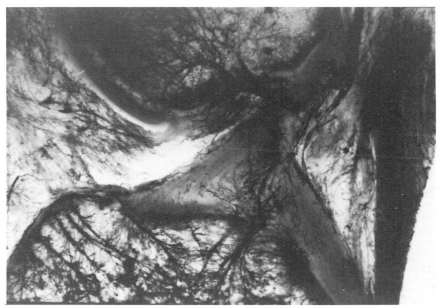

Fig. 6.3 Dye study using fresh cadaveric specimen demonstrating the circulatory supply of the anterior and posterior cruciate ligaments.

instability may occur. Such an instability is usually described by the patient as the knee 'slipping' or 'giving way'. This is particularly common during vigorous pivoting-type manoeuvres. Most often it is expressed by the patients by rotating their clenched fists on one another.

6.3.3 PATHOMECHANICS

Anterior cruciate insufficiency represents the *reduction* of the anteriorly subluxed tibia as weight-bearing occurs on the affected side just following heel strike. The mechanism of this phenomenon has been demonstrated to be as follows: during the first 10% of the normal gait cycle following heel strike, there are several forces acting to anteriorly displace and internally rotate the tibia, (1) the inertial extension moment of the leg driving the knee into extension; (2) an anteriorly directed quadriceps pull; (3) an internal rotational torque; and (4) an anteriorly directed sheer stress at the joint line in the plane of progression. If the anterior cruciate is stretched or torn, the stability of the knee will necessarily depend upon the remaining structures that serve to restrain the tibia against excessive anterior and internal rotation displacement. However, as the knee approaches the position of full extension these secondary restraints become less effective than they are in the flexed position. The hamstring musculature becomes less mechanically efficient, the lateral femoral condyle abruptly presents a relatively flat distal surface to the lateral plateau of the tibia, and the purchase of the lateral meniscus is reduced so that the posterior horn of the lateral meniscus begins to be wedged beneath the lateral femoral condyle. This widens the lateral compartment of the knee joint; which ultimately is sufficiently widened to allow the tibia and posterior horn of the lateral meniscus to suddenly sublux anteriorly beneath the femoral condyle. As the gait cycle continues through mid-stance the increasing vertical load of weight-bearing approaches its maximum but the forces responsible for anterior displacement of the tibia have abated. The extension moment has ceased, the quadriceps pull has ended, the direction of the internal rotational torque and anterior sheer stress have been reversed. The result is spontaneous reduction of the subluxated tibia and the lateral meniscus, perceived by the patient as the knee 'slipping' or 'giving way'.

This subluxation–reduction slipping motion can easily be observed during cineradiographic examination of an affected knee. This sequence has been termed the 'pivot shift'. It can be reproduced clinically as follows: the patient is rotated 20° from supine onto the unaffected side; the affected knee is flexed 70° and the ipsilateral hip 20°; the examiner applies a valgus stress to the knee by pressing down on the lateral aspect of the distal part of the thigh; simultaneously an internal rotational torque is applied at the ankle while the knee is brought towards extension. During this manoeuvre the examiner will feel a sudden slip or jog to occur within the knee during the final 20° of extension; and a similar sensation will be appreciated on passive return of the knee into flexion. This technique is a modification of the method described by Galway and McIntosh (1980), who first coined the term 'pivot shift'.

Over the longer period (2–10 years) postinjury, depending upon the conditioning maintained in limb musculature and the stresses applied, this instability will result in an insidious and pernicious decompensation of the secondary restraints against anterior displacement and internal rotation. This will be associated with progressive functional compromise due to more frequent episodes of 'giving way' and increasing clinical signs of knee joint senescence (osteophyte formation, recurrent effusions, and meniscal degeneration and failure). As such, it is not unusual to have a patient present with 'acute' meniscal pathology only to discover before or at the time of surgery that there is absence of the anterior cruciate ligament. In such a case histological examination of the meniscal material will demonstrate stigmata of chronic degenerative change rather than acute laceration. These changes (mucoid degeneration, cloning of intrameniscal cells, horizontal fissuring, and loss of hyaluronic acid from meniscal substance) (Fig. 6.4(a) and (b)) indicate

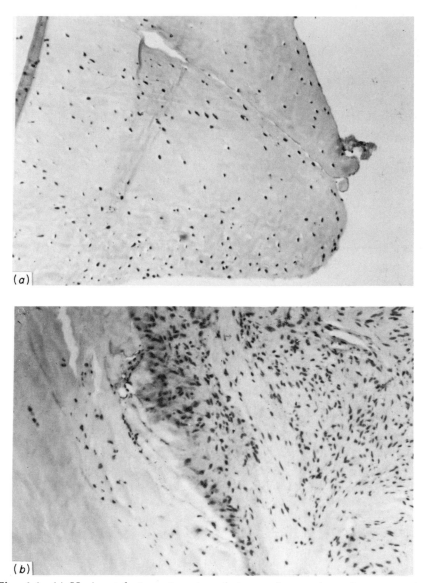

Fig. 6.4 (*a*) Horizontal stress tear in substance of a meniscus in an anterior cruciate deficient knee. (*b*) Higher magnification demonstrating the cellular infiltration, mucoid degeneration, and stigmata of fatigue failure of the meniscus.

chronic and excessive sheer stresses as being the aetiology of meniscal failure. A fatigue type of failure develops in the meniscus as it tries to act as a stabilizer against anterior and internal rotational displacement in the absence of an anterior cruciate ligament. It is noteworthy to mention that in such cases following meniscectomy the knee may become significantly more unstable, thus rendering a previously compensated knee functionally compromised much to the dismay of both the patient and the physician. Therefore, although showing apparent early recovery, the ultimate functional prognosis of untreated uncompensated anterior cruciate ligament insufficiency is premature functional and structure deterioration of the knee joint.

6.3.4   MECHANISM OF INJURY

The anterior cruciate ligament may be most commonly ruptured by one of three mechanisms of injury. The first hyperextension–internal rotation will produce an 'isolated anterior cruciate ligament injury'. As defined above this means that although it is not usually possible to injure only one structure, an 'isolated injury' means that there is *clinically appreciable* compromise of only a single static stabilizer. In such a case together with the anterior cruciate ligament there will be usually found on surgical exploration haemorrhage within the posterolateral capsule of the knee. Therefore presentation of a knee injury with haemoarthrosis and posterolateral pain should strongly direct the examiner's attention towards an assessment of anterior cruciate ligament integrity. The second mechanism of injury, flexion–valgus–external rotation will result in compromise of the anterior cruciate ligament only after medial collateral ligament compromise has occurred, and may be accompanied by medial meniscus damage creating an O'Donoghue triad. Further valgus angulation may extend the sequence of injured structures to include compromise of the posterior cruciate ligament. These injuries are so devastating to knee stability as to render the joint unstable under weight-bearing stress even when pain is relieved. Hyperflexion as the third mechanism of injury is by far a much less commonly encountered manner of anterior cruciate ligament compromise. Rupture of the anterior cruciate ligament may also, but infrequently, occur with varus stress after lateral ligament compromise. A history which includes any of the described mechanisms of injury should raise the examiner's index of suspicion of anterior cruciate ligament compromise.

The anatomic site of rupture along the ligament has a significant effect on prognosis. Avulsion injuries have a much better prognosis under surgical repair than do 'mid-substance' tears. Studies seem to indicate that the speed of ligament loading may influence the location of structural failure, such that rapid loading (downhill skiing) will cause intraligament failure whereas a slow loading situation will result in terminal bone–ligament failure. In this regard the history may be of assistance in preparing the physician for the appropriate course of treatment and possibly anticipate the type of injury to be encountered if surgery is chosen.

6.3.5 DIAGNOSIS

So characteristic is the history of anterior cruciate ligament injury and insufficiency that diagnosis may be strongly suspected on it alone. *Acute* anterior cruciate ligament injury will present usually with a very specific mechanism of injury. Rupture may be associated with an audible 'pop' as reported by patients in 80% of the cases studied. There will be an acute onset of swelling (haemoarthrosis); and ability to bear weight will be variable depending upon the presence or absence of additional ligaments having been compromised. Likewise late or chronic anterior cruciate ligament insufficiency has a characteristic history. The patient usually presents with repeated episodes of knee 'giving way' and swelling or with apparent acute meniscal injury. Careful investigation will uncover a previous history of one or more injuries in which the mechanism of injury may raise suspicion of previous anterior cruciate ligament compromise. The patient will usually relate a pattern of gradual, insidious functional deterioration prior to this latest event. Dysfunction is most often blamed upon a lack of confidence in the 'stability of the knee' on change of direction, landing from a jump, or quick pivoting manoeuvres. It is usually compensated for by change in activity or modification of the patient's degree of participation. This modification may be subtle; and be uncovered only through meticulous investigation of the patient's history. Just as the history is specific for anterior cruciate ligament injury, so too are the signs observed during physical examination specific for anterior cruciate ligament compromise. Manual stability tests which demonstrate *increased* anterior displacement of the tibia on the femur (that is, anterior drawer sign) indicate probable anterior cruciate ligament disruption. However it has been demonstrated that compromise of the medial collateral ligament or menisci may slightly increase anterior displacement in the presence of an intact anterior cruciate ligament. Therefore anterior displacement alone may be *insufficient* to accurately assess anterior cruciate ligament integrity. For this reason the concept of 'endpoint resistance' was introduced. Endpoint resistance refers to the quality of the resistance appreciated at the terminus of passive anterior displacement of the tibia. Anatomic and functional integrity of the anterior cruciate ligament is implied when this endpoint has a discrete and firm quality. If the quality of the endpoint is 'soft', 'spongy', or 'ill-defined', it may be inferred that there is anterior cruciate ligament compromise. These endpoint evaluations may be employed when anterior displacement is attempted with the knee flexed at 90° (the anterior drawer test) (Fig. 6.5) or when the knee is flexed 10–30° (Lachman test). The latter test has the dual advantage over the anterior drawer test of being more easily applied to the acutely injured knee, and also it negates the potential false-negative resistance to anterior displacement produced by hamstring spasm or guarding. There are additional methods of clinically assessing anterior cruciate ligament integrity. They fall into two categories. The first is a modification of the classic anterior drawer test in which rotation of the tibia is performed prior to the application of the anterior displacement force. This test (Slocum test) assesses capsular integrity. The second category of tests is comprised of those manoeuvres which attempt to clinically reproduce the patient's 'pivot shift phenomenon'. These may be termed the pivot shift test, the jerk test or sign, or flexion–rotation drawer test. The basic premise of each of these is to reproduce the relative anterior–internal rotation subluxation of the tibia in the face of anterior cruciate ligament insufficiency. These tests do have a significant percentage of false-positive and false-negative results (approximately 15%). This is due to

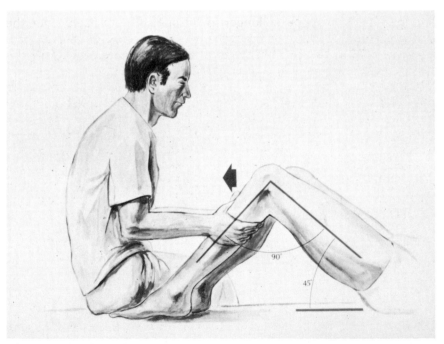

Fig. 6.5 Proper positioning and performance of the classic anterior drawer test.

their reliance upon intact menisci and absence of generalized ligamentous laxity.

In addition to clinical stress testing, ancillary tests may be of significant assistance in developing an accurate diagnosis of anterior cruciate ligament injury. In the acute or chronic anterior cruciate ligament insufficient knee single contrast arthrography (Fig. 6.6(a) and (b)) and stress films will define anterior cruciate ligament integrity by outlining in the intact ligament or documenting anterior translation of the tibia respectively. Routine anteroposterior, lateral, and particularly 'tunnel' views of the knee will demonstrate the stigmata of chronic instability (periarticular and intracondylar osteophyte formation) (Fig. 6.7(a) and (b)). More recently investigations employing CAT scanning techniques have been utilized in order to visualize the anterior cruciate ligament. To date these have produced equivocal success at best. However NMR technology does hold much promise. In all, anterior cruciate ligament injury, whether acute or chronic, does have a characteristic presentation, which when familiar will greatly enhance the diagnostic accuracy of the examining physician.

6.3.6 TREATMENT OPTIONS

For the past 80 years, and longer in Europe, the argument over the superiority of closed versus operative management of anterior cruciate ligament injuries has raged in America. European literature prior to the turn of the century, and on both sides of the Atlantic since, have strongly indicated the importance of an intact anterior cruciate ligament for physiological knee kinematics. Originally, the demands of meticulous technique during what could prove to be long operative exposures without benefit of antibiotic coverage mitigated against acceptance of operative repair of anterior insufficiency (acute or chronic). Later due to the lack, until recently, of standardized evaluation technqiues, it had been difficult to definitively assert the superiority of one technique of repair and/or reconstruction over another. These factors together with the *apparent* early initial functional recovery of anterior cruciate ligament with non-operative treatment resulted in the continued sinusoidal oscillation between operative and non-operative treatment modalities being employed for anterior cruciate ligament injuries during the first third of this century.

The work of Palmer in 1938 definitively underscored for the first time, in a documented fashion, the long-term consequences of unresolved anterior cruciate ligament compromise. His work reinforced the concepts of Smith, Hey Groves, and others before him who argued for surgical repair; and it laid the foundation for those who followed. These workers

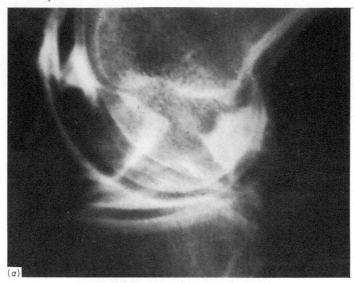

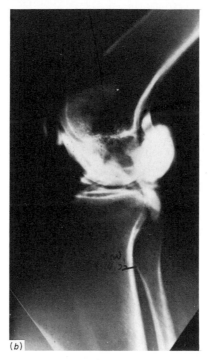

Fig. 6.6 (*a*) Single contrast arthrography with demonstration of intact anterior and posterior cruciates. (*b*) Single contrast arthrogram demonstrating compromise of the anterior cruciate ligament and presence of intact posterior cruciate ligament.

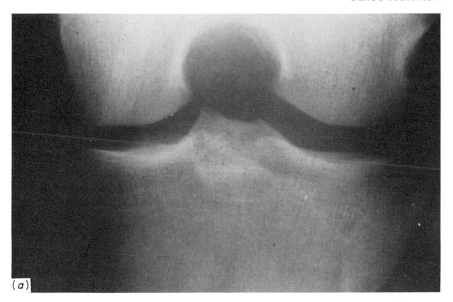

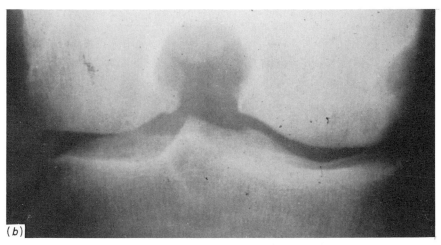

Fig. 6.7 (*a*) Anteroposterior projection tunnel view of a knee diagnosed as having an anterior cruciate injury. (*b*) Same knee similar projection demonstrating the periarticular changes which have occurred in a 2-year period. Specifically the changes demonstrate erosions of the articular surfaces with periarticular osteophyte formation at the intercondylar and pericondylar margins.

suggested various techniques of primary surgical repair and/or reconstruction for anterior cruciate ligament compromise, they advocated techniques which utilized primary anastomosis or augmentation/substitution of the anterior cruciate ligament with fascial, tendonous or

129

meniscal material. These latter procedures require the borrowed structure to be an anatomically correct counterfeit of the original ligament and to remain firmly attached to both the femur and the tibia. Long-term retrospective and prospective studies seem to indicate that tendonous substitution whether harvested from the medial hamstrings or a segment of quadriceps mechanism provide the most successful method of reconstructing a compromised anterior cruciate ligament. Although differences of opinion exist on the timing of 'safe' return to activity, the most recent research suggests that following surgical repair, ligament strength requires 12–18 months to attain full recovery.

An average postoperative course would be 6 weeks cast immobilization to allow primary ligament healing; 2–4 weeks of physical therapy to re-establish a functional range of motion; and 3–6 months of progressive strength and endurance training and return to previous physical activities not permitted until demonstration of recovery of 75% of strength as compared to the opposite unaffected leg. This return is usually protected by the use of a protective brace during the periods of participation.

In spite of this preponderance of evidence for the desirability of an intact anterior cruciate ligament, surgery is not the only available alternative in the physician's treatment armamentarium. And certainly if surgery is chosen there is a great variability in terms of the magnitude of the procedure which may be undertaken. The determinants of which course of treatment might be chosen should be examined and understood. First it is important to realize that primary or reconstructive surgery for anterior cruciate ligament insufficiency will entail a major surgical undertaking together with a protracted period of intensive postoperative rehabilitation. By definition this demands a patient who:

(1) requires *full* functional stability and not someone who may choose or require less for his or her daily needs;

(2) has comprehension of the available alternatives; and understands there exists an option for late reconstruction (albeit with probable less total function return than with early primary repair);

(3) does not present an unacceptable medical risk under surgical treatment; and

(4) is willing and able to comply with the time and discipline a period of protracted rehabilitation requires.

Given these considerations a middle-aged or sedentary individual may choose to be treated symptomatically with a 4–6 week period of cast immobilization; and employ exercise and bracing post casting (knee cage or derotational-type brace) as an alternative to surgery. Or if reluctant to undergo a major intra-articular reconstruction, a patient may choose a less extensive extra-articular procedure (pes anserine transfer or

McIntosh lateral transfer). The treatment options are therefore manifold and dependent upon individual needs.

However the underlying principles and concepts do remain. They are:

(1) anterior cruciate ligament integrity is critical for physiological knee kinematics;

(2) the anterior cruciate ligament has not been observed to *usually* heal spontaneously;

(3) the best long-term functional results appear to follow early (less than 2 weeks postinjury) primary surgical repair of the injured ligament.

6.3.7 SUMMARY

The anterior cruciate ligament is the primary static stabilizer against anterior–internal rotational displacement of the tibia. It has three specific mechanisms of injury. When injured, the patient with an acute, or chronic anterior cruciate ligament insufficiency will present with characteristic signs and symptoms. This ligament's integrity is critical to proper knee joint mechanics and function. Compromise of this ligament will doom the joint to eventual functional and structural compromise. The magnitude of this is dependent upon the patient's ability to compensate with secondary static and dynamic stabilizers and the tolerance of these stabilizers to withstand the stresses to which the knee is subjected. Treatment of anterior cruciate ligament insufficiency (acute or chronic) is strictly dependent upon patient needs. However, the best prognosis does follow early primary surgical anastomosis of the ruptured ligament.

6.4 Posterior cruciate ligament (PCL)

6.4.1 ANATOMY

The posterior cruciate ligament, like the anterior cruciate ligament, is a dense collagenous band which lies extrasynovially within the knee joint. It originates at the posterior third of the intercondylar aspect of the medial femoral condyle. It is directed inferiorly in an almost vertical line (Fig. 6.8) to insert on the posterior midline intracondylar sulcus of the proximal tibia 1.5 cm distal to the tibial plateau (Fig. 6.9). Its appearance resembles a vertical axle within the knee joint. The posterior cruciate ligament has approximately a 30% (13 mm) greater diameter than does the anterior cruciate ligament. Its vascular supply arises primarily posteriorly from the middle geniculate artery after that vessel pierces the oblique popliteal ligament.

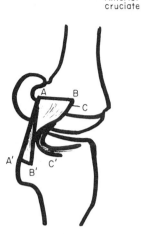

Fig. 6.8 Schematic representation of the alignment of the posterior cruciate ligament emphasizing its anatomical direction as nearly vertical in the posterior part of the knee joint.

A–A′ posterior bundle of PCL.

B–B′ anterior bundle of PCL.

C–C′ meniscal attachment to posterior cruciate.

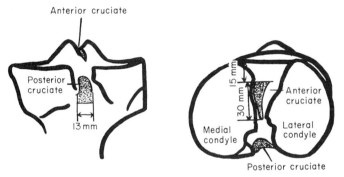

Fig. 6.9 Attached points of both the anterior and posterior cruciate ligaments at the intercondylar eminence and posterior aspect of the proximal tibia.

6.4.2 FUNCTION

Experimental cuttings have demonstrated the posterior cruciate ligament to be the primary restraint against posterior translation of the tibia on the femur. It also functions as a secondary stabilizer after the medial collateral ligament and anterior cruciate ligament against valgus angulation. As a stabilizer against anterior gliding of the femur the posterior cruciate

132

ligament is vitally important in descending an incline. In such a situation gravity acts to accentuate the anterior glide stress on the femur. Without an intact posterior cruciate ligament the body supported by the femur would sublux forward on the fixed tibia. This would result in potential collapse of the supporting limb. The quadriceps muscle is the dynamic counterpart of the posterior cruciate ligament against posterior tibial subluxation. For this reason the posterior cruciate ligament is critically necessary to knee mechanics during that portion of the gait cycle when resultant stresses of anterior translation of the femur on the fixed tibia (relative posterior translation of the tibia) must be checked and the quadriceps are less active (that is, midstance through toe-off). In this manner posterior cruciate instability causes greater distortion of joint mechanics during normal ambulation than does any other ligament injury. Because unlike the situation of other ligament compromise where episodes of instability result due to the insufficient compensation of dynamic counterparts at times of stress, the posterior cruciate ligament's dynamic counterpart (the quadriceps) is not insufficient but rather inhibited at those times when there is tensile stress applied to the posterior cruciate ligament. Therefore, in the face of posterior cruciate ligament insufficiency the joint is left with neither static nor dynamic stabilizers to prevent tibiofemoral posterior subluxation. As such, this fundamental instability will deter an individual from stressful activity much more certainly than will anterior cruciate ligament insufficiency. Isolated posterior cruciate ligament insufficiency is rarely observed. This is due to two factors: first, its more massive size; and second, its central location within the knee. Both afford a greater protection against injury except during more violent types of stress (such as posterior dislocation of the knee). As such posterior cruciate injury presents much more often in the presence of multiple ligament compromise.

6.4.3   MECHANISM OF INJURY

The most frequent mechanism of posterior cruciate ligament rupture is forceful posterior translation of the tibia in a flexed knee, that is, posterior dislocation of the knee. Such an incidence occurs most often in high speed injuries: falling from a motorcycle; or a passenger's flexed knee striking the dashboard during a motor vehicle accident. A second mechanism of injury is continued valgus angulation after rupture of the medial collateral and anterior cruciate ligaments has occurred. The posterior cruciate ligament as the last major static stabilizer against valgus angulation will then be compromised. This is usually together with an avulsion of the vastus medialis obliquis muscle from its femoral origin and extension of capsular damage into the posteromedial aspect of the knee.

6.4.4 DIAGNOSIS

History, mechanism of injury and amount of force sustained should raise suspicion of posterior cruciate ligament injury due to the massive extent of soft tissue damage usually coincident with posterior cruciate ligament rupture. Manual testing for acute posterior cruciate ligament insufficiency may be most difficult. However under general anaesthesia, posterior displacement of the tibia can be demonstrated in two ways. First is the 'drop-back sign'. In this test the hip and knee are flexed to 90° and the foot is supported off the table. In this position the anterior profile of the tibia is observed. If there is posterior cruciate ligament damage this profile, usually a straight or slightly convex line, will demonstrate a *concavity* along the proximal tibial border and patellar tendon. The second means of evaluating posterior cruciate ligament integrity is the posterior Drawer sign. With the patient supine the ipsilateral hip and knee are flexed 45° and 90° respectively. In this position a posteriorly directed force is applied to the proximal tibia. Posterior translation of the tibia without a firm endpoint resistance is taken as inferential evidence of posterior cruciate ligament insufficiency. Care must be taken to guard against misinterpretation of the direction of tibial instability. In the initial position the tibia may, due to gravity, spontaneously assume a posteriorly subluxed attitude giving a false-negative interpretation to the test; as such a false-positive anterior drawer sign may be recorded as the tibia is brought forward and reduced to the true neutral position. Ancillary testing such as single contrast arthrography may be of use, but more so in the chronic posterior cruciate ligament insufficiency rather than the acutely injured knee, because extensive capsular disruption may make outlining of the posterior cruciate ligament by intra-articular contrast media impossible due to the extravasation of dye from the joint space.

CAT scanning has proven effective and reliable as a diagnostic tool with which to assess posterior cruciate ligament integrity. The ligament's relatively larger diameter and vertical alignment make posterior cruciate ligament imaging an easier task than can be accomplished with the anterior cruciate ligament. The posterior cruciate ligament stands out as a distinct soft tissue structure surrounded by less dense fatty tissue in the posterior intracondylar fossa and tibial sulcus.

6.4.5 TREATMENT OPTIONS

Conservative management has been advocated by some authors who believe posterior cruciate ligament insufficiency to pose no significant compromise to knee kinematics. However longer-term observations seem to indicate that severe disruption of normal gait mechanics, particularly in descending an incline, occur due to the presence of posterior cruciate ligament insufficiency. This posterior subluxation instability will classically be worsened by a conventional derotational brace. However, a reversal of this brace has been designed to accommodate such an instability.

Animal models and sufficiently long-term clinical follow-up of posterior cruciate ligament insufficiency have not been reported in great number. Also, the relative infrequency of this injury and rarity of isolated posterior cruciate ligament compromise make long-term prognosis and consequences of posterior cruciate ligament insufficiency uncertain at this time. It can only be inferred that such an instability, as with any pathological instability, will eventually result in premature articular senescence.

Early surgical repair of the posterior cruciate ligament may be accomplished by primary anastomosis with or without augmentation using tendonous or fascial tissue. Exposure of the posterior cruciate ligament is most readily and safely achieved through a medial approach utilizing the interval between the pes anserine and medial gastrocnemius. Tenotomy and retraction posteriorly of the medial head of the gastrocnemius will provide soft tissue protection of the posterior neurovascular structures while also providing excellent exposure of the posterior proximal tibia and posterior oblique ligament under which lies the posterior cruciate ligament. Late reconstruction of the posterior cruciate ligament may be accomplished by tendon transfer. This may be harvested as a distally based portion of the quadriceps–patellar tendon, or medial hamstring, of which sufficient proximal length has been taken to allow the harvested structure to course posteriorly through the tibia, superiorly through the joint, medially through a drill hole in the medial femoral condyle at the original attachment point of the posterior cruciate ligament, and be fixed to the medial aspect of the medial femoral condyle with a staple. An alternative method of reconstruction is to transplant the medial head of the gastrocnemius onto the posterior margin of the lateral face of the medial femoral condyle.

At repair and/or reconstruction, the knee joint should be stabilized by a transarticular Steinman pin at 30° of flexion. This will prevent posterior tibial subluxation and tensile stress at the surgical repair site due to gravity during the period of cast immobilization. Postoperative immobilization rehabilitation is carried out similarly to that following anterior cruciate ligament surgery. Initially postimmobilization, little emphasis is placed on active hamstring exercise so as to reduce the tensile loading at the repair site. As in the case of the anterior cruciate ligament, function of the knee following primary repair or reconstruction of the posterior cruciate ligament is superior to that of a posterior cruciate ligament insufficient knee. However, there is insufficient data available to state whether primary or late reconstruction is the optimum course of treatment to be undertaken. Prognosticating the results following posterior cruciate ligament injury is also made most difficult by the large amount of soft tissue damage usually coincident with posterior cruciate ligament injury.

6.4.6 SUMMARY

The posterior cruciate ligament is a larger, more centrally located structure than is the anterior cruciate ligament within the knee. It acts as the central pivot of the knee. It is the primary static stabilizer against posterior subluxation of the tibia on the femur. It requires considerable force to be ruptured. As such it is rarely found as an isolated lesion. Diagnosis is made by history of significant force applied in a posteriorly directed fashion resulting in, for example, posterior dislocation of the knee, together with specific signs (posterior drawer sign, 'drop-back', arthrography). The posterior cruciate ligament is critical to normal ambulation kinematics. It is amenable to surgical repair and/or reconstruction by primary anastomosis or substitution techniques.

6.5 Lateral collateral ligament (LCL)

6.5.1 ANATOMY

The lateral collateral ligament is a firm cordlike structure. It measures approximately 40 mm in length × 5 mm in diameter. It originates at the lateral femoral epicondyle and is directed inferiorly and posteriorly to insert onto the superior aspect of the fibular head. It lies deep to the iliotibial band, superficial to the popliteus tendo/arcuate ligament complex, and is distally invested within the biceps femoris insertion at the fibular head. Unlike the medial collateral ligament, the lateral collateral ligament cannot be divided into two component segments.

6.5.2 FUNCTION

The body's centre of gravity falls medial to the knee joint. Therefore unlike the medial compartment of the knee, the lateral compartment is usually exposed to a tensile loading. This tensile load will occur during both dynamic and static activities. Therefore the lateral side of the knee must be constructed so as to resist *constant* tensile loading throughout the range of motion. As such, rather than having subdivisions within a single static stabilizer (that is, the medial collateral ligament), which vary in response depending upon the degree of flexion or extension present, the lateral compartment is stabilized by a network of static stabilizers which crisscross the lateral side of the knee joint (Fig. 6.10(a) and (b)). The lateral collateral ligament may be visualized as a guywire spanning the lateral joint line taut throughout the range of knee motion. Its function is to resist varus angulation of the knee. In this capacity it is the primary varus stabilizer of the knee joint. Its thin cordlike structure in stark contrast to the thin broad fan of the medial collateral ligament makes it aptly suited for this task. At full extension the lateral collateral ligament lies beneath the iliotibial band. The two structures enhance each other's ability to resist the varus moment acting across the knee. As the knee proceeds towards 90° of flexion, the iliotibial band becomes less mechanically effective against varus stresses leaving the lateral collateral ligament as the lone static restraint against varus stress. Without a compensatory lateral shift of the centre of gravity, the lateral collateral ligament insufficient knee will spontaneously angulate towards a varus alignment during weight-bearing activity. Secondary restraints (iliotibial band, arcuate ligament complex, lateral and posteriolateral capsule, popliteus tendon,

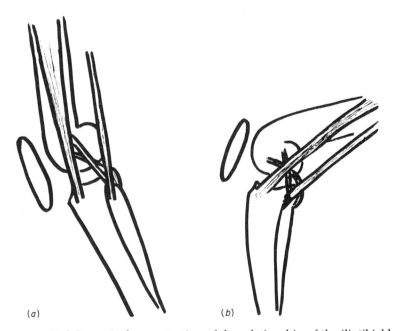

(a)　　　　　　　　　　　(b)

Fig. 6.10 (a) Schematic demonstration of the relationship of the iliotibial band, lateral collateral ligament, popliteus tendon and biceps tendon at the lateral aspect of the knee in extension. (b) Same structures in an approximate 90° flexion attitude.

and biceps tendon) will attempt to compensate for this insufficiency. However due to their orientation and size, none of these structures are as mechanically efficient throughout the range of motion as is the lateral collateral ligament. The end result therefore is an increased varus loading of the medial compartment due to insufficient lateral restraint.

6.5.3 MECHANISM OF INJURY

Although under a tensile load throughout the range of motion, the lateral collateral ligament is much less frequently subjected to sudden excessive varus angular stresses analogous to the valgus stress on the medial collateral ligament at 'push-off'. Its thicker cordlike structure makes it more resistant to the tensile loading to which it is subjected. Also, externally applied varus angular stresses are unusual at the knee. Therefore, fewer lateral collateral ligament injuries are encountered as compared with the relatively more commonly seen medial collateral ligament sprains. The usual scenario of lateral collateral ligament injury when it does occur involves a violent incident in which an object being straddled falls onto the medial aspect of the affected knee (a motorcycle, for example). A continuation of the varus stress which caused lateral collateral ligament compromise may lead to rupture of the anterior cruciate ligament.

6.5.4 TREATMENT

The relative infrequency of lateral collateral ligament injury as compared with that of the medial collateral ligament and anterior cruciate ligament make definitive prognostic statements about these lesions difficult. However, due to the potential support of surrounding soft tissue structures it appears that the lateral collateral ligament does have an excellent opportunity for full recovery with conservative treatment. As emphasized above, this ligament is critical to knee function. Therefore attempt at primary surgical repair is not unreasonable. Its unique shape, however, does make attempts to suture this ligament typically less satisfying than one would hope. Chronic lateral collateral ligament insufficiency usually has a poor response to bracing alone. Late reconstruction of that ligament is best afforded by substitution with half of the biceps femoris tendon transferred to the lateral femoral epicondyle. Postinjury or postsurgery the knee should be protected with cast immobilization for 6 weeks and later with a hinged support (knee cage). Expectation is for full functional return.

6.5.5 SUMMARY

The lateral collateral ligament is the primary static stabilizer against varus angulation of the knee throughout the range of motion. It is supplemented by the iliotibial band, popliteus tendon, arcuate complex, capsular ligament, and biceps tendon. It functions as a lateral guywire resisting the constant varus moment occurring at the knee. It crosses the knee joint but does not attach onto the tibia. It is less commonly injured than is the medial lateral ligament and anterior cruciate ligament and even the posterior cruciate ligament. The most common mechanism of injury is excessive varus angulation. This may in extreme cases be accompanied by anterior cruciate ligament rupture. Acute lateral collateral ligament injury is amenable to either closed or operative management. Chronic lateral collateral ligament insufficency is best treated surgically by reconstruction through staple attachment of one-half of the biceps femoris tendon to the lateral femoral epicondyle.

6.6 State of the art: a look ahead

As outlined above both traditional closed and operative (early and reconstructive) treatments are matters of discussion, preference, and to be individualized to a given patient's needs. There are however certain definitive statements which can be made:

(1) Isolated medial collateral ligament injuries can be treated with good expectation of full recovery by either closed or open techniques.

(2) Anterior and posterior cruciate ligament ruptures do best with primary repair (with or without augmentation).

(3) Repair of midsubstance anterior and posterior cruciate ligament and reconstruction of anterior and posterior ligament injuries are technically demanding and less certain than those involving avulsion injuries of these ligaments.

(4) No anterior and posterior cruciate ligament reconstructive procedure has been proved to provide better than 80% of effectiveness in providing full return to normal function.

(5) Extra-articular substitution for cruciate insufficiency is a less effective and more temporary solution for joint instability than are intra-articular procedures.

(6) Postinjury or postsurgery immobilization requires prolonged rehabilitation.

The future directions of treatment are towards the development of answers to these problems. First, injury prevention; second, the facilitation of soft tissue healing; third, development of better materials (biological, synthetic) for reconstructive procedures. The first category will be accomplished through better education and conditioning of athletes together with the development of better equipment designed to afford protection against excessive stresses while not compromising function. The second area of investigation has expanded to research means of facilitating and enhancing fibroblastic/collagen activity and synthesis. The question of beneficial *long-term* effects of early motion on static stabilizer function has yet to be decided. It appears, however, that under laboratory control collagenous healing in animal models can be beneficially affected through the application of anodal current. The mechanism of this response is hypothetical and poorly understood at this time; but its effectiveness has been demonstrated. It remains to further discern the nature of this response and its applicability to clinical medicine. With regard to the third area of research, to date attempts have been made to substitute various synthetic materials for compromised ligament structures. These have nearly universally met with failure due to insufficient strength, durability, fixation, or biocompatibility. Attempts at biocompatible/bioresorbable fibrous ingrowth implants is being pursued. However, longer-term follow-up assessment will be required before endorsement of such techniques for general usage may be made.

The key to success still remains in an intermarriage of a thorough understanding of knee joint anatomy, kinematics and physiology together with available technology.

Bibliography

Abbott, L. *et al.* (1944), Injuries to the ligaments of the knee joint. *J. Bone Joint Surg.*, **26**, 503–15.

Alm, A. *et al.* (1974), The anterior cruciate ligament. *Acta Chirurg. Scand.* **Suppl. 445–78**.

Alm, A. *et al.* (1976), Clinical and experimental experience in reconstruction of the anterior cruciate ligament. *Orthop. Clin. N.Am.*, **7**, 181–200.

Bosworth, D. (1952), Transplantation of the semitendinosus for repair of laceration of the medial collateral ligament of the knee. *J. Bone Joint Surg.*, **34A**, 196, 208.

Brantigan, A., *et al.* (1943), The tibial collateral ligament: its function, bursae and relation to the medial meniscus. *J. Bone Joint Surg.*, **25**, 121–32.

Bristow, W. R. (1939), Internal derangement of the knee joint. *Am. J. Surg.*, **43**, 458–67.

Campbell, W. C. (1939), Reconstruction of the ligaments of the knee. *Am. J. Surg.*, **43**, 473–90.

Clancy, W. (1982), Anterior cruciate ligament injuries. *Mediguide Orthop.* **1**, 1–21.

Cowan, D. J. (1965), Reconstruction of the anterior cruciate ligament by the method of Kenneth Jones. *Proc. Roy. Soc. Med.*, **58**, 336–45.

Cubbins, W. *et al.* (1939), Cruciate ligaments. *Am. J. Surg.*, **43**, 481–90.

Dandy, D. J. (1982), Arthroscopy and the management of the ruptured ACL. *Clin. Orthop.*, **167**, 43–50.

Dandy, D. J. (1982), The long term results of unrepaired tears of the PCL. *J. Bone Joint Surg.*, **64**, 92–9.

DuToit, G. (1967), Knee joint cruciate ligament substitution. The Lindemann operation. *S. Afr. J. Surg.*, **5**, 25–38.

Edwards, A. (1925), Operative repair of cruciate ligaments in severe trauma of the knee. *Br. J. Surg.*, **13**, 432–49.

Feagin, J. and Abbott, H. (1972), The isolated tear of the anterior cruciate ligament. *J. Bone Joint Surg.*, **54A**, 1340–51.

Fetto, J. and Marshall, J. (1979), Injury to the anterior cruciate ligament producing the pivot shift sign: an experimental study on cadaver specimens. *J. Bone Joint Surg.*, **61**, 710–14.

Fick, R. (1911), Anatomie und medhanik der gelinke unter berucksich-tigung der bewegenden muskelen. Band II, Teil III, in *Handbuch des Anatomie des Menschen*. Karl von Bardeleben.

Firooznia, H. *et al.* (1983), Computerized tomography in the detection of joint disorders. *Orthop. Rev.*, **12**, 69–80.

Franke, K. (1976) Clinical experience in 130 cruciate ligament reconstructions. *Orthop. Clin. N.A.*, **1**, 191–208.

Frankel, A. *et al.* (1971), Biomechanics of internal derangement of the knee. *J. Bone Joint Surg.*, **53A**, 945–52.

Galway, H. R. and MacIntosh, D. L. (1980), The lateral pivot shift: A symptom and sign of anterior cruciate ligament insufficiency. *Clin. Orthop.*, **147**, 45–46.

Girgis, F., Marshall, J. L. and Monagem, A. R. S. (1975), The cruciate ligaments of the knee joint. *Clin. Orthop.*, **106**, 216–20.

Graves, E. W. (1920), The cruciate ligaments of the knee joint: their function, rupture, and the operative treatment of the same. *Br. J. Surg.*, **7**, 505–11.

Hughston, J. (1962), Acute knee injuries in athletes. *Clin. Orthop.*, **23**, 114–28.

Hughston, J. C. (1969), The posterior cruciate ligament in knee joint stability. *J. Bone Joint Surg.*, **51A**, 1045–52.

Insall, J. N. (1982), Bone-block transfer of the medial head of the gastrocnemius for PCL insufficiency. *J. Bone Joint Surg.*, **64**, 691–708.

Jack, E. A. (1950), Experimental rupture of the MCL of the knee. *J. Bone Joint Surg.*, **32B**, 396–403.

Jacobsen, K. (1981), Gonylaxometry. Stress radiographic measurements of pass-ive stability in the knee joints. *Acta Orthop. Scand.*, **52**, 1–18.

Jacobsen, K. and Rosenkilde, P. (1976), A clinical and stress radiographical follow-up investigation after Jones' operation for replacing the anterior cruciate ligament. *Injury*, **8**, 221–32.

Jones, K. (1963), Reconstruction of the anterior cruciate ligament. *J. Bone Joint Surg.*, **45A**, 925–41.

Jones, R. and Smith, A. (1913), On rupture of the cruciate ligaments of the knee and on fracture of the spine of the tibia. *Brit. J. Surg.*, **1**, 70–81.

Kaplan, E. B. (1962), Some aspects of the functional anatomy of the human knee joint. *Clin. Orthop.*, **23**, 18–32.

Ligament Injuries and their Treatment

Kennedy, J. C. (1982), The use of the medial head of the gastrocnemius muscle in the PCL deficient knee. *Am. J. Sports Med.*, **10**, 63–70.

Kennedy, J. *et al.* (1974), The anatomy and function of the anterior cruciate ligament. *J. Bone Joint Surg.*, **56A**, 223–32.

Liljedahl, S. *et al.* (1965), Early diagnosis and treatment of acute ruptures of the anterior cruciate ligament. *J. Bone Joint Surg.*, **47A**, 1503–20.

Liljedahl, S. O., Linduall, N. and Wettertors, J. (1969), Roentgen diagnosis of rupture of anterior cruciate ligament. *Acta Radiol.*, **4**, 225–31.

Loos, W. C. *et al.* (1981), Acute PCL injuries. *Am. J. Sports Med.*, **9**, 86–97.

Lysholm, J. *et al.* (1982), Long term results after early treatment of knee injuries. *Acta Orthop. Scand.*, **53**, 109–30.

Marshall, J. L. (1969), Periarticular osteophytes. *Clin. orthop.*, **62**, 37–43.

Marshall, J. *et al.* (1975), The anterior drawer sign: what is it? *Am. J. Sports Med.*, **3**, 152–64.

Marshall, J. *et al.* (1982), Primary surgical treatment of ACL lesions. *Am. J. Sports Med.*, **10**, 103–24.

Marshall, J. L., *et al.* The Anterior Cruciate Ligament: Its Current Status. Submitted for publication.

Mauch, H. (1942), Severe acute injuries of the knee. *Am. J. Surg.*, **56**, 54–71.

McIntosh, D. (1974), *Acute tears of the anterior cruciate ligament: over-the-top-repair*, unpublished.

McMaster, J. *et al.* (1974), Diagnosis and management of isolated anterior cruciate ligament tears. *J. Trauma*, **14**, 230–42.

Noyes, F. R. *et al.* (1980), Knee ligament tests: what do they really mean? *Phys. Ther.*, **60**, 1596–1610.

O'Donoghue, D. (1950), Surgical treatment of fresh injuries to the major ligaments of the knee. *J. Bone Joint Surg.*, **32A**, 721–40.

O'Donoghue, D. (1955), An analysis of end results of surgical treatment of major injuries to the ligaments of the knee. *J. Bone Joint Surg.*, **37A**, 1–24.

O'Donoghue, D. (1960), Surgical treatment of injuries to the knee. *Clin. Orthop.*, **23**, 11–31.

Palmar, I. (1938), Injuries to the ligaments of the knee joint. *Acta Orthop. Scand.* **Suppl. 53**.

Paulos, L. *et al.* (1981), Knee rehabilitation after ACL reconstruction and repair. *Am. J. Sports Med.*, **9**, 140–47.

Pringle, J. (1907), Avulsion of the spine of the tibia. *Ann. Surg.*, **46**, 169–175.

Richman, R. and Barnes, K. (1946), Acute instability of the knee ligaments as a result of injuries to parachutists. *J. Bone Joint Surg.*, **28A**, 473–86.

Robichon, J. (1968), The functional anatomy of the knee joint with special reference to the MCL and ACL. *Can. J. Surg.*, **11**, 36–50.

Rubin, R., Marshall, J. and Wang, J. (1975), Prevention of knee instability. *Clin. Orthop.*, **113**, 212–19.

Slocum, D. and Larson, R. (1968), Pes anserinus transplantation. *J. Bone Joint Surg.*, **50A**, 226–43.

Slocum, D. *et al.* (1973), Late reconstruction procedures used to stabilize the knee. *Orthop. Clin. N.Am.*, **4**, 679–94.

Smith, S. A. (1918), The diagnosis and treatment of injuries to the cruciate ligaments. *Br. J. Surg.*, **6**, 176–85.

Wang, J. and Marshall, J. (1975), Acute ligamentous injuries of the knee. Single contrast arthrography – a diagnostic aid. *J. Trauma*, **15**, 431–50.

Wang, J. *et al.* (1975), A mechanism of isolated anterior cruciate rupture. *J. Bone Joint Surg.*, **57A**, 411–21.

Warren, F. and Marshall, J. L. (1974), The prime static stabilizer of the medial side of the knee. *J. Bone Joint Surg.*, **56A**, 665–75.

Witt, A. N. *et al.* (1977), Das instable Kriegelenk-aklulle. Gesichhspunkte in Grundlagen-forschung, Diagnostick and Therapie. *Archiv Orthop. Unfall-Chirurg.*, **88**, 49–70.

7 Knee lesions II: Anterior instability

A. E. ELLISON

7.1 Introduction

It is axiomatic that one cannot treat symptomatic instability of the knee without an understanding of the biomechanics and pathodynamics of the instability. In spite of this obvious truth, there are a myriad of procedures for the multiplicity of instabilities encountered, many of which suggest lack of understanding of underlying principles.

Stability of the knee, indeed, any joint, demands appropriate bone and cartilage geometry, integrity of the primary static stabilizers as well as their several back-up structures referred to as the secondary static stabilizers, plus an intact and well-conditioned, dynamic musculo-tendinous support system. The major controversy in knee ligament surgery is the relative contribution of each of these components, and the most efficacious way to repair, reinforce or substitute for them when they do not possess normal integrity.

When our concern is restricted to anterior instability, the problem is somewhat more simple. Here, the anterior cruciate ligament (ACL) clearly plays a role. Depending upon one's point of view, it is felt to be primary or secondary. It either assists, or is assisted by, the capsular structures in resisting anterior displacement of the tibia on the femur when such a force is applied in neutral rotation.

Virtually all acknowledge that the intact meniscus also aids stability. Menisci function in concert with their capsular relationships, particularly posteromedially and posterolaterally. It is this role of the meniscus resisting instability and late arthrosis that has largely fuelled the recent interest in meniscal repair.

Another, lesser controversy is the natural history of anterior cruciate insufficiency. This is more a matter of degree, since virtually all concede that if there is sufficient laxity, with the tibia regularly subluxating anteriorly on the femur, degenerative changes will occur. Some hold that this is virtually inevitable (Jacobsen, 1977). Others feel that the knee can

145

be a highly satisfactory and, indeed, a relatively high performance joint that does not go on to significant degenerative disease even in the face of the absent cruciate (Feagill and Curl, 1976).

7.2 History

The historical background of the anterior cruciate is pertinent to our understanding of the controversy surrounding it. As early as 1920, Hey Groves clearly stated that the anterior cruciate ligament was a 'check upon the forward movement' of the tibia (Hey Groves, 1920). In the same paper, he clearly described an active pivot shift test and noted the important contribution of the anterior cruciate in this type of subluxation. In 1938, in the landmark paper 'On the Injuries to the Ligaments of the Knee Joint', Ivar Palmer also was remarkably clear in his analysis of the function of the anterior cruciate. He concluded that 'a strongly pronounced drawer sign presupposes injury to the cruciate' (Palmer, 1938).

The 1940s saw two outstanding works on contributions of the ligaments of the knee, both published by Americans. Brantigan and Voshell (1941) again confirmed the work of Hey Groves and Palmer, and concluded that the 'anterior cruciate ligament prevents forward gliding of the tibia on the femur, because such force is directed in the line of the attachment of the anterior cruciate ligament'. The second paper was published in 1944 by Leroy Abbott and associates (Abbott et al., 1944), and again was unequivocal that 'if the anterior cruciate ligament has been torn, the tibia can be displaced forward on the femur'.

The early 1950s witnessed a dramatic increase in the awareness and treatment of knee ligament instability, largely because of the pioneering writings of O'Donoghue (1959). Faced with the resumption of North American football after the Second World War and a significant increase in the awareness of orthopaedic surgeons to the 'triad' of deficits that resulted from an illegal clip, consisting of medial capsular tears, medial meniscal lesions and anterior cruciate ligament ruptures, orthopaedic surgeons the world over embarked on a far more aggressive surgical approach to these problems.

In the course of treating these injuries, a dilemma appeared. Surgeons observed knees that appeared to have an intact anterior cruciate but an anterior drawer sign elicited both preoperatively and at the operating table. There were other cases in which the anterior cruciate was obviously ruptured, with an apparent absence of anterior drawer. These observations ultimately seemed resolved when Slocum (1968) delineated the spectrum of anteromedial rotatory instability, and pointed out that, with a mid-third capsular tear without anterior cruciate involvement, one could obtain a rotational drawer in which the medial tibial condyle rotated anteriorly, seemingly to give a positive drawer sign, but that this did not represent a true anterior displacement of the tibia on the femur. It was this specific delineation of the spectrum of ligament and meniscal loss of integrity that directly led to the concept that the capsule represented the primary stabilizer and that the anterior cruciate functioned as the accentuator of these deficits.

In 1972, Galway and McIntosh described the lateral pivot shift that was attributed to anterior cruciate ligament deficiency. This was subsequently countered by Hughston (Hughston *et al.*, 1976) in which it was his contention that anterolateral rotatory instability was the mirror image of anteromedial, with the primary deficit in the capsular ligament, and again, the degree of instability accentuated or enhanced by anterior cruciate ligament insufficiency. Although a host of authors have subsequently vigorously confirmed the primacy of the anterior cruciate ligament in anterior instability, Hughston and Barrett (1983) have recently published a series of cases with excellent results, purporting to 'prove' that knees stable in an anterior plane, and without developing the stigmata of instability, can be achieved through restoration of the meniscocapsular complex alone.

7.3 Function of the anterior cruciate ligament

At this time, it is reasonable to state that the overwhelming majority of knee surgeons regard the anterior cruciate ligament as the primary stabilizer of the tibia on the femur resisting anterior displacement in a neutral rotational axis. In addition, from historic times to the present, it has been consistently taught that critical secondary stabilizers exist. These consist of the capsular ligaments both medially and laterally, and particularly posteromedially in the form of the posterior oblique ligament, and posterolaterally in the form of the arcuate ligament. In addition, on the medial side, there is the major contribution of the medial collateral ligament and laterally the iliotibial band and tract. The dynamic stabilizers – most importantly the semimembranosus and biceps, but consisting of all of the intregrated functioning of the musculotendonous units as well as both the medial and lateral menisci – are vital in assisting the anterior cruciate in maintaining anteroposterior stability.

In addition to their role in anteroposterior stability, the cruciates also provide a significant secondary role in stabilizing the joint from both valgus and varus forces, contributing a varying degree of resistance depending on the amount of flexion of the joint. There is also an obvious role played by the cruciate in resisting rotation, both medially as its helical fibres tighten and wind about the posterior cruciate, and laterally, as it initially unwinds but ultimately is buttressed against the lateral femoral condyle.

Ultimately, it may be demonstrated that one of the most significant functions of the anterior cruciate ligament is to act as a guidance mechanism for the screw-home motion of the knee. The screw-home is the critical element of knee stability as the joint approaches terminal extension, ultimately to achieve its maximum in a locked, rigid joint. It carries out this function by going from a position of tension in 90° of flexion to maximum relaxation between 30° and 40° of flexion, after which tension again begins to increase. Because of knee geometry and the ability of the tibia to glide and rotate as tension builds within the cruciate, there comes a point where there is less force required to produce this screw-home motion than to further stretch the anterior cruciate itself.

This function of the anterior cruciate is important in our consideration of surgical approaches to restore the anterior cruciate deficient knee. Since it is relatively easier to resist rotation at the rim of a wheel than at the hub, the rotational functions of the ligament in an anterior cruciate deficient knee can be more effectively restored extra-articularly. Similarly, if rotation medially and laterally is resisted by extra-articular procedures both laterally and medially, the vector of anterior instability can also be addressed in a purely extra-articular manner. This, in association with a functional meniscus and good musculotendonous reconditioning, is Hughston's basic thesis.

The contribution of the anterior cruciate to both valgus and varus stresses is, as mentioned, only the role of a secondary stabilizer and, again, restoration of the integrity of both the medial and lateral collaterals and capsules with their surrounding structures can more than adequately address this need, as well.

It is in the area of guidance of the terminal rotation of the screw-home, however, that one requires an intra-articular structure and is a major indication for intra-articular restorative procedures. When one considers that an effective structure through the notch also provides additional resistance to anterior subluxation of the tibia on the femur, intra-articular substitutions take on a major importance and account for the dramatic increase in recent surgical advances to effectively substitute intra-articularly.

If, however, we wish to achieve the 'physiological knee' (Larson, 1983), it is essential that we obtain both intra-articular and extra-articular restoration as well as preservation of normal joint geometry with the important, additional contributions of a physiological meniscus in both compartments and good musculotendinous rehabilitation.

7.4 Surgical considerations

The choice of specific surgical procedures utilized to restore the anterior cruciate deficient knee will be directly determined by one's understanding of the deficits to be addressed. If one believes in the primacy of the meniscocapsular complex, the bulk of one's efforts will be directed at these structures whereas, if one feels that the anterior cruciate ligament is the *sine qua non*, some appropriate type of repair or substitution of this ligament will be required. Ultimately, it is to be hoped that most surgeons will consider these interrelated and mutually interdependent and thus address both.

For the purpose of this discussion, our consideration of surgical approaches will be divided into two parts: extra-articular and intra-articular.

7.4.1 EXTRA-ARTICULAR

Anteromedial rotatory instability with associated anterior cruciate insufficiency has historically been the best understood and the most successfully treated (Slocum and Larson, 1968b; Slocum, Larson and James, 1974; Perry *et al.*, 1980; Freeman, Beaty and Haynes, 1982). There has been relatively little controversy, although some have held that the mid-third capsular ligament, particularly the meniscotibial portion of it, was the first line of defence, whereas others such as Marshall (Warren, Marshall and Girgis, 1974; Fetto and Marshall, 1978) have maintained that it is consistently torn not because it is the first line of defence but because it is the weakest ligament. For it to be torn, there must be some deformation of collagen in the medial collateral ligament that may or may not be within its capacity to heal.

There has been virtual unanimity in the importance of the postero-medial corner, and particularly the posterior oblique ligament (Hughston and Eilers, 1973). There is no need, however, to be a member of either the capsular primacy or the anterior cruciate primacy school to recognize that the function of the knee joint will be diminished if there is pathological laxity in these structures and, irrespective of the area of primacy, they must be restored to physiological function if we are to obtain uniformly good results.

The importance of the medial meniscus has been repeatedly emphasized (Hsieh and Walker, 1976; Hughston *et al.*, 1976), and within the last few years has been felt by many to be critical. Some authors now advise attempted repair, even though the lesion is in the substance rather than at the meniscosynovial junction (Henning, 1982).

Ligament Injuries and their Treatment

The dynamic secondary restraints of the medial hamstrings, and particularly the semimembranosus, have been emphasized by a host of authors and is non-controversial in the sense that improved function of these units is universally felt to be critical (Paubs *et al.*, 1981; McDaniel and Damerou, 1980). The precise method of utilization, whether in a pes anserinus transfer or through rerouting of the semimembranosus and its multiple attachments will depend largely upon the author's preference.

The critical structure to be restored to gain medial stability and to enhance its function as a co-worker with the anterior cruciate ligament is the medial collateral ligament. The consensus at this time is that the medial collateral ligament should be advanced on the tibial face where this is possible, and a slightly more anterior direction of its fibres further enhances its mechanical ability to resist anterior displacement of the tibia, thus improving its function as a co-stabilizer with the anterior cruciate ligament.

Since the recognition of anterolateral rotatory instability and the fact that this instability is probably more pernicious and ultimately more incapacitating than anteromedial rotatory instability (Ellison, 1979), major investigative work has been directed at its restoration. On rare occasions, a Segund fracture (Losee, Johnson and Southwick, 1978; Fetto and Marshall, 1979) or the so-called lateral capsular sign (Ellison, 1979; Insall *et al.*, 1981; Losee *et al.*, 1978; Ireland and Trickery, 1980; Arnold *et al.*, 1979; Fetto and Marshall, 1979) will facilitate an excellent repair, since this avulsion of bone can be replaced with ease, or perhaps advanced slightly more anteriorly and distally if there appears to be deformation in the iliotibial band.

In the chronic case, an enormous amount of work has been done in regard to the iliotibial band (Slager, 1982). The bulk of this work has been to produce a tenodesis, with or without a cam effect, by passing the iliotibial band transfer below the fibulocollateral ligament. Although the dynamic principles vary, the underlying surgical objective is to reproduce anterior cruciate ligament function by essentially paralleling its fibres and limiting the anteromedial excursion of the lateral tibial condyle on the femur.

It is the consensus of all authors that a simple iliotibial band transfer alone is probably not sufficient to resist the enormous forces of anterior displacement of the tibia, particularly in an active athlete. Thus, all of these procedures require back-up, perhaps medially and intra-articularly as well as restoring the integrity of the posterolateral corner. This is not unlike the importance of the posteromedial corner in anteromedial rotatory instability. The anterior and middle thirds of the lateral capsular ligament are considered by most to be weak and probably not worthy of

150

significant attempts to reconstruct them, although Hughston has strongly disagreed with this.

Although the fibulocollateral has been advanced by some authors as a technique to directly combat anterolateral rotatory instability (Losee, Johnson and Southwick, 1978; Ellison, 1979; Arnold *et al.*, 1979), the majority of authors 'relatively' shorten the fibulocollateral by double vesting the capsule beneath it (Marshall, Girgis and Zelko, 1972), passing additional tissue such as the iliotibial band and/or the biceps femoris below it, or wrapping other soft tissue structures (Ellison, 1980) around it. All of these procedures have essentially the same objective, reducing the functional length of the fibulocollateral and thus making an additional contribution to varus stability, although this has relatively little effect on anterior instability.

There are critical elements in virtually all extra-articular lateral procedures that utilize the iliotibial band as a transfer. The width of the band removed from the tract (band is the condensed or narrow portion; tract is the area) is often too narrow to be effective. A lateral retinacular release should be done to permit a wider transfer. The capsule, especially posterolaterally, must be plicated to remove all laxity. Finally, the tract must be closed at the conclusion of the reconstruction to prevent varus instability (Kennedy, 1980; James *et al.*, 1979).

The musculotendonous unit most importantly involved with anterolateral rotatory instability is the biceps femoris. It is a major back-up in most of the procedures utilizing an iliotibial band transfer or tenodesis. The majority of procedures involve a biceps advancement in an attempt to improve the mechanical leverage of the biceps as an external rotator of the tibia on the femur, as well as the dynamic resister of anterior displacement of the tibia, *per se*. Some authors believe that the biceps should not be completely removed, but rather its superficial portion advanced anteriorly. If the entire biceps is removed to reroute it and obtain improved mechanical advantage, it must have restitution of its reinsertion into the site of the normal attachment of the deep head of the biceps (Norwood and Cross, 1977).

The popliteus is essentially uninvolved in the reconstructive procedures designed for anterolateral rotatory instability.

7.4.2 INTRA-ARTICULAR

Intra-articular procedures can be divided into acute and chronic.

(a) Acute

In the acute case, there is unanimity that any anterior cruciate rupture with attached avulsed bone, either femoral or tibial, should be repaired

151

either arthroscopically or through open procedures. Chances for success in these cases are very high. There is less than unanimity but growing concensus that avulsion, and particularly the classic avulsion from the femur, without explosive deformation of the collagen fibres should also be repaired. The success of these procedures undoubtedly is less satisfactory.

There is considerable controversy in regard to the treatment of mop end tears. In the high performance athlete or the young person with physiologically lax joints, with major dependence upon the anterior cruciate ligament to prevent crippling instability, there is a growing feeling that repair should be undertaken and accompanied by augmentation. The structure used for augmentation, whether it be iliotibial band, semitendonosus or some form of artificial stint or prosthesis, is an area of active research. Many of the authors utilizing such augmentation also advocate this for the non-bony avulsion injury, particularly when the ligament is off the femur. Here the stint is usually passed over the top, and the ligament itself reinserted at its physiological posterior insertion on the medial face of the lateral femoral condyle.

It cannot be overemphasized that, in the acute anterior cruciate tear, the ligament has been stretched approximately 20% of its length, or about an additional centimetre. Damage to other ligamentous structures in the form of deformation of collagen, if not in visible residuals, must be accepted and appropriately treated. Where there are visual deficits, either medially or laterally and where medical indications and criteria for surgical repair exist, such deficits must be repaired in addition to the anterior cruciate itself. Even in those cases where operative intervention is not felt to be indicated, the treatment protocol must permit healing for complete restoration of the secondary stabilizers, even if the anterior cruciate is accepted as a total loss. Thus, treatment of the acute anterior cruciate lesion, even in an older, non-athletic patient, unaccompanied by other signs or symptoms of ligamentous or meniscal deficits, must be aggressive even though not necessarily surgical. This would include appropriate postoperative programmes to be described.

(b) Chronic

It is in the area of surgical treatment of chronic anterior cruciate deficient knees that the major controversies surrounding this ligament exist: specifically, when considering intra-articular procedures, what is to be used and how it is to be placed. Although many authors strongly disagree, it is probable that placement of an intra-articular substitution for the anterior cruciate at approximately the anatomical site or slightly anteromedial to it is the position of choice in the tibia, and that modest variation will be of relatively little effect. An angle of inclination of 40° from the tibial plateau may also be of importance.

The femoral attachment of any intra-articular anterior cruciate substitute is far more critical, and subjected to far greater stresses. It is probable that the over-the-top route, perhaps slightly rounded or flared, providing a somewhat funnel-like access to the physiological attachment site, or slightly grooved below the traditional over-the-top approach, will stand the test of time.

The structure to be used and the precise technique of using it are still highly debatable. Many feel that the iliotibial band is of such an enormous importance to the lateral stability of the knee, and has other critical functions and uses as to reduce its desirability as an intra-articular substitute. Although there have been some disquieting reports in the literature (Alm and Gillquist, 1974; Arnoczky, Tarvin and Marshall, 1982; Clancy *et al.*, 1982; Jones, 1963; Lam, 1968), at the present time the majority of knee surgeons utilize some form of the patella tendon, either medial or central third, in the majority of instances. Precise techniques vary with every author, and the basic surgical premise of meticulous attention to a specific technique carefully worked out in the laboratory and applied with sufficient frequency to ensure consistency and ability to compensate for multiple variables is a *sine qua non*.

There still is a large body of surgeons who believe that, since the enzyme systems of the synovium differ from the enzyme systems of vascularized tissue, and both differ from those of cartilage, the so-called 'hostile environment' of the knee will continue to frustrate a significant percentage of all procedures barring dramatic improvement in our understanding of the biology of healing. To this end, prosthetic replacement of the anterior cruciate, not only for augmentation of acute tears, and thus with a relatively limited life but, hopefully, for permanent preservation in chronic deficits, is a major area of current research and hoped-for success in the future.

7.5 Rehabilitation

In no area of surgery is appropriate postoperative care and rehabilitation more critical than in the postoperative anterior cruciate deficient knee. Sound healing, maturation of collagen, restoration of function in structures that have frequently been moved or asked to perform new functions, such as biceps transfers, restoration of the kinaesthetic sense and restoration of dynamic strength and power all require protection and rehabilitation far longer than was initially anticipated.

The majority of knee surgeons currently utilize immobilization in a fixed cast for a relatively short period of 2–3 weeks, followed by 4–6 weeks in some form of moveable cast. Upon removal of the cast, the knee should be actively mobilized with heavy emphasis on hydrotherapy until an essentially full range of motion is achieved. Complete extension is not essential early, and may be contraindicated.

When good active motion has been achieved, the knee should be further stabilized with appropriate bracing and resistance exercises instituted. It is well recognized that the quadriceps exerts an anterior displacing force upon the proximal tibia. Quadriceps exercises should be deferred until hamstring power on the operative side has been restored.

Our own protocol calls for progressive resistance exercises for the hamstring group until they achieve parity both in regard to strength and power with the quadriceps on the opposite side. At this time, quadriceps exercises are introduced, and both hamstrings and quadriceps are strengthened until they achieve essential parity with the non-operative side. At this juncture all muscle groups, including hip abductors, adductors, plantar flexors and dorsiflexors of the foot as well as muscle groups about the knee, are vigorously developed until both quadriceps groups begin to pull ahead on the basis of sheer muscle bulk alone.

When this state has been achieved, coordination exercises, running, endurance programmes and, ultimately, acceleration, cutting and deceleration manoeuvres are carried out. The athlete is then ready to return to his or her sport.

7.6   Conclusion

The knee joint is a magnificently complex, biomechanical structure that continues to challenge the finest efforts of knee surgeons. Its basic stability is predicated upon its ingenious geometry, aided by the primary and secondary static stabilizers, menisci and appropriate, coordinated inputs from the well-conditioned, musculotendonous dynamic stabilization system. Deprived of any of its integral parts, the knee can function only at a level inferior to its ultimate capability. Once injured, it must be restored to this highly coordinated state.

Although anterior instability secondary to anterior cruciate ligament insufficiency continues to be the most consistent and significant of its disabling ligamentous insufficiencies, an understanding of the contributions of its multiple components and surgical procedures predicated upon restoration of the sum of the individual parts will probably provide us with the most rewarding results.

References

Abbott, L. C., Saunders, J. B., Bost, F. C. and Anderson, G. E. (1944), Injuries to the ligaments of the knee joint. *J. Bone Joint Surg.*, **26A**, 503–21.

Alm, A. and Gillquist, J. (1974), Reconstruction of the anterior cruciate ligament by using the medial third of the patellar ligament. Treatment and results. *Acta Chir. Scand.*, **140**, 289–96.

Arnold, J. A. , Coker, T. P. and Heaton, L. M., *et al.* (1979), Natural history of anterior cruciate tears. *Am. J. Sports Med.*, **7**, 305–13.

Arnoczky, S. P., Tarvin, G. B. and Marshall, J. L. (1982), Anterior cruciate ligament replacement using patellar tendon. An evaluation of graft revascularization in the dog. *J. Bone Joint Surg.*, **64A**, 217–24.

Brantigan, O. C. and Voshell, A. F. (1941), The mechanics of the ligaments and menisci of the knee joint. *J. Bone Joint Surg*, **23A**, 44–66.

Clancy, W. G. Jr, Nelson, D. A., Reider, B. *et al.* (1982), Anterior cruciate ligament reconstruction using one-third of the patellar ligament, augmented by extra-articular tendon transfers. *J. Bone Joint Surg.*, **64A**, 352–59.

Ellison, A. E. (1979), Distal iliotibial-band transfer for anterolateral rotatory instability of the knee. *J. Bone Joint Surg.*, **61A**, 330–39.

Ellison, A. E. (1980), The pathogenesis and treatment of anterolateral rotatory instability. *Clinical Orthop.*, **147**, 51–5.

Feagin, J. A. Jr and Curl, W. W. (1976), Isolated tear of the anterior cruciate ligament: 5-year follow-up study. *Am. J. Sport Med.*, **4**, 95–100.

Fetto, J. F. and Marshall, J. L. (1978), Medial collateral ligament injuries of the knee. *Clinical Orthop.*, **132**, 206–18.

Fetto, J. F. and Marshall, J. L. (1979), Injury to the anterior cruciate ligament producing the pivot-shift sign. An experimental study on cadaver specimens. *J. Bone Joint Surg.*, **61A**, 710–14.

Freeman, B. L. III, Beaty, J. H. and Haynes, D. B. (1982), The pes anserinus transfer. A long-term follow-up. *J. Bone Joint Surg.*, **64A**, 202–07.

Galway, R., Beaupre, A. and McIntosh, D. L. (1972), Pivot-shift: A clinical sign of symptomatic anterior cruciate insufficiency. *J. Bone Joint Surg.*, **54B**, 763.

Henning, C. (1982), Presentation, AOSSM. Osage Beach, Missouri, July 19.

Hey Groves, E. W. (1920), The crucial ligaments of the knee-joint: their function, rupture, and the operative treatment of the same. *Br. J. Surg.*, **7**, 505–15.

Hsieh, H. and Walker, P. S. (1976), Stabilizing mechanisms of the loaded and unloaded knee joint. *J. Bone Joint Surg.*, **58A**, 87.

Hughston, J. C. and Eilers, A. F. (1973), The role of the posterior oblique ligament in repairs of acute medial (collateral) ligament tears of the knee. *J. Bone Joint Surg.*, **55A**, 923–40.

Hughston, J. C., Andrews, J. R., Cross, M. J. (1976), Classification of knee ligament instabilities. Part I. The medial compartment and cruciate ligaments. *J. Bone Joint Surg.*, **58A**, 159–72.

Hughston, J. C., Andrews, J. R. and Cross, M. J. (1976), Classification of knee ligament instabilities. Part II. The lateral compartment. *J. Bone Joint Surg.*, **58A**, 173–79.

Ligament Injuries and their Treatment

Hughston, J. C. and Barrett, G. R. (1983), Acute anteromedial rotatory instability. *J. Bone Joint Surg.*, **65A**, 145–53.

Insall, J., Joseph, D. M. and Aglietti, P. (1981), Bone-block iliotibial-band transfer for anterior cruciate ligament insufficiency. *J. Bone Joint Surg.*, **63A**, 560–69.

Ireland, J. and Trickey, E. L. (1980), MacIntosh tenodesis for anterolateral instability of the knee. *J. Bone Joint Surg.*, **62B**, 340–45.

Jacobsen, K. (1977), Osteoarthrosis following insufficiency of the cruciate ligaments in man. A clinical study. *Acta Orthop. Scand.*, **48**, 520–26.

James, S. L., Woods, G. W., Homsy, G. A. (1979), Cruciate ligament stents in reconstruction of the unstable knee: a preliminary report. *Clin. Orthop.*, **143**, 90–96.

Jones, K. G. (1963), Reconstruction of the anterior cruciate ligament. A technique using the central one-third of the patellar ligament. *J. Bone Joint Surg.*, **45A**, 925–932.

Kennedy, J. C. (1980), Intraarticular replacement in the anterior cruciate ligament deficient knee. *Am. J. Sports Med.*, **8**, 1–8.

Lam, S. J. S. (1968), Reconstruction of the anterior cruciate ligament using the Jones procedure and its Guy's Hospital modification. *J. Bone Joint Surg.*, **50A**, 1213–24.

Larson, R. L. (1983), The knee – the physiological joint. *J. Bone Joint Surg.*, **65A**, 143–44.

Losee, R. E., Johnson, T. R. and Southwick, W. O. (1978), Anterior subluxation of the lateral tibial plateau. A diagnostic test and operative repair. *J. Bone Joint Surg.*, **60A**, 1015–30.

McDaniel, W. J. Jr and Dameron, T. B. Jr (1980), Untreated ruptures of the anterior cruciate ligament. A follow-up study. *J. Bone Joint Surg.*, **62A**, 696–705.

Marshall, J. L., Girgis, F. G. and Zelko, R. R. (1972), The biceps femoris tendon and its functional significance. *J. Bone Joint Surg.*, **54A**, 1444–50.

Norwood, L. A. Jr and Cross, M. J. (1977), The intercondylar shelf and the anterior cruciate ligament. *Am. J. Sports Med.*, **7**, 171–76.

O'Donoghue, D. H. (1959), Surgical treatment of injuries to ligaments of the knee. *JAMA 169*, 1423–31.

O'Donoghue, D. H. (1963), A method for replacement of the anterior cruciate ligament of the knee. Report of twenty cases. *J. Bone Joint Surg.*, **45A**, 905–24.

Palmer, I. (1938), On the injuries to the ligaments of the knee joint. *Acta Chir. Scand.* **81**, (Suppl. 53).

Paulos, L., Noyes, F. R. and Grood, E. (1981), Knee rehabilitation after anterior cruciate ligament reconstruction and repair. *Am. J. Sports Med.*, **9**, 140–49.

Perry, J., Fox, J. M. and Boitano *et al.* (1980), Functional evaluation of the pes anserinus transfer by electromyography and gait analysis. *J. Bone Joint Surg.*, **62A**, 973–80.

Slager, R. S. (1982), Presentation, Annual Meeting, American College of Sports Medicine. Tar-Tara, Lake of the Ozarks, Missouri. July 12.

Slocum, D. B. and Larson, R. L. (1968), Pes anserinus transplantation. A surgical procedure for control of rotatory instability of the knee. *J. Bone Joint Surg.*, **50A**, 226–42.

Slocum, D. B. and Larson, R. L. (1980), Rotatory instability of the knee. Its pathogenesis and a clinical test to demonstrate its presence. *J. Bone Joint Surg.*, **50A**, 211–25.

Slocum, D. B., Larson, R. L. and James, S. L (1974), Pes anserinus transplant: impressions after a decade of experience. *Am. J. Sports Med.*, **2**, 123–36.

Warren, R. F., Marshall, J. L. and Girgis, F. (1974), The prime static stabilizers of the medial side of the knee. *J. Bone Joint Surg.*, **56A**, 665–74.

8 Knee lesions III: Diagnostic aids and meniscal reconstruction

F. M. IVEY

8.1 Introduction

Normal function of the knee depends upon coordinated interaction among all joint components (Table 8.1). When one or several components are abnormal, either from disease or injury, symptoms arise and patients seek medical assistance. Proper treatment and prognosis depend upon obtaining complete and accurate diagnosis. This precise diagnosis is not always easy to obtain with routine history, physical examination and plain roentgenograms. When indicated, diagnostic aids such as stress views, aspiration, arthrography, examination under anaesthesia and diagnostic arthroscopy will increase diagnostic accuracy near to 100%. Obtaining a complete diagnosis acutely helps minimize long-term disability.

Table 8.1 Components of normal knee function

Extensor mechanism
Articular cartilage
Ligamentous restraints
Menisci
Synovium

8.2 History

Data should include age, occupation, recreational interests and general medical condition. Previous injury or symptoms may signify recurrent problems with progressive deterioration. Patients with on-the-job injuries frequently embellish their complaints in the absence of significant objective findings since they receive compensation while unable to work.

159

Ligament Injuries and their Treatment

If previous surgery on the knee was performed, exact details should be available including the examination under anaesthesia, intraoperative findings and the procedure details.

The majority of complaints with ligamentous instability are related to previous injury. Some exceptions would be from ligamentous laxity due to chronic joint distension as in rheumatic diseases or recurrent bleeding in haemophilia. The mechanism of injury is important to document. A history of hyperextension indicates initial injury to the posterolateral bundle of the anterior cruciate ligament whereas a valgus and external rotation stress to a flexed knee may first injure medial ligamentous structures. Many injuries are non-contact in nature and result from cutting or deceleration.

(a) Pain

Pain is a subjective complaint and at times difficult to quantitate. Its effect on the patient's activity and function should be evaluated. In acute injury, pain is primarily due to capsular disruption or distension. Generalized pain often reflects an effusion whereas localized pain denotes underlying injury to ligaments, bone or menisci. Pain at the extremes of motion is commonly due to meniscal abnormality or muscle spasm. Acute injuries may not produce severe pain if the capsule is completely disrupted. Pain with activity in the absence of injury or at rest pain may be related to articular cartilage damage from degenerative arthritis. Anterior peripatellar pain aggravated by stair climbing and bent knee positions is typical of extensor mechanism abnormalities.

(b) Swelling or joint effusion

Swelling or joint effusion can be present in acute injury or with chronic recurrent instability. Swelling that occurs within 2 hours of an injury, being maximal by 12 hours, should be considered to be the result of acute haemarthrosis until proven otherwise. Swelling which is first noticed after 12 hours is most commonly due to serous effusion. Chronic swelling in the presence of instability generally reflects articular cartilage damage with synovial hypertrophy.

(c) Popping, clicking and grinding

Popping, clicking and grinding may be related to meniscal abnormalities, loose bodies, articular cartilage damage or rarely, ligament stumps. Unstable meniscal fragments may momentarily displace with a popping feeling or sound and then return to their normal position. Capsular traction from this abnormal motion of the meniscus produces pain. When a meniscus remains in a displaced position, as with a bucket handle tear, motion is impaired at the extremes of flexion and extension. Loose bodies

160

generally cause locking associated with pain but the defect at their site of origin may be the source of crepitus.

(d) Buckling

Buckling or giving away can be a difficult symptom to evaluate. It may be due to ligamentous instability described as a joint 'coming apart' or 'feeling loose' with activity. Muscular weakness after injury, immobilization or inadequate rehabilitation can cause giving away especially in bent knee activities. A painful stimulus such as a displacing meniscal fragment, impinging loose bodies, periarticular osteophytes or a subluxating patella may cause momentary reflex atony of the limb's antigravity muscles giving a feeling of buckling.

(e) Locking

True locking of the knee occurs when a mobile object such as a loose body or displacing meniscal fragment becomes interposed between the tibia and femur. Manipulation by the patient using flexion, extension and/or rotation may relieve the locked position.

An audible or palpable *pop* at the time of initial injury is highly suggestive of anterior cruciate ligament injury, but it can also be associated with meniscal damage or fracture.

(f) Stiffness

A feeling of *stiffness* or loss of full motion commonly noted by patients with acute injury may be due to intraligamentous haemorrhage, reflex muscle spasm or joint effusion. Patients with chronic ligamentous instability may develop loss of terminal flexion or extension due to soft tissue or capsular contracture or to bony block from osteophytes.

8.3 Physical examination and diagnostic aids

One should systematically move from a general evaluation to more specific areas in the physical examination (Tables 8.2 and 8.3). Points in the general and regional examination may influence the physician to choose one method of treatment over another. For example – an overweight patient with generalized ligamentous laxity and varicose veins may be treated with anti-inflammatory medication, physical therapy and orthotic support for recurrent patella dislocation, rather than accept the higher risk and recurrence rate of surgery as an initial procedure.

Ligament Injuries and their Treatment

Table 8.2   General and regional examination

General Examination
   Height/weight
   Gait
   Use of lateral support
   Ligamentous laxity (generalized)

Regional examination
   Distal motor and sensory exam
   Peripheral pulses
   Signs of venous stasis
   Joint effusion
   Scars/tibial tubercle sensation
   Quadriceps/calf atrophy
   Localized tenderness/swelling/ecchymosis
   Popliteal swelling/masses

Table 8.3   Specific tests for joint function

Extensor mechanism
   Active range of motion
   Foot progression angle
   Hamstring tightness
   Extremity alignment (Q angle)
   Femoral rotation
   Tibial torsion
   Subtalar mobility
   Patellar mobility
   Patellar facet tenderness
   Patellofemoral crepitus with motion
   Apprehension on lateral motion of
      patellar (Fairbanks test)
   Vastus medialis obliquus atrophy/
      dysplasia
   Patella alta
Articular cartilage
   Effusion
   Palpable osteophytes
   Boggy synovium
   Crepitus with compartment com-
      pression (Varus/Valgus) through
      range of motion
   Abnormal extremity alignment

Meniscal
   Pain at extremes of motion
   Loss terminal 'screw-home' external
      rotation
   Joint line pain to palpation
   McMurray's Test
   Apley's compression test
Ligamentous
   Tibial dropback
   External rotation recurvatum
   Varus/Valgus instability in extension
   Abnormal Varus/Valgus laxity in 30°
      flexion
   Anterior/Posterior drawer abnor-
      malities
   Lachman test
   Tests for anterolateral rotatory
      instability

8.3.1 EXTENSOR MECHANISM

Extremity alignment in all planes is important to the health and function of the extensor mechanism. Static measurement of subtalar mobility, tibial torsion and hip rotation combine to produce the dynamically observed foot progression angle. Standing static alignment in the frontal plane give an indication of the limb's anatomical axis which is directly related to the Q angle. In the extended relaxed position, the patella should easily move medially and laterally 1 cm. Palpation of medial and lateral retinacular attachments to the patella should be examined along with the patellofemoral motion during flexion and extension of the knee. As the knee is actively flexed and extended, one can feel patellofemoral crepitus and should document the degree of flexion in which it occurs in order to correlate with the contact surfaces. A positive apprehension or Fairbank's test is fairly reliable evidence of patellar subluxation. Patella alta can be clinically diagnosed when the knee is flexed to 90°. In this position the anterior surface should be perpendicular to the thigh; if tilted anteriorly, patella alta is clinically present and is associated with an increased incidence of recurrent subluxation and dislocation.

8.3.2 MENISCUS

The majority of knees with acute and chronic ligamentous instability have meniscal abnormalities. Frequently the development of an unstable meniscal tear in a chronically unstable knee will first cause a patient to seek medical attention. Loss of terminal flexion or extension, joint line pain to palpation and a positive McMurray's test are helpful physical signs. Displaced bucket-handle tears of the meniscus can restrict terminal external rotation of the tibia. Apley's compression test in the prone position helps differentiate joint line pain due to acute ligamentous tears versus meniscal pathology.

8.3.3 ARTICULAR CARTILAGE DAMAGE

Articular cartilage damage is common in both acute and chronic ligamentous instability involving the anterior cruciate ligament. Chondral and osteochondral fractures occur with 15–20% of these acute injuries. If the bony fragment is small it may not be apparent on routine roentgenograms. Additional aids such as arthroscopy may be necessary for diagnosis. The delicately balanced motion of a normal knee becomes disrupted with ligamentous instability. This frequently causes chondromalacic changes in the articular cartilage leading to gonarthrosis involving especially the weight-bearing surfaces of the femoral condyles.

Ligament Injuries and their Treatment

Periarticular osteophytes alone can cause pain through capsular irritation. They may be palpable at the joint margins. Articular cartilage debris within the joint helps initiate and propagate joint effusion which can be palpable in chronic cases.

The physician may find in acute knee injuries that examination of ligaments is difficult because of pain, muscle spasm or apprehension. The examination should, nevertheless, be as complete as possible within the limits of pain. It is generally easier to perform an examination for chronic ligamentous instability. Certain manoeuvres which seek to demonstrate momentary subluxation of the knee may still be uncomfortable and the patient may guard against these tests. In circumstances where the examination is incomplete because of muscle guarding, consideration should be given to an examination under general anaesthetic.

8.3.4 LIGAMENTOUS EXAMINATION

Ligamentous instability is classified according to type and degree of severity. Instability can be classified as either straight or rotational depending on which direction the tibia moves away from the femur with applied stress (Hughston *et al.*, 1976). By definition, straight instability exists when the posterior cruciate is non-functional and rotational instability exists when it is functionally intact. Combined instability is common, especially in chronic anterior cruciate deficient knees. Instability is graded I to III depending on degree of injury to ligaments. A grade I injury results in pain on palpation and stress of the ligament, but there is no abnormal motion of the tibia in relation to the femur. A grade II injury shows 5–10 mm greater laxity compared to the normal side but a good stop. A grade III injury (complete disruption) demonstrates greater than 10 mm laxity with a soft endpoint. The techniques for examining the knee for ligamentous instability and for classifying the types of instability are well described in the literature (Hughston *et al.*, 1976).

The most disabling component of anterior cruciate injury is anterolateral rotatory instability which occurs during the last 20–30° of extension. The anterolateral portion of the tibial plateau subluxates forward on the femur giving the sensation that the knee is 'coming apart' or buckling. Several tests (Hughston *et al.*, 1976; Losee, Johnson and Southwick, 1978; MacIntosh, 1973; Noyes *et al.*, 1980; Slocum *et al.*, 1976) have been described to demonstrate anterolateral rotatory instability and each examiner uses one or more of them depending upon his preference and the patient's ability to cooperate. It is common, especially in acute injuries, to be unable to perform these tests without anaesthesia.

The Lachman test is the most sensitive test for anterior cruciate ligament deficiency (Torg, Conrad and Kalen, 1976). It is generally positive with anterior cruciate ligament injury even without anaesthesia. With the knee flexed to 20° and the femur stabilized with one hand, an anterior drawer stress is applied to the proximal tibia. Anterior motion of the tibia on the femur is detected by the thumb and index finger of the stabilizing hand and also by the increasing prominence of the tibial tubercle.

A complete thorough ligament examination is essential to the treatment plan. Keypoints in the history and physical examination should alert the examiner to the possibility that severe, or potentially severe, injury has occurred (Table 8.4). Additional diagnostic aids may then be necessary.

Table 8.4 Key points in history and physical exam alerting examiner to possibility severe injury

---

History
Hearing or feeling a 'pop' at time of injury
Timing of swelling compatible with haemarthrosis
Immediate disability, inability to walk
Knee buckles, locks, feels stiff

Physical
Abnormal neurovascular exam
Inability to perform complete exam due to pain, spasm or apprehension
Large joint effusion
Signs of patellar dislocation, meniscal abnormality or ligamentous instability

---

8.3.5 X-RAY

Roentgenographic evaluation routinely includes anteroposterior, lateral, tunnel, and patellar sunrise views. Additional views may be necessary depending on the patient's age and the clinical impression. Oblique views help define fracture patterns and stress views help rule out epiphyseal injury in the skeletally immature (Kennedy, 1979) (Figs. 8.1 and 8.2 (a), (b), (c) and (d)).

Any fleck of bone about the knee suggests a potentially severe injury (Woods, Stanley and Tullos, 1979). It is not so much the size of bone that is important but the ligament or capsular structure which is attached to it plus commonly associated ligamentous injuries (Figs. 8.3 and 8.4).

An arteriogram may be indicated when distal pulses are unequal, signs or symptoms of a compartment syndrome are present or when a knee dislocation has occurred (Green and Allen, 1977; Jones, Smith and Bone, 1979) (Fig. 8.5).

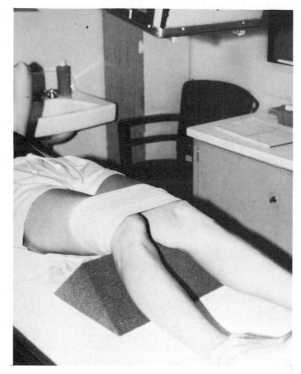

Fig. 8.1   Valgus stress roentgenogram of the knee.

In a chronically unstable knee, radiographic findings associated with degenerative arthritis may be present. These include cartilage space narrowing, periarticular osteophytes, subchondral sclerosis and cyst formation. A defect in the lateral femoral condyle on oblique views is occasionally seen in knees with chronic anterolateral rotatory instability (Losee, Johnson and Southwick, 1978).

8.3.6   ASPIRATION

Joint aspiration can be used to confirm the clinical impression as to the possibility of severe injury. If serous fluid is aspirated and no alarming points are elicited in the history or physical examination, a short trial of crutch protection and physical therapy may be indicated. Bloody aspirate suggests a serious injury (Table 8.5).

In knees with chronic instability, joint fluid may contain cartilage flakes in the absence of radiographic abnormality or symptoms of degenerative arthritis (Sedgwick *et al.*, 1980).

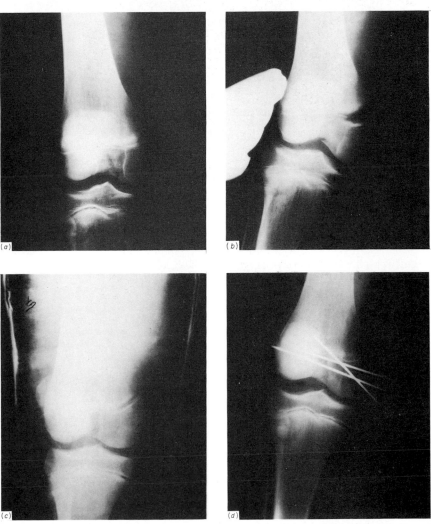

Fig. 8.2 (a) Anteroposterior roentgenogram of the knee with mild widening of the medial epiphyseal plate. (b) Valgus stress roentgenogram demonstrating a Salter III epiphyseal fracture of the medial femoral condyle. (c) Residual displacement of the medial femoral condyle after stress views. (d) Intraoperative roentgenogram demonstrating anatomical positioning of the medial femoral condyle.

Some authors advocate evaluation of haemarthrosis fluid qualitatively and quantitatively. 'Cruciate blood' as such is not a valid determination and severe injuries may yield little or no blood aspirate as fluid leaves the joint through large capsular rents. Droplets of fat in the aspirate may indicate interarticular fracture, fat pad injury or synovial disruption.

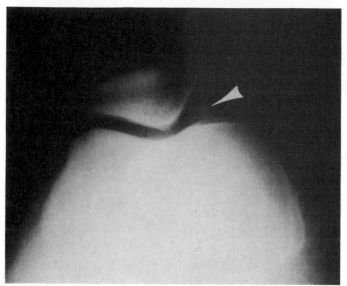

Fig. 8.3 Sunrise view of the patella (30°), pointer indicates medial osseous fragment highly suggestive of capsular avulsion from patellar dislocation.

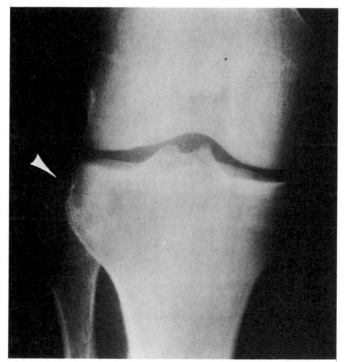

Fig. 8.4 Anteroposterior roentgenogram with pointer indicating the 'lateral capsular sign'. This indicates avulsion of the mid-third lateral capsular ligament and in a high percentage of cases associated injury to the anterior cruciate ligament and menisci.

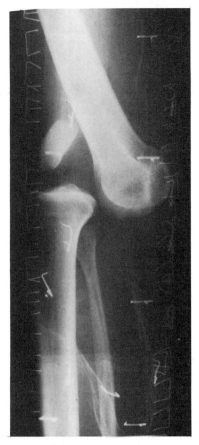

Fig. 8.5 Anterior dislocation of the knee; subsequent anteriogram demonstrated intimal injury to the popliteal artery requiring vascular repair.

Table 8.5 Causes of bloody effusion

Patellar dislocation
Intraligamentous tears
Peripheral meniscal injury
Osteochondral fracture
Penetrating injury/contusion

Ligament Injuries and their Treatment

8.3.7 ARTHROGRAPHY

The technique of double contrast arthrography is well established (Freiberger, Robert and Kaye, 1979). Under fluoroscopic control the X-ray beam is positioned tangential to the joint surfaces and multiple exposures are made while the extremity is rotated. Important information is primarily obtained regarding meniscal structures. Cruciate ligament shadows, articular cartilage contour and capsular integrity can also be evaluated. Accuracy is dependent upon a technically well-done procedure and upon which structure is being evaluated. The lateral meniscus is generally not as well visualized as the medial meniscus due to overlying shadows of the popliteus tendon and the distal sloping of the lateral tibial plateau. Medial meniscal accuracy with a technically well-done arthrogram is generally greater than 95% (Fig. 8.6). Cruciate ligament integrity should be ascertained by manual ligament testing and not by the appearance of a shadow on the lateral view of an arthrogram.

Athrography and arthroscopy should be considered complementary procedures. In relatively 'tight' knees the posteromedial corner is difficult to see arthroscopically, even with the use of a small-diameter scope, a second puncture probe and the posteromedial portal. Arthrograms give important information in this area. The lateral meniscus is best evaluated

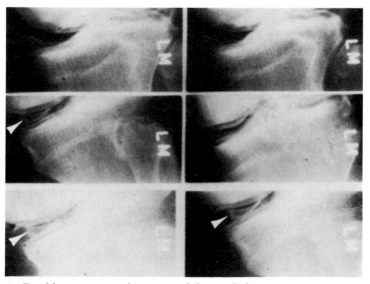

Fig. 8.6 Double contrast arthrogram of the medial compartment; pointer indicates dye within the meniscal substance on three different views – a longitudinal vertical tear.

arthroscopically from anterior portals plus the use of a second puncture probe.

To improve diagnostic accuracy with the use of various diagnostic tests, physicians on an interval basis should compare their preoperative diagnosis with arthrographic and arthroscopic findings and interpretations. The majority of knees with acute and chronic instability involving the anterior cruciate ligament have abnormalities affecting one or both menisci. Any diagnostic aid that gives information regarding these structures helps the physician obtain a complete diagnosis and facilitates preoperative discussions and long-term planning.

8.3.8 EXAMINATION UNDER ANAESTHESIA

Acute knee injuries are associated with pain, swelling, limitation of motion, involuntary muscle spasm and patient apprehension. It is not surprising that clinical examination of the ligaments of these knees is difficult and often incomplete. Knees previously operated upon for meniscus or ligament pathology, and knees that are unstable on clinical examination have a significant incidence of unrecognized classes and grades of instability unless the examination is performed under anaesthesia (Ivey *et al.*, 1980). The most commonly overlooked abnormality is anterolateral rotatory instability due to anterior cruciate ligament deficiency. Tests demonstrating the sudden anterior subluxation of the lateral tibial plateau on the femur cause pain or patient apprehension and unanaesthetized patients commonly resist these manoeuvres (Ivey *et al.*, 1980). Displaced meniscal tears and large joint effusions may give false-negative findings under anaesthesia (Johnson, 1979).

8.3.9 ARTHROSCOPY

Diagnostic arthroscopy adds to, refines or changes preoperative impressions in a significant number of patients. It should be considered complementary to other diagnostic aids. Arthroscopy using local anaesthesia should be used only in selected patients having known extensor mechanism abnormalities or articular cartilage degeneration, as arthroscopy rarely allows a complete comprehensive ligament examination unless performed under regional or general anaesthetic.

In acutely injured joints, arthroscopy should not be performed when local skin infection or a bleeding diathesis is present. Arthroscopy is contraindicated when a major capsular disruption exists because extravasated fluid may compress neural and vascular structures (Noyes *et al.*, 1980). Acute injuries generally require a large-bore arthroscope with a good irrigation system to clear blood from the joint. A tourniquet should be placed on the thigh but it is rarely necessary to inflate it. After a few minutes of irrigation and pressure distention of the joint, a clear view can be obtained of all structures. The physician should be familiar with multiple puncture sites and with the use of a second puncture probe to completely evaluate all regions and structures within the joint. Difficulty in examining one area can be remedied by changing portals, using a different angle scope or by the use of a probe. Certain surgical procedures may be performed with the arthroscope such as loose body removal and partial meniscectomy as indicated.

8.3.10 DISCUSSION

Treatment of the acute and chronic anterior cruciate deficient knee is highly debatable and depends upon many factors. Associated pathology such as meniscal injury and chondral damage, patient expectations and type of athletic activity are all factors in the decision-making process. Obviously not all patients with anterior cruciate ligament damage require early surgical treatment; however, it is likely that a significant number of patients who are not operated upon with time develop disabling symptoms. In fact, interest in determining natural history of these injuries has uncovered certain patients who may very well have benefited from early surgical repair, reconstruction or augmentation of the damaged anterior cruciate ligament. These patients include those with associated complete grade III tears of peripheral capsular-ligamentous structures, those with injury to both menisci and those with grade III instability of the anterior cruciate ligament in a highly competitive athlete (Noyes, 1982). Surgical treatment in these patients is chosen rather than early protection, guarded careful rehabilitation and brace-protected return to activity.

Chronic anterior cruciate ligament instability can lead to meniscal tears, progressive combined instability, articular cartilage damage, and extensor tracking problems (Ivey et al., 1980). These patients may complain of pain, swelling, buckling and progressive disability related both to athletics and to activities of daily living. Should a comprehensive rehabilitation programme, moderation of activities and brace protection not result in significant functional improvement, reconstructive surgery may be indicated.

The anterior cruciate ligament is the primary restraint to anterior displacement of the tibia on the femur (Butler, Noyes and Grood, 1980). It also limits excessive tibial rotation and hyperextension. For disabling mild (grade I) cruciate instability, appropriate extra-articular reconstructive procedures have an acceptable success rate both objectively and functionally (Fox et al., 1980). Moderate and severe anterior cruciate

172

ligament laxity generally requires direct reconstruction of the anterior cruciate ligament to provide full objective stability. Ideal replacement of the anterior cruciate ligament should be compatible in the joint, provide adequate strength, become securely attached to bone at each end, and remain viable. The surgical procedure must, of course, be technically feasible. Autogenous tissue from about the knee used for anterior cruciate reconstruction should be functionally expendable.

8.4 Meniscal reconstruction for anterior cruciate ligament deficient knees

The meniscus meets all of the previously mentioned criteria. It is readily accessible and surgical exposure to mobilize it need not be extensive. Technically it is not a difficult surgical operation to perform and the meniscus usually survives quite well within the joint. Experimentally the meniscus used as a cruciate substitute becomes attached to bone, gains a blood supply and undergoes metaplasia with time looking more like a ligament (Bullough et al., 1970; Collins et al., 1974). Tensile strength studies show the meniscus to be generally equal in strength to a normal anterior cruciate ligament with variations primarily due to age-related changes (Bullough et al., 1970; Kennedy, personal communication, 1979; Mathur, McDonald and Ghormley, 1949). A normal meniscus should not be used for reconstruction. Ideally the meniscus should be irreparable, and should require excision due to its injury. Many menisci in chronically unstable knees have multiple tears and are unsuitable for use as an anterior cruciate ligament substitute.

8.4.1 SURGICAL PROCEDURE

All patients undergo clinical examination and diagnostic arthroscopy under general or regional anaesthetic. With tourniquet haemostasis and prophylactic antibiotic coverage, the meniscus chosen for reconstruction is detached except for its anterior horn. The lateral meniscus requires only an anterolateral capsular incision for preparation whereas the medial meniscus requires both anteromedial and posteromedial capsular incisions. A heavy non-absorbable suture is placed in the free end of the meniscus (Fig. 8.7(a) and (b)). A guide pin is placed from the flare of the lateral femoral condyle entering the intercondylar notch just posterior and superior to the exact origin of the anterior cruciate ligament (Fig. 8.7(c)). A cannulated reamer is placed over the guide pin to prepare an interosseous tunnel in the lateral femoral condyle (Fig. 8.7(d)). The anterior edge of the hole in the intercondylar notch is bevelled with a curved curette to prevent a sharp edge from contacting the meniscus (Fig. 8.7(e)). A rubber catheter facilitates passage of the sutures through the condyle, care being taken not to twist the meniscus (Fig. 8.7(f)). With the meniscus snugly held in position (Fig. 8.7(g)), the knee is moved through its full range of motion. No telescoping or impingement of the meniscus should occur with motion. The positioning should therefore be isometric

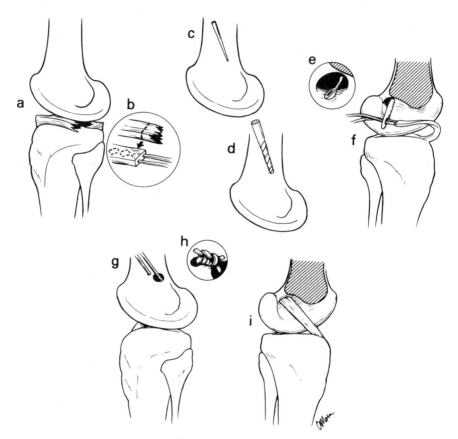

Fig. 8.7 Meniscal reconstruction of the anterior cruciate ligament. (*a*) The meniscus is detached except for its anterior bony attachment. (*b*) The torn edge is trimmed and a heavy non-absorbable suture placed in its free end. (*c*) A guide pin is placed from the flare of the lateral femoral condyle entering the intercondylar notch just superior and posterior to the exact origin of the anterior cruciate ligament. (*d*) A cannulated reamer over the guide pin prepares an interosseous tunnel in the lateral femoral condyle. (*e*) A curved curette bevels the anterior edge of the intercondylar hole (*f*) Rubber catheter assisting passage of the meniscus into lateral femoral condyle. (*g*) Lateral bone bridge preparation. (*h*) Non-absorbable suture tied over bone bridge. (*i*) Positioning of the meniscus after completed transfer.

and excellent stability should be demonstrated when performing the Lachman, anterior drawer test, and flexion rotation drawer. When positioning has been demonstrated to be correct, the non-absorbable sutures are tied over a cortical bone bridge laterally (Fig. 8.7(h)). Additional procedures for articular cartilage lesions, meniscal or extensor mechanism abnormalities are accomplished before closure. Extra-articular procedures for specific components of instability are performed as indicated during closure. The limb is held with a plaster cast in 45° of flexion and in neutral rotation.

Postoperatively patients received antibiotics for 48 hours. Subcutaneous and intra-articular drains are discontinued on the second postoperative day. Bed exercises for the involved extremity are begun the day following surgery. Isometric exercises for all muscle groups of the lower extremity are continued until the incisions have healed. Usually in 2 weeks the extremity can be placed in a limited motion brace to allow for range of motion exercise which excludes the terminal 30° of extension. It is in the final degrees of extension that the quadriceps exerts maximum stress on the newly reconstructed anterior cruciate ligament substitute. Touchdown weightbearing with crutches is allowed at approximately 6 weeks to minimize non-weight-bearing effects on the extremity. Rehabilitation continues along accepted principles (Paulos et al., 1981) with discontinuation of the brace at approximately 4 months and of crutches at 5 months, and with return to functional activity at 7 months. Brace-protected return to full sporting activities is allowed 12 months after surgery when full motion, strength and neuromuscular coordination are demonstrated.

8.4.2 RESULTS

A previous retrospective analysis of 76 patients with disabling anterior cruciate deficiency treated only by extra-articular stabilization revealed disappointing results in those with moderate to severe instability (Fox et al., 1980). A direct reconstruction of the anterior cruciate ligament was then initiated. Analysis of results clinically showed it to be at least as good as a patellar tendon reconstruction (Ivey et al., 1980) and to have some distinct advantages. Exposure was not as extensive, terminal flexion was not impaired and operative time was shortened. Improper positioning, poor lateral condyle fixation and improper tension on the meniscus were technical errors early in this series that were thought to be responsible for failures of the procedure in approximately 20% of patients.

Several menisci broke at the entrance to the femoral bone canal. This was remedied by isometric positioning and by bevelling the anterior edge of the hole. Improper anterior positioning (especially for the lateral meniscus) is remedied by using the meniscus as a free graft and placing the anterior horn within a tibial bone canal. Postoperative fibroarthrosis is being noted by more and more investigators after this type of extensive surgery. Early protected motion in a brace appears to be effective in preventing this problem but results are still preliminary. Fixation, thus, must be initially secure, early graft degeneration must not result in a dangerously weakened reconstruction and guarded range of motion must not stress the meniscus during the last 30° of extension. Clinically, early motion is beneficial and objective results have not deteriorated.

The decision for reconstruction must not be based on preoperative pain complaints. Pain relief is unpredictable with this procedure and relates primarily to articular cartilage damage found at surgery. Functional results are related to the absence of buckling, to the ability to participate in recreational sports with brace protection and to realistic preoperative expectations. Objective results depend on technical factors at the time of surgery and on guarded postoperative rehabilitation.

Chronic disabling symptoms of anterior cruciate ligament deficiency may persist in spite of brace protection and an extensive rehabilitation programme. Reconstruction of the damaged anterior cruciate ligament may be indicated in selective patients acutely and in chronic disabling instability. The meniscus used as an anterior cruciate ligament substitute has demonstrated good to excellent objective, functional and subjective results with a 42-month follow-up (Ferkel, 1985). This preliminary evidence is encouraging. Continued basic research and clinical evaluation continues to demonstrate that the meniscus is yet another autogenous tissue that can give satisfactory clinical results in selected patients with acute and chronic deficiency of the anterior cruciate ligament.

References

Bullough, P. G., Munuers, L., Murphy, J. and Weinstein, A. M. (1970), The strength of the menisci as it relates to their fine structure. *J. Bone Joint Surg.*, **52B**, 564–70.

Butler, D. L., Noyes, F. R. and Grood, E. S. (1980), Ligamentous restraints to anterior-posterior drawer in the human knee. A biomechanical study. *J. Bone Joint Surg.*, **62A**, 259–70.

Collins, H. R., Hughston, J. L., DeHaven, K. E., Bergfield, J. A. and Evarts, C. M. (1974), The meniscus as a cruciate ligament substitute. *Am J. Sports Med.*, **2**, 11–21.

Ferkel, R. D. (1985), Private communication.

Fox, J. M., Blazina, M. E., DelPizzo, W., Ivey, F. M. and Broukhim, B. (1980), Extra-articular stabilization of the knee joint for anterior instability. *Clin. Orthop.*, **147**, 56–61.

Freiberger, R. H. and Kaye, J. J. (1979), *Arthrography*, Appleton-Century-Crofts, New York, pp. 5–30.

Green, N. E. and Allen, B. L. (1977), Vascular injuries associated with dislocation of the knee. *J. Bone Joint Surg.*, **59A**, 236–9.

Hughston, J. C., Andrews, J. R., Cross, M. J. and Moschi, A. (1976), Classification of knee ligament instabilities. Part I: The medial compartment and cruciate ligaments. Part II: The lateral compartment. *J. Bone Joint Surg.*, **58A**, 159–79.

Ivey, F. M., Blazina, M. E., Fox, J. M. and DelPizzo, W. (1980), Intra-articular substitution for anterior cruciate insufficiency. *Am. J. Sports Med.*, **8**, 405–10.

Ivey, F. M., Blazina, M. E., Fox, J. M. and DelPizzo, W. (1980), Arthroscopy of the knee under general anesthesia: an aid to the determination of ligamentous instability. *Am. J. Sports Med.*, **8**, 235–8.

Johnson, L. L. (1979), Lateral capsular ligament complex: Anatomical and surgical considerations. *Am. J. Sports Med.*, **7**, 156–60.

Jones, R. E., Smith, E. C. and Bone, G. E. (1979), Vascular and orthopaedic complications of knee dislocation. *Surg. Gynecol. Obstet.*, **149**, 554–8.

Kennedy, J. C. (1979), *The Injured Adolescent Knee*, p. 82. Williams and Wilkins Co., Baltimore, p. 82.

Losee, R. E., Johnson, T. R. and Southwick, W. O. (1978), Anterior subluxation of the lateral tibial plateau. *J. Bone Joint Surg.*, **60A**, 1015–30.

MacIntosh, D. L. (1973), *The Lateral Pivot Shift. Symposium on Treatment of Injuries of the Knee.* American College of Surgeons Clinictypes, C72–0R3.

Mathur, P. D., McDonald, J. R. and Ghormley, R. K. (1949), A study of the tensile strength of the menisci of the knee. *J. Bone Joint Surg.*, **31A**, 650–4.

Noyes, F. R., Bassett, R. W., Grood, E. S. and Butler, D. L. (1980), Arthroscopy in acute traumatic hemarthrosis of the knee. *J. Bone Joint Surg.*, **62A**, 687–95.

Noyes, F. R. (1982), *The Anterior Cruciate Deficient Knee.* AAOS Instruction Course, Aspen, Colorado.

Paulos, L., Noyes, F. R., Grood, E. and Butler, D. L. (1981), Knee rehabilitation after anterior cruciate ligament reconstruction and repair. *Am. J. Sports Med.*, **9**, 140–9.

Sedgwick, W. G., Gilula, L. A., Lesker, P. A. and Whiteside, L. A. (1980), Wear particles: their value in knee arthrography. *Radiology*, **136**, 11–14.

Slocum, D. B., Jones, S. L., Larson, R. L. and Singer, K. M. (1976), Clinical test for anterolateral rotatory instability of the knee. *Clin Orthop.*, **118**, 63–9.

Torg, J. S., Conrad, W. and Kalen, V. (1976), Clinical diagnosis of anterior cruciate instability in the athlete. *Am. J. Sports Med*, **4**, 84–93.

Woods, G. W., Stanley Jr., R. F. and Tullos, H. S. (1979), Lateral capsular sign: X-ray clue to a significant knee instability. *Am. J. Sports Med.*, **7**, 27–33.

9 Knee lesions IV: Acute anteromedial rotatory instability

LYLE A. NORWOOD AND JACK C. HUGHSTON

9.1 Introduction

Anteromedial rotatory instability is a medial knee ligament injury producing an anterior and external rotation of the medial tibial condyle and a valgus laxity. The term 'rotatory' implies posterior cruciate ligament integrity; a condition not found in straight medial rotatory instability. A torn posterior cruciate ligament allows medial tibial femoral joint opening without external tibial rotation and may produce abduction looseness in full extension when compared with the uninjured knee (Hughston, 1976a; Hughston, 1976b; Hughston, 1980b).

The ligament healing response divides injuries into acute and chronic reactions. Injured ligaments surrounded by haematoma begin healing by reorganization and revascularization. Synovial fluid provokes a phagocytic response. If injured ligaments are surgically repaired prior to onset of the ligament softening stage, 10 days after injury, the ligaments then heal by a primarily healing response – acute. Surgical repair 10 days after injury progresses by phagocytosis, reorganization and revascularization; the same response found in ligament reconstructions – chronic. Thus, the immediate 10 days following knee ligament injury determine the healing response of surgical repair. A knee evaluated 12 days after injury is acute in terms of recentness, and chronic in terms of surgical healing.

9.2 Clinical examination and diagnosis

Examination of the acutely injured knee includes tests which detect posterior cruciate ligament integrity: the abduction stress test and the anterior drawer test (Hughston, 1976a; Hughston, 1976b; Hughston, 1980a). During the abduction stress test the patient is supine with head resting on the examining table. The patient's thigh rests on the table, and the examiner grasps the injured extremity forefoot, and abducts the leg

179

slightly. The examiner rests his proximal hand against the lateral distal femur which stabilizes the femur and eliminates hip motion. Abduction stress at 30° of flexion is applied in a gentle, swinging manner, avoiding forced abduction. The examiner can see and feel the abduction opening. Some knees do not demonstrate external tibial rotation during the abduction stress test, due to specific ligament injury. A relative joint opening of less than 5 mm is a 1+, or mild injury; 5 mm to 1 cm represents a 2+, or moderate injury; and 1 cm or more of opening represents a 3+, or severe medial compartment injury. Abduction forces are not applied at the heel or distal tibia, because this controls or prevents external tibial rotation, and produces more force and discomfort: the resulting protective muscle contraction may conceal the instability, or prevent appropriate injury grading.

Intact posterior cruciate ligaments eliminate abduction opening at 0°, or relative full extension. Abduction examination in relative full extension detects torn posterior cruciate ligaments and changes the diagnosis from anteromedial rotatory instability to straight medial instability (Hughston, 1976a; Hughston, 1976b; Hughston, 1980b). A common error occurs when the examiner tests the knee at 0°, rather than in the appropriate amount of hyperextension. Abduction opening at 0° degrees is correlated with posterior cruciate ligament injury, and the examiner diagnoses straight medial instability, when the posterior cruciate ligament is intact and the diagnosis is anteromedial *rotatory* instability. This mistake may be avoided by careful assessment of contralateral extension prior to abduction stressing in maximum extension.

The anterior drawer test is also performed in the supine position; ipsilateral foot resting on the table and knee in 80–90° flexion (Hughston, 1976a; Hughston, 1976b). The examiner stabilizes the patient's foot and controls the joints proximal and distal to the knee by resting his thigh on the patient's foot. At the same time, he has two hands for the anterior drawer test; using one hand in the test hampers detection of external tibial rotation in the pull phase. The test is performed in neutral, external, and internal tibial rotation. With both hands around the proximal tibia, the examiner gently pushes and pulls the lower limb, grading anterior tibial motion as in the abduction stress test. In anteromedial rotatory instability the anterior and external rotation of the medial tibial condyle occurs during the pull phase.

The test may be positive in neutral position, but is more pronounced in external tibial rotation. In maximum internal rotation, the posterior cruciate ligaments, anteromedial and posterolateral bundles tighten. An intact posterior cruciate ligament, even in a 3+ acute anteromedial rotatory instability will completely stabilize the anterior drawer test with the tibia in full internal rotation. Therefore, a knee which demonstrates a

180

positive anterior drawer test with maximum internal rotation, has at least a partial posterior cruciate ligament injury (Hughston, 1980b; Hughston, 1980a). As in abduction stress test, errors in test interpretation are possible. If the tibia is not completely internally rotated, the examiner may detect a positive anterior drawer test and incorrectly diagnose a posterior cruciate ligament injury. The arthrotomy reveal an uninjured posterior cruciate ligament, and the examiner regards the test as worthless. The inadequacy, however, lies with the examiner's inattention to detail, and not with the test itself.

The clinical examination tells the examiner which knees require medial ligament repair. Rehabilitated knees with grade I, or mild anteromedial rotatory instability, will be as stable as grade I injuries repaired surgically. Grade III injuries are repaired surgically, as are most grade II injuries. The specific sites of puffiness and tenderness provide additional information in grade II injuries. Injuries from the femur, posterior oblique ligament or tibial collateral ligament, heal better than injuries from the medial meniscus or tibia. Some grade II injuries with tenderness only at the femur are treated non-operatively. Conversely, grade II injuries with specific tenderness over the medial meniscus, tibial attachment of the mid-third medial capsular ligament, or posterior oblique ligament, are surgically repaired.

9.3 Surgical repair

The first steps of acute medial ligament injury repair are determining the ligament injury site, and whether the ligaments require surgical repair. Careful clinical examination provides this information. When surgical repair is indicated, the injured ligaments are identified through a medial knee exposure (Fig. 9.1). This exposure should also permit evaluation of medial and lateral intra-articular structures and the patella femoral joint: a medial utility incision (Hughston, 1973a) fulfils these requirements. The subcutaneous fat remains with the posterior and distal skin flap. Joint entry is an anteromedial capsular incision beginning at the patella xyphoid process. The intra-articular structures are examined prior to ligament evaluation or repair. Hip external rotation, with the lateral foot resting on the operating table, creates a varus posture and lateral knee opening. Operative examination of the lateral intra-articular structures is accomplished with a modified fat pad retractor, placed posterior to the patellar tendon. This leg position and retractor facilitate lateral meniscus evaluation by direct visualization and nerve hook palpation. The cruciate ligaments are carefully examined. If there is haemorrhage beneath the posterior cruciate ligament synovium, the synovium is incised

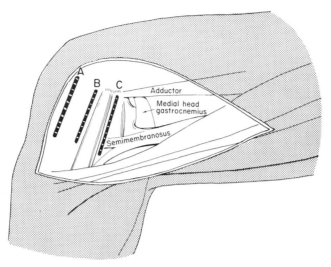

Fig. 9.1 Medial utility incision: surgical approach to the right knee. (*a*) Anteromedial arthrotomy incision. (*b*) Anterior retinacular incision; for examination of midthird medial capsular ligament with intact tibial collateral ligament. (*c*) Posteromedial capsular incision; between posterior oblique ligament and tibial collateral ligament.

longitudinally for ligament fibre examination. When changing knee position to open the medial joint, a Smiley-type retractor is placed at the medial joint line, and abduction force is gently applied at 30° flexion. The medial compartment opens, secondary to injury, and the medial meniscus can be directly palpated and examined with the meniscus hook.

Hip flexion and external rotation facilitate surgical medial ligament examination. The ipsilateral foot once again rests on the operating table (Hughston, 1973a). Haemorrhage indicates the areas of injury. However, it is possible to have a complete ligament tear with little or no haemorrhage. Tenderness detected in the preoperative examination also helps identify the injured ligaments. The surgeon completely evaluates the tibial collateral ligament, mid-third medial capsular ligament, posterior oblique ligament, anterior cruciate ligament, and the semimembranosus.

Some knees require an additional longitudinal incision anterior to the tibial collateral ligament for mid-third medial capsular ligament evaluation (see Fig. 9.1). Ligament integrity to the femur and tibia must be confirmed. If these are intact, the ligament may be torn at the meniscus or in the meniscal femoral or meniscal tibial portions. All knees with acute anteromedial rotatory instability have a torn mid-third medial capsular ligament, and/or posterior oblique ligament (Hughston, 1973b; Nor-

182

wood, 1980). Tibial collateral ligament injury alone does not produce operative instability. When the tibial collateral ligament is torn from the tibia, the surgeon must look deep to the tibial collateral ligament for mid-third medial capsular ligament injury. The posterior oblique ligament must also be evaluated at its osseous attachments, meniscal edges, meniscal femoral, and meniscal tibial aspects. Semimembranosus injury may be easily overlooked. Intact capsular and tibial arms of the semimembranosus are essential for dynamic ligament stability in flexion, and pull on the peripheral medial meniscus.

The tourniquet is deflated after identifying and correcting intra-articular injury, and exposing medial ligamentous injury, always prior to ligament repair. Deflation in this manner decreases postoperative pain, haematomas, and infection. After obtaining haemostasis, systematic medial closure begins with the knee in 60° flexion. Towels placed under the lateral forefoot keep the tibia internally rotated. Closure and repair progress from anterior to posterior; in the opposite direction, the surgeon may be unable to close the anterior incision after posterior and medial ligament repair. Thus, the anteromedial incision is closed first, and if incision was made anterior to the tibial collateral ligament it is then closed.

Staples are not used in ligament repair. They were employed early in this series, but their use was discontinued when the difficulties of ligament–bone fixation became apparent. Staple ligament–fixation produces an avascular portion of ligament around the staple. Since the healing process requires a vascular supply to bone and ligament, staples are contraindicated. They stabilize the knee at surgery, but the ligament does not heal, and instability subsequently redevelops. Our only indication for staple ligament fixation involves fractures. Fractures with ligament–fragment attachment may require staple fixation to maintain fracture reduction for bone healing. Small fractures are replaced and held by direct suture fixation.

Ligament repair begins with the mid-third medial capsular ligament, using mattress sutures and passing the needle through the periosteum, if the ligament is torn from the femur or tibia. We then repair peripheral medial meniscal tears by passing sutures through the meniscal rim and back through the ligament (Fig. 9.2). The medial meniscus is sutured prior to repairing the posterior oblique ligament, because there is no space for proper placement of the sutures after posterior oblique ligament repair. The posterior oblique ligament may be torn from the femur or tibia, or horizontally at the joint line. The posterior oblique ligament is advanced onto the mid-third medial capsular ligament through the tibial collateral ligament and mid-third medial capsular ligament; with the proximal portion advanced anteriorly and superiorly onto the femur's

Ligament Injuries and their Treatment

References

Andrews, J. R., Norwood, L. A., and Cross, M. J. (1976), The double bucket handle tear of the medial meniscus. *Am. J. Sports Med.*, **3**, 232–7.

Andrews, J. R., McLeod, W. D., Ward, T., and Howard, K. (1977), The cutting mechanism. *Am. J. Sports Med.*, **5**, 111–21.

Hughston, J. C. (1973a), A surgical approach to the medial and posterior ligaments of the knee. *Clin. Orthop.*, **91**, 29–33.

Hughston, J. C. and Eilers, A. F. (1973b), The role of the posterior oblique ligament in repairs of acute medial (collateral) ligament tears of the knee. *J. Bone Joint Surg.*, **55A**, 923–40.

Hughston, J. C., Andrews, J. R., Cross, M. J., and Moschi, A. (1976a), Classification of knee ligament instabilities. Part I: The medial compartment and cruciate ligaments. *J. Bone Joint Surg.*, **58A**, 159–72.

Hughston, J. C., Andrews, J. R., Cross, M. J., and Moschi, A. (1976b), Classification of knee ligament instabilities. Part II: The lateral compartment. *J. Bone Joint Surg.*, **58A**, 173–9.

Hughston, J. C. and Norwood, I. A. (1980a), The posterolateral drawer test and external rotational recurvatum test for posterolateral rotatory instability of the knee. *Clin. Orthop.*, **147**, 82–7.

Hughston, J. C., Bowden, J. A., Andrews, J. R., and Norwood, L. A. (1980b), Acute tears of the posterior cruciate ligament. *J. Bone Joint Surg.*, **62A**, 438–50.

Norwood, L. A. and Cross, M. J. (1977), The intercondylar shelf and the anterior cruciate ligament. *Am. J. Sports Med.*, **5**, 171–6.

Norwood, L. A. and Cross, M. J. (1979a), Anterior cruciate ligament: Functional anatomy of its bundles in rotatory instabilities. *Am. J. Sports Med.*, **7**, 23–6.

Norwood, L. A., Andrews, J. R., Meisterling, R. C., and Glancy, G. L. (1979b), Acute anterolateral rotatory instability of the knee. *J. Bone Joint Surg.*, **61A**, 704–9.

Norwood, L. A. and Hughston, J. C. (1980), Combined anterolateral–anteromedial rotatory instability of the knee. *Clin. Orthop.*, **147**, 62–7.

10 Knee lesions V: Fresh injuries and postoperative treatment

G. HELBING

10.1 Introduction

The treatment of injuries to the knee joint ligaments has changed within the last 20 years. The Vienna school advocated a purely conservative treatment of acute ligament injuries up until the early 1960s. According to the degree of instability, the period of immobilization was determined and considered necessary for as long as 16 weeks. Negative effects of long periods of immobilization, such as major quadriceps atrophy and long-lasting joint stiffness, were not reported provided that the patients walked with the cast and performed isometric exercises.

Based on the experience of American and later on French orthopaedic surgeons, a tendency towards operative treatment grew as the results of conservative treatment were not considered satisfactory in major lesions. In particular, either mobility was poor when stability was fair or vice versa.

Today it is rather accepted worldwide that surgical management is indicated when there is evidence of loss of stability in injury to an active patient's knee. Less severe trauma with stability present, usually called distortion, is considered suitable for conservative treatment. As patient's demands on the surgeon have increased, the therapeutic aim in ligamentous injury is complete anatomic and functional reconstruction; that is, stability, mobility and strength of the extremity should be restored as completely as possible. In order to achieve full functional regeneration, early reconstruction is better than late plastic surgery which presents major problems. For plastic surgery to be effective a detailed knowledge of the instability is required whereas with fresh injuries the obvious anatomical damage can be repaired.

Whatever the timing of surgery, further postoperative treatment is also essential. In the surgical treatment of fractures, experience indicated that at least functional stability should be achieved by an osteosynthesis in order to avoid additional immobilization with all its negative effects described by the term 'fracture disease'. Following ligament injuries similar alterations occur which in analogy could be called 'rupture disease'. In contrast to operative fracture treatment immediate post-operative functional stability is not achieved in ligament reconstruction.

Premature exercise would cause damage to the freshly repaired ligaments and thus would not provide stability in the long term. On the other hand, longer immobilization is harmful to a joint with a certain risk of causing accelerated occurrence of osteoarthritis.

10.2 Effects of immobilization

Meanwhile the effects of immobilization are well known. Experimental findings fit into the pattern of clinical experience. Four components, most of them adding to the stability are involved in the 'rupture disease'. These are the muscles, particularly the quadriceps femoris muscle with the vastus medialis, the intact ligaments, the capsule, and the cartilage.

10.2.1 MUSCLES

In the knee in particular the tone of the thigh muscles contributes considerably to stability of the joint (active stabilization), while the ligaments alone are mainly responsible for the correctly guided motion but have little resistance to mechanical forces (passive stabilization). Thus muscular atrophy is extremely unfortunate when it occurs after ligament injuries.

Nevertheless, a rapid loss of the quadriceps muscles can be observed after injuries and during postoperative immobilization. Rebuilding of the original amount of muscles, however, takes a long time and may be rather demanding for the patients (Fig. 10.1).

The loss of muscular substance is accompanied by enzymatic alterations due to the lack of motion (Eriksson, 1976). With full function permitted, enzyme activity will only approach normal levels slowly. There is no way to completely avoid muscular atrophy as it occurs even in highly active athletes within several days after trauma.

10.2.2 LIGAMENTS

Immobilization does not only result in muscular atrophy but also involves the intact ligaments of the joint as well as the bony components. A significant loss of strength in the knee ligaments of dogs after immobilization for as little as 6 weeks was found experimentally (Laros, Tipton and

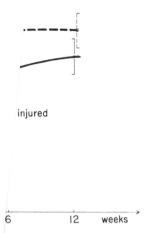

injured

6 12 weeks

Fig. 10.1 Average atrophy of the quadriceps muscles in 50 patients.

Cooper, 1971) thus indicating the disadvantages of immobilization and the importance of exercises.

In biomechanical and histological studies in primates 'functional properties of knee ligaments and alterations induced by immobilization' were tested (Noyes, 1977). The effect of immobility on the biomechanical properties of an anterior cruciate bone–ligament–bone unit of rhesus monkey is reported and the long-term effects of disuse have been investigated for 5 months following total-body immobilization.

A significant decrease in maximum failure load and energy absorbed to failure occurred after 8 weeks of immobilization. This was accompanied by an increase in ligament compliance but it required up to 12 months for the complete recovery of ligament strength parameters.

Additional bone resorption in the cortex immediately beneath the ligament insertion site was found to be the mechanism of failure of the ligament unit observed as an increase of osseous avulsion fractures after immobilization. A comparison between the immobilized and the non-immobilized side in another group of animals showed no evidence of disuse effects on the free motion side (Noyes, 1977).

10.2.3 CAPSULE

Although the importance of the different parts of the capsule, particularly the posterior parts, has only been realized recently, it is known that long-term immobilization leads to a loss of mobility. The main reason is shrinking of the capsule under conditions of non-function in connection with adhesion of the superior recessus of the joint by fibrin and later connective tissue. Joint stiffness does not occur only following ligament injuries but is also the consequence of immobilization for other reasons, for instance conservatively treated fractures. The effects of immobilization can be observed best when older patients with injuries of the shoulder are treated. Free motion even after minor lesions is often never regained. Depending on the age of the patient – younger individuals being less prone – and the duration of disuse, there is evidence of acclerated degeneration following immobilization.

10.2.4 CARTILAGE

The chronic and probably irreversible effects of disuse are associated with the articular cartilage itself. The influence of single factors is not yet clear, but the result from a combination of mechanical stress and biochemical changes is always the same. The sum of all the influences leads to osteoarthritis.

As the cartilage is avascular, nutrition of the chondrocytes is provided by diffusion of synovial fluid from the articular surface towards the deeper layers. Physiological pressure changes and shearing forces are supposed to be important mechanisms influencing the metabolism of articular cartilage. Thus the steady state of nutrients is decreased by immobilization. Additional changes in the composition of the synovial fluid as a result of a trauma or a haemarthrosis are cumulative factors. The matrix and chondrocytes, beginning on the superficial layers are destroyed by the enzymatic activities of either the synovial fluid or of plasmatic or granulocytic origin. Proteolytic activities derived from destroyed chondrocytes or synovial cells may also contribute to damage of the articular cartilage. Another contributing factor may be a reduced blood circulation in the synovial capillaries when joint function is impaired (Cotta, 1973).

The influence of a haemarthrosis on later-occurring osteoarthritis was investigated experimentally by electron microscopy (Dustmann, Puhl and Schneitz, 1971). Superficial fibrillation was found in the cartilage of rabbits following autologous intra-articular blood injections. The effect was amplified when the joints were immobilized and seemed to be less severe by using proteinase inhibiting agents at the same time.

If there is one conclusion that can be drawn from all these findings it is that, from every aspect, immobilization of a joint is harmful in the long term and should be avoided as far as possible.

10.3 Therapy of fresh ligament injuries

Minor injuries of knee ligaments with sufficient stability present do not need surgical management. Neither do they need immobilization. If necessary, an elastic bandage is applied and the patient is advised not to stress it for a few days but to move as far as painlessly possible. Ligament injuries with apparent or suspected instability, however, should be repaired immediately. This should be undertaken keeping the negative consequences of long-term immobilization in mind.

If for any reason immediate reconstruction is not possible, immobilization is avoided preoperatively by encouraging the patients to bend their knees within a painfree range. A 20° dorsal splint is made preoperatively for the sole purpose of positioning the leg immediately after the operation. Intraoperatively the torn or damaged structures are carefully identified and according to the situation sutured or reattached beginning with the central complex, that is, the menisci and the cruciate ligaments. At the end of the operation, the leg is positioned in elevation on the prepared 20° dorsal cast splint. Motion should be encouraged as long as the reconstructed ligaments are not endangered during further treatment.

10.4 Theoretical considerations for avoiding immobilization effects

Postoperative treatment after reconstruction of injured ligaments must be a compromise between the demands of not risking early or late secondary instability and the consciousness of avoiding long-term immobilization effects. There is no suture or reattachment method which provides enough stability for unlimited postoperative exercises compared with an extremity stabilized by an osteosynthesis.

In order to determine the postoperative range of knee motion in which the reconstructed ligaments were not endangered, simple experiments on human knee preparations were performed. The single ligaments were cut and reattached by elastic sutures. The specimens then were moved. The ends of the ligaments came under tension and came apart depending on the angle of flexion. The tension-free range was determined for each ligament. It varied from an average of 20–60° of flexion for the medial collateral ligaments to 20–130° of flexion for the lateral collateral ligaments, the cruciates being somewhere in between (Fig. 10.2(a)). An uncritical 20–60° range was established with no pulling force exerted on the mass of the fibres of all ligaments (Fig. 10.2(b)).

More sophisticated experiments were performed later using measuring

Ligament Injuries and their Treatment

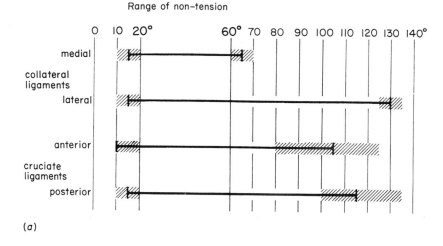

Range of non–tension

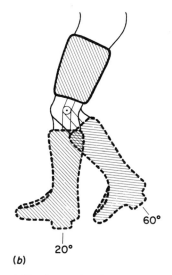

Fig. 10.2 (*a*) Experimentally determined range of motion with the mass of the fibres of the single ligaments not extended, when reattached with elastic sutures. (*b*) Motion to be used for postoperative treatment for all ligaments.

cells to test the biomechanical properties of the collateral ligaments again with human knee preparations (Claes *et al.*, 1979).

Measurements of absolute strain and stress on collateral ligaments of human knees were made. The medial collateral ligament was found to have three functional different parts, the most important of which was the ventral. During motion of the knee, tensile forces amounted to about

194

20 N when the lateral ligament was in full extension and the medial ligament in full flexion. Moments of abduction and adduction increased strain and stress (Fig. 10.3(a)). These experiments revealed a mobility between 25–80° of flexion to be used in therapy, if abduction and adduction motion is avoided (Fig. 10.3(b)).

The lack of adverse effects on functional stress on repaired ligaments was demonstrated by experiments with rabbits (Burri, Pässler and Radde, 1973). Two-thirds of the collateral ligaments were dissected and the animals treated in two different ways. One group was allowed to run free, the other group immobilized by plaster fixation, the functional results as well as the histological findings of the ligaments in animals without limited motion were superior to those ligaments subjected to plaster fixation. Sufficient stability of the collaterals was found in the series of knee joints with free function, whereas insufficiency occurred in the plaster group. Histological sections of the ligaments showed longitudinal collagen formation in the scar after free motion, but this was not seen in the group of previously immobilized knee joints (Fig. 10.4(a) and (b)).

The results of the experiments indicate that there is a range of motion which can be used for therapeutic means following surgery of the knee ligaments without endangering the repaired structures. Furthermore, they demonstrate that function is useful even in regard to the effectiveness of regeneration. With a limited motion permitted the extent of trophic disorders subsequent to knee injuries and reconstructive surgery should be minor compared to complete immobilization. The possibility of early functional treatment, however, depends on the actual kind of lesion and must be regarded entirely individually. Lesions involving the posterior complexes especially probably need extra treatment due to the resulting forces on these structures.

10.5 Translating theory and experimental findings into a therapeutical concept

There is more than one aspect to be considered in the treatment of fresh ligament injuries of the knee joint.

(1) There is a trauma which damages a different and not always well-defined number of ligamentous, capsular, cartilagenous and sometimes tendon structures.

(2) There is the need for an operation with additional unfortunate side-effects despite a skilful technique; it is, however, necessary in order to prevent long-term instability.

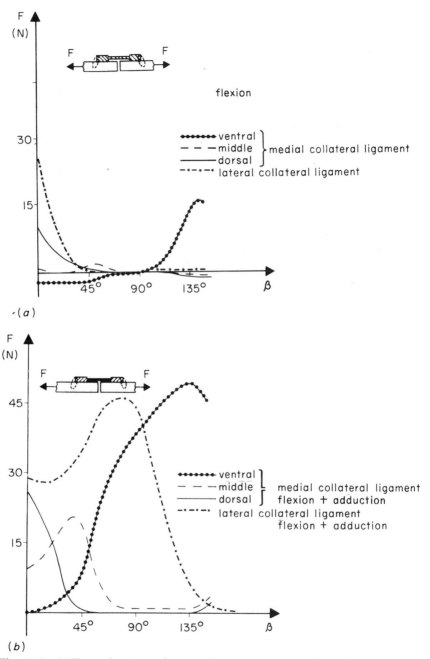

Fig. 10.3 (*a*) Typical pattern of tension forces on normal collateral knee ligaments depending on the angle of flexion β. (*b*) Same experiment with additional abduction respective adduction stress of 400 N/cm applied.

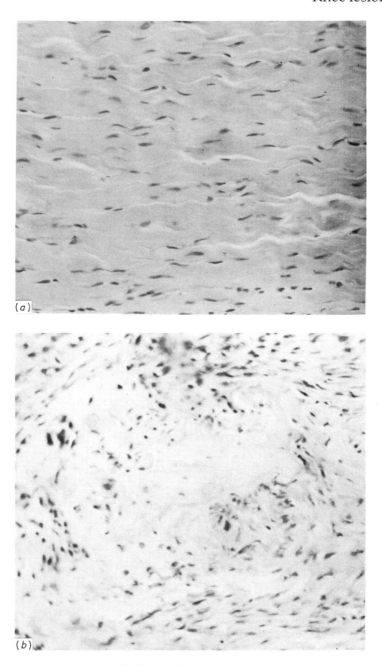

Fig. 10.4 (*a*) Longitudinal collagen formation after two-thirds dissection of the medial collateral ligament of a rabbit followed by no immobilization (*b*) Multidirectional fibres after cast immobilization with no function possible.

(3) The benefit of the operative procedure cannot be effective, when the joint is afterwards immobilized to shield the sutured or reattached structures from early stress, which in a controlled degree is useful for good regeneration.

(4) The reaction patterns of the different patients, such as tendency of swelling or some patients getting Sudeck's dystrophy, must be taken into consideration.

In this sense we feel that early restoration of function is necessary for both the physical and psychological well-being of the patient. The earlier a patient uses his operated leg the sooner full function can be achieved. Athletes are good examples which support this view.

The idea of permitting a tension-free range of motion in early post-operative treatment is not a new one. It needs, however, a well-trained staff of physiotherapists. With guided exercises, and avoiding excessive flexion or extension with no varus, valgus or rotation stress applied, early mobilization may be realized. But a few exercise sessions twice or even three times a day are not sufficient. Using a hinged cast, axial instabilities and to a certain extent rotational instabilities can be excluded. Flexion and extension can also be limited to a degree appropriate for the repaired ligaments.

Since we routinely use a limited motion cast (LMC) for the aftertreatment of ligament injuries even weight-bearing is permitted. Meanwhile the benefits for muscles and ligaments are being monitored with a large number of patients. Initial applications of a similar cast to ligamentous elbow and ankle injuries have not proved useful in a comparable way, as the anatomy and therapeutic problems are different and generally minor to those of the knee joint.

10.6 Principles of postoperative treatment

As mentioned before, we feel that preoperative immobilization is not necessary as no further trauma is likely to occur because of the patient's pains and fear. On the other hand, the patients are encouraged to do painless exercises. Rapid atrophy of the quadriceps muscles can be reduced but not completely avoided. A 20° dorsal splint is prepared preoperatively for the sole purpose of positioning the leg after the operation. With this splint immediate isometric quadriceps training is permitted. It is supplemented by guided flexion up to 60° after removal of the drains on the 2nd or 3rd postoperative day. A limited motion cast is applied on the 10th day postoperatively when the sutures are removed and an elastic bangage is tailored to avoid swelling of the knee region. The patients are advised to make full use of the available motion, to simulate kneebends and to exercise with resistance. Full weight-bearing is allowed (Fig. 10.5(a) and (b)). Depending on the site of the repaired lesion, the cast can be applied in more varus or valgus position, thus reducing pulling forces from the ligaments. Based on experiments with lower extremities of cadavers an improved model was proposed (Daniel and Rice, 1979) with more axial stability, particularly valgus stability, ascertained by carefully modelling the femoral condyles (Fig. 10.6). Even with the diameter of the thigh and lower leg decreasing during the limited motion cast period with subsequent loosening of the cast, it is expected to provide sufficient stability. The cast is removed after 5 weeks and the aim is full function under physiotherapeutic supervision, if necessary (Burri, Helbing and Spier, 1978).

This is our routine procedure for the main number of ligament injuries involving the collateral ligaments and the capsule alone, or in combination with the anterior cruciate and/or the menisci. Instabilities involving the posterior cruciate require different treatment with unfortunate

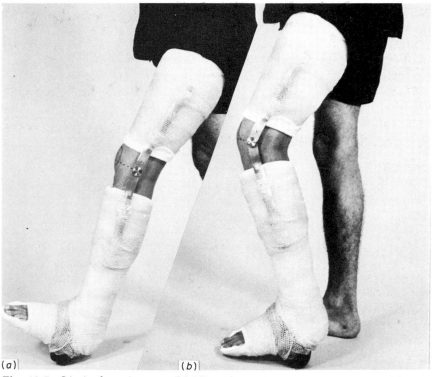

(a) (b)

Fig. 10.5 Limited motion cast (LMC) with maximum extension (*a*), and flexion (*b*) possible.

Ligament Injuries and their Treatment

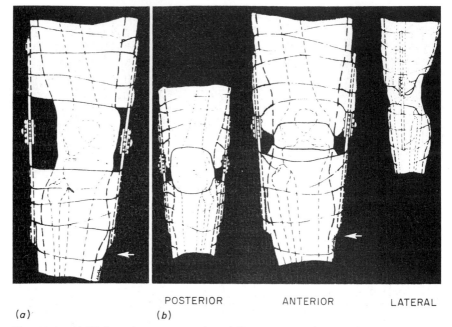

POSTERIOR   ANTERIOR   LATERAL

(a)   (b)

Fig. 10.6 (a) Slight valgus or varus instability can occur despite the cast, with the cast-brace, and in particular the hinges, not correctly modelled. (b) Extension of the thigh portion over the femoral condyles protects the joint more securely against axial stress (from Daniel and Rice, 1979).

restrictions on mobility. Due to lack of experience with these lesions the optimal treatment is still being developed.

In the present situation immobilization versus early functional treatment is determined by the surgeon. Depending on the extent of the trauma and the ease of refixation, immobilization may vary from 3–6 weeks with the knee bent at least 30°. Even temporary transfixation of the patella with a Steinmann pin is considered useful for resisting the pulling forces of the posterior muscles of the thigh which have a hamstring effect.

Immobilization exceeding 6 weeks is not necessary even in severe lesions, as healing of ligamentous structures does not require more time and exercises then are most important to restore function. After the removal of any cast, either the limited motion cast or a splint with 30° or more flexion, further treatment is tailored to the individual until normal mobility is regained. When in some patients, despite early function, excessive stiffness of the joint results due to adhesions of the recessus and muscles and no progress is evident during physiotherapy within another 6 weeks, we recommend early hospitalization again with the aim of

200

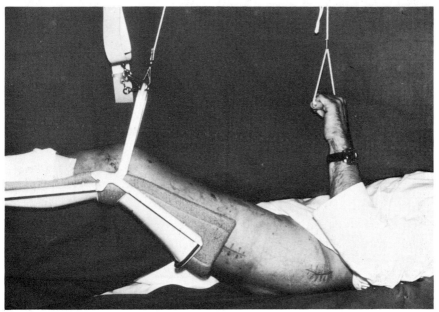

Fig. 10.7 Passive motion of the knee and hip joint after osteosynthesis of the femur and reconstruction of knee ligaments.

mobilization when implants such as fixating screws or wire sutures must be removed anyway.

As these patients usually have more than average pain local anaesthesia with a peridural catheter has proved useful thus enabling painfree mobility over a period of several days. With active motion impossible because of the anaesthesia a special splint that can be moved by the patient himself is useful (Fig. 10.7).

A more expensive but also more effective device is a motor splint with variable range and cycles of motion (Fig. 10.8). The machine is also available for the purpose of elbow motion.

10.7 Experience with early functional treatment

Getting the patient back to early physical activities, in particular using the injured extremity, is the best approach. Another argument neglected till now because of the lack of evidence, is that the incidence of obscure embolism respective to thromboembolic complications seems to be lower. Mild thrombosis of the deep veins of the lower leg is suspected in up to 30% of immobilized extremities. An increase in activities may therefore

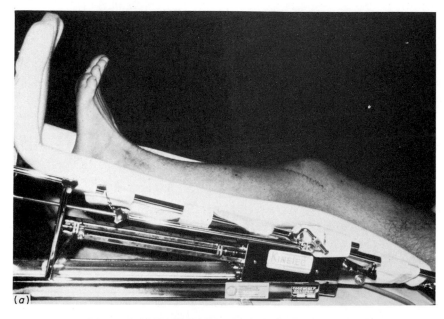

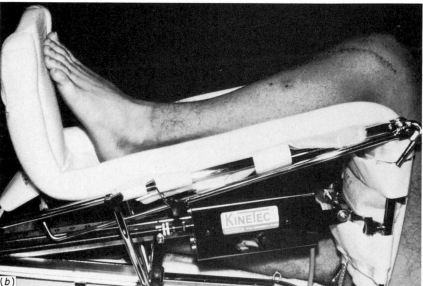

Fig. 10.8 Motor splint with variable range and cycles of motion; it is only used in late joint stiffness after complete healing of the ligaments.

help to minimize the risk. After removal of the limited motion cast a range of motion of almost 10° (extension) and over 80° (flexion) is usually possible. As a rule, the average time necessary for rehabilitation is little more than 3 months. Within this time, free motion is achieved by four-fifths of the patients, another eighth making progress towards completely free function within the following 3 months. In one out of 20 patients treated for a fresh injury of the knee joint, final stability is not achieved, the contralateral joint serving as a reference.

It is certainly worth noting that some patients were able to work wearing a limited motion cast, naturally depending on the kind of work. When the cast is made using waterproof materials, swimming and muscle training under water is possible with a positive effect upon trophic disorders.

A comparison of ten athletes scheduled for surgery for chronic ruptures of the anterior cruciate ligament and randomly assigned into two groups was performed using a standard fixed cast after surgery and a moveable cast (Gollnick *et al.*, 1974). The main criteria were the times for total convalescence, return of the normal range of motion of the knee, and return to athletic participation.

The patients fitted with a moveable cast had less muscle atrophy on removal of the cast than those with the 'closed cast' (−0.5 cm versus −3 cm). The return of normal mobility of the knee joint also occurred faster in those patients fitted with the moveable cast (Fig. 10.9). Furthermore, they were able to resume athletic training after less convalescence than those with the closed cast (1.5 versus 3.75 months); 4 months after surgery all patients were judged to have experienced a successful reconstruction of

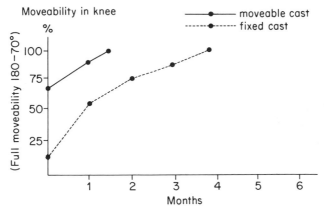

Fig. 10.9 Complete restoration of mobility after immobilization and following early functional treatment (from Gollnick *et al.*, 1974).

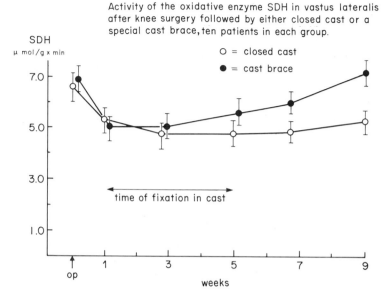

Fig. 10.10 Succinic dehydrogenase (SDH) activity following injury of knee ligaments (from Eriksson, 1976).

the cruciate ligament with no or minimal 'drawer sign'. No differences in knee stability were evident between the two groups.

Enzymatic activities of the vastus lateralis also revealed differences between the two kinds of treatment, the limited motion and a fixed cast. Succinic dehydrogenase returned faster to normal values after employment of the mobile cast-brace. (Eriksson, 1976, Fig. 10.10).

10.8   Long-term results

Since we recommend functional postoperative treatment the results have been judged critically. The benefits of early mobility, in terms of avoiding or at least decreasing the 'rupture disease', are evident. But what about protection against long-lasting effects, in other words prevention of osteoarthritis?

Follow-ups in an average interval of 7 years after reconstructive surgery revealed satisfying joint function; stability was still as sufficient as it was at the end of the treatment. No patient developed additional weakening of the ligaments unless because of a new trauma. In contrast to the early findings there was almost no quadriceps atrophy to be measured. Besides, the long-term results after plastic surgery were less satisfying concerning stability and muscular atrophy. With injured ligaments reconstructed operatively and stability present, there is a minor risk of getting osteoarthritis due to the ligament lesion. If osteoarthritis did occur in the injured knee joint, it seemed to be related to the meniscus. With a meniscus removed because of contusion or tear, four out of five patients showed osteoarthritis of the involved joint or a significantly higher degree compared with the contralateral joint. Two out of five patients with menisci intact or reattached had signs of degeneration apparent in the X-ray pictures of their injured joint. In 40% of patients, average age 36 years, no osteoarthritis was found at all.

10.9 Conclusions

It is accepted worldwide that fresh ligament injuries with instability present should be treated operatively. Only the operation can show the extent of the lesion and offer a chance of complete reconstruction with subsequent healing and full rehabilitation. With inadequate or delayed treatment chronic insufficiency is likely to occur but the results of plastic surgery are often inferior to those of reconstructive surgery (Helbing and Burri, 1977). Even with sutures of freshly injured ligaments performed or the structures anatomically reattached, joint function is not restored because the fibres need stress protection over the healing period. If immobilization is used, a number of disadvantages including muscular atrophy, the weakening of all other ligamentous structures, joint stiffness due to the shrinking of the capsule and the trophic disorder to the cartilage resulting from insufficient nutrition must be taken into consideration. Additional haemarthrosis is considered to be an important aetiological factor leading to arthrosis.

In order to minimize these established negative effects of immobilization an early functional aftertreatment is recommended, based on experimental findings which demonstrate that a range of motion between 20° and 60° of flexion is harmless to all knee ligaments. Valgus or varus stress or malrotation of the lower leg must be avoided absolutely. Based on these conditions functional treatment is possible and very useful. It may be performed by a physiotherapist or other means. To exclude the risk of harmful movements and to encourage the patients to do active exercises, a limited motion cast has proved beneficial. Functional treatment is also possible by means of a passively moved splint or a motor splint.

The time necessary for complete rehabilitation after fresh injuries of the ligaments is shortened and mobility regained earlier with sufficient stability. A future possibility of providing even more function

Ligament Injuries and their Treatment

postoperatively is by internal stabilization of an injured joint using carbon fibres instead of a limited motion cast (see Section III).

References

Burri, C., Helbing, G. and Spier, W. (1978), The rehabilitation of knee ligament injuries progress in orthopedic surgery, in *The Knee: Ligament and Articular Cartilage Injuries*, Vol. 3 (ed. D. E. Hastings), Springer-Verlag, Berlin, Heidelberg, pp. 53–8.

Burri, C., Pässler, H. and Radde, J. (1973), Experimentelle Grundalgen zur funktionellen Behandlung nach Bandnaht und -plastik am Kniegelenk. *Z. Orthop.*, **111**, 378–9.

Claes, L., Burri, C., Mutschler, W. and Plank, E. (1979), Experimentelle untersuchungen zur Biomechanik der Seitenbänder a Knie. *Langenbecks Arch. Chir.*, **Suppl.**

Cotta, H. (1973), Die Pathogenese der Gonarthrose. *Z. Orthop.*, **111**, 490–94.

Daniel, D. and Rice, T. (1979), Valgus-varus stability in a hinged cast used for controlled mobilization of the knee. *J. Bone J. Surg.*, **61A**, 135–6.

Dustmann, H. O., Puhl, W. and Schneitz, K. P. (1971), Knorpelveränderungen beim Hämarthros unter besonderer Berücksichtigung der Ruhigstellung. *Arch. Orthop. Unfall-Chirurg.*, **71**, 148–59.

Eriksson, E. (1976), Sports injuries of the knee ligaments: their diagnosis, treatment, rehabilitation, and prevention. *Med. Sci. Sports*, **8**, 133–44.

Gollnick, B., Eriksson, E., Hägmark, T. and Saltin, B. (1974), Recovery with a movable or standard cast following intra-articular reconstruction of the anterior cruciate ligament. *Nat. conference on the Medical Aspects of Sports*, Vol. 15, pp. 56–60 (ed. T. T. Craig) Chicago, 1974.

Helbing, G. and Burri, C. (1977), Functional postoperative care after reconstruction of knee ligaments, in *Injuries of the Ligaments and their Repair* (ed. G. Chapchal), Georg Thieme, Stuttgart.

Helbing, G. and Burri, C. (1980), Die Nachbehandlung nach Bandnähten und Plastiken am Kniegelenk. *Unfallheilkunde*, **83**, 426–30.

Laros, G. S., Tipton, C. M. and Cooper, R. R. (1971), Influence of physical activity on ligament insertions in the knees of dogs. *J. Bone Joint Surg.*, **53A**, 275–86.

Noyes, F. R. (1977), Functional properties of knee ligaments and alterations induced by immobilization. *Clin. Orthop.*, **123**, 210–42.

11 Knee lesions VI: Peripheral reconstruction for anterior cruciate loss

JOHN KING

11.1 Introduction

The field of surgery for the unstable knee is bedevilled by the variety of the terms used to describe a relatively small number of abnormal physical signs, and the complexity of and dispute about their interpretation in terms of the pathological anatomy.

I do not believe that debate about the pathological anatomy is helpful in a chapter such as this although a clearer understanding of the abnormal motion allowed by weakness of particular structures is important on theoretical grounds and research must continue. I shall merely take as common ground that damage to the anterior cruciate ligament (ACL) allows abnormal anterior motion of some part of the tibia in respect of the femur, while adding that not all anterior motion implies damage to that structure.

The physical signs will be described and some of the less controversial anatomical defects will be associated with them. This latter point may, however, not apply any further than the fact that surgical correction is directed to these areas. Despite the fact that surgery at a particular point corrects the patient's complaint it is not always justified to assume that this area had failed and was the cause of symptoms. An understanding of this last point may make it easier to comprehend the debate which continues to rage between the 'pivot centrale' school from Lyon, France and the 'peripheral school' mainly American; in other words, it is possible that the failure is in the centre of the joint (the anterior cruciate ligament) but in certain circumstances (congenital or post-traumatic) excessive excursion of the peripheral tissues allows instability to be superimposed on the laxity deriving from the anterior cruciate ligament loss.

It is apposite at this moment to clarify these terms. Laxity is a clinical finding and may be minimal or severe. Instability is the patient's complaint. It must *never* be assumed that a demonstrated laxity is the root cause of the patient's complaint and can only be said to be so when the patient recognizes the manoeuvre which demonstrates the laxity as being the same sensation which to him is instability. Re-examination on a number of occasions, and after getting the patient's confidence, or even assessment by a therapist in the gym, may be necessary to confirm this.

Examination under anaesthesia is to be abhorred in the assessment of the chronically unstable knee (compare the acute situation where it is vital). A facile assumption that the laxity demonstrated in the anaesthetized relaxed patient is the cause of the instability has surely produced more confusion as to the indication and results of operative treatment than anything else. Equally the habit of performing two operations to correct instability, namely meniscectomy and some form of reconstruction, gives an entirely erroneous impression of the efficacy of either procedure.

It is assumed that any surgeon who professes himself confident to embark upon this sort of operation is aware of the needs of a conservative rehabilitation programme and only on the failure of this will he embark upon surgical management. However, it is very distressing to find how frequently the 'rehabilitation' programme for an anterior cruciate lesion is a quadriceps programme.

As stated above it is common ground that anterior cruciate instability is represented by some form of abnormal *anterior* motion of the tibia on the femur in the *flexed* knee. The only muscles capable of stopping or controlling this motion are the hamstrings which insert on either side of the top of the leg and act exactly as the reins on a horse's head. Contraction will stop abnormal anterior motion. Paying out appropriately controls this motion. Controlled motion is not instability.

It must only be after a failure of this sort of rehabilitation that operation can be contemplated. Even then the first step of that operation may only be meniscectomy (if the cartilage is torn in such a way as could be expected to give instability) or the removal of an equally troublesome loose body. Not only must the muscle be strengthened but the co-ordination must be improved and the use of the wobble board for re-education at this level seems as appropriate as its use at the ankle where its success is well established (Freeman, 1965). With this regime only about one-fifth of patients need to have a second operation for reconstruction.

Before getting into the surgical techniques it is important to acknowledge that this chapter is about peripheral reconstructions for anterior cruciate instability. It must not be thought to exclude consideration of the intra-articular reconstructions such as the Erikson and Trillat modification of the Jones procedure (Erikson, 1976; Jones, 1963) and there are recent suggestions that intra-articular and extra-articular reconstructions may need to be combined to get the best results (Deacon, 1981).

Finally, no surgery will ever succeed if done for the wrong reasons or if only part of the problem is dealt with. Posterolateral instability must be excluded in abnormal anteroposterior motion of the lateral tibial plateau and may be difficult because of its comparative rarity and the difficulty of defining the mid-neutral point. And it remains salutory that every now and again a patient is referred for 'failed' anterior cruciate reconstruction and examination reveals that a passively produced posterior drawer sign has been corrected and interpreted as an anterior drawer sign. These operations fail.

11.2 The physical signs and the tests commonly used to demonstrate them

11.2.1 ABNORMAL ANTERIOR MOTION OF THE TIBIA IN THE FLEXED KNEE

(a) Anterior drawer sign

The foot is stabilized by the weight of the examiner's haunch, with the foot pointing forwards. The tibia is grasped with the middle, ring and little fingers of each hand behind the upper leg and pulled forwards. The index fingers are extended onto and assess spasm of the hamstrings. If this is present the test is non-contributory. Unless the resting position of the tibia is assessed by looking across both similarly flexed knees, correction of a passive posterior drawer sign cannot be excluded.

The sign is useful to demonstate laxity. Instability is rarely reproduced unless the mobile posterior horn of the meniscus is pulled forward beneath the femoral condyle. This can lead to locking and is recognized by the patient.

The anterior cruciate is divided into two main functional bands. The anteromedial seems more important in resisting anterior motion in the flexed knee, and it is probably this component which is being tested.

(b) Slocum–Larsen sign

The examiner and patient are in similar positions for the anterior drawer sign (Slocum and Larsen, 1968). The abnormal anterior motion is assessed with the foot in neutral, internal and external rotation.

When positive the amount of abnormal motion increases as the foot is externally rotated, thus relaxing the posterior cruciate and posterior capsule and emphasizing the insufficiency of the posteromedial structures, often referred to as the posterior oblique ligament, which is reinforced by reflected fibres of semimembranosus which run downwards and forwards. The anterior motion decreases in internal rotation as the posterior structures are tightened.

Ligament Injuries and their Treatment

The sign can be present to some extent in the absence of injury to the anterior cruciate ligament. Its main importance is to emphasize weakness of the posteromedial structures.

11.2.2 ABNORMAL ANTERIOR MOTION IN THE VERY SLIGHTLY FLEXED KNEE

If the knee is small or the examiner has big hands it is possible to hold the thigh and proximal leg in different hands and attempt anteroposterior motion. An abnormal degree of anterior motion is difficult to assess and greater emphasis should be placed on the quality of the 'stop' at the end of the motion. A soft stop is abnormal. This test is attributed to Lachman in the United States and to Trillat in France. It is probable that it is most sensitive to ruptures of the posterolateral fibres of the anterior cruciate (compare the anterior drawer sign).

11.2.3 ABNORMAL OPENING OF THE MEDIAL SIDE OF THE KNEE JOINT

With the knee flexed enough to relax the posterior structures (about 25°) a valgus force is applied. The variations for doing this are extensive and designed to eliminate rotation, which mimicks abnormal opening. The implication of the sign is damage to the longitudinal ligaments on the medial side of the knee. Its main use is when combined with one or more of the tests of abnormal rotation (see below, p. 211). In isolation it is infrequent and infrequently associated with instability.

11.2.4 ABNORMAL OPENING ON THE LATERAL SIDE OF THE KNEE JOINT

With the knee as for medial testing a varus force is applied, again with control or recognition of rotation. The implication is damage to the longitudinal lateral structures. On the whole it is important when associated with some form of rotatory laxity (see below, p. 212). However, pure varus is more frequently a cause of instability than pure valgus. It is a matter of observation that more high-class athletes have varus knees than would be proportionate in the general population (although cause, effect and functional advantage are debatable). In an already varus-aligned knee, varus laxity may represent a rather greater disability.

11.2.5 ABNORMAL ANTERIOR DISPLACEMENT OF THE LATERAL TIBIAL PLATEAU WITH A RAPID UNCONTROLLED REPOSITION OR DISPLACEMENT

(a) Initial displacement with a rapid uncontrolled relocation

The affected limb is held in extension. The lower leg is held by the examiner's distal (in respect of patient) hand and internally rotated. The knee is supported with the proximal hand, fingers up, palm down and with direct pressure to produce a valgus force. The knee is then flexed and the test is positive if there is an abrupt posterior translation of the lateral tibial plateau at around 30–40° of flexion. To label this an instability the patient must recognize the sensation. They are not usually in doubt!

This type of test is usually associated with the name of MacIntosh from Toronto (Galway, Beaupre and MacIntosh, 1972) but was called by him the 'lateral pivot shift test'. Confusion with this latter title has arisen because it is a demonstration of *lateral* hypermobility, associated with a *medial* shift of the pivot point from the centre of the joint to the medial capsular structures.

(b) Abrupt anterior subluxation of the lateral tibial plateau

With the knee flexed a valgus force is applied at the knee with the foot held initially in internal rotation. When the knee is extended and the foot allowed to rotate in and at about 30° there is an abrupt anterior translation of the lateral plateau to the subluxed position. The name of Losee (Losee *et al.*, 1978) is usually associated with this test.

The importance of the relaxed hamstrings needs emphasis, as it can be blocked by a tight biceps femoris.

Both these tests demonstrate, most sensitively, loss of the anterior cruciate. This ligament runs not only downwards and forwards but it is directed medially so that it resists internal rotation of the tibia to a significant extent as well as pure anterior motion.

A third test described by Hughston (Hughston *et al.*, 1976) and called the 'jerk' test seems similar. The knee is held in flexion and valgus force and internal rotation of tibia applied. As the knee is extended the tibia is said to sublux at 30° and to relocate as extension is completed, the relocation producing the 'jerk'. Hughston claims that there must be an injury to the mid one-third of the lateral capsule, and has demonstrated this lesion in *some* acutely injured knees.

It is difficult to explain the jerk test and having watched it on film from Hughston's clinic on many occasions I remain to be convinced that it does not show what Losee has demonstrated. Losee suggests that the final few degrees of extension relocate the tibial plateau and it may simply be that these few degrees have been 'unlocked' at the commencement of the MacIntosh test to allow one to feel a subluxation as a starting point.

There is no doubt that these signs can occur immediately in anterior cruciate lesions in which there is no evidence at all of capsular lesions. I have yet to find a rupture of the anterior cruciate ligament which does not demonstrate this type of *laxity*. I am sure the variation in instability depends upon the underlying 'normal' anterior excursion allowed by the lateral structures (see above).

Accepting this as the most sensitive test of anterior cruciate dysfunction I have found the most useful test is described by Casey (personal communication). In this the manoeuvre is commenced as for the conventional pivot shift. The difference is that as the proximal hand supports the knee the thumb is extended and placed behind the fibular head. As the valgus force is applied with that hand the internal rotation of the other hand can be augmented by forward pressure from the thumb. When the abrupt posterior translation of the lateral plateau takes place it can be controlled by the thumb (or recognized by it in very mild cases). As this movement is controlled it allows the test to be done in otherwise very apprehensive patients and the vital requisite of patient recognition can be achieved even if they say that it is 'nearly what they feel'. With careful repeated use of this test I feel examination under anaesthetic to be unnecessary to establish the diagnosis of instability secondary to anterior cruciate loss.

An alternative to this is to lay the patient on the good side with the affected foot supported on the couch and the hip and good knee flexed so it is not under the bad one.

Gravity produces the valgus force and the patient is asked to flex and extend the knee producing alternately the 'pivot shift' and the 'Losee'! The greatest use is in the apprehensive patient who goes rigid the moment he is touched by the surgeon; this was described by Slocum.

During all these tests of a rather limited set of possible laxities it remains vital to remember that torn or loose menisci, or anything else free within the joint, can become trapped in the course of any of them and mimic a ligamentous instability. The knee may actually be blocked from achieving the neutral position on occasions so the regularity of the positive test may be variable. As in all cases of tests with the knee flexed and relaxed it is important to make sure of the starting position.

The risk of confusing the passive posterior drawer correction with anterior laxity has been mentioned. Equally, posterolateral laxity (although rare) has been confused with anterolateral laxity. The cause seems to be loss of integrity of the popliteus, the fibular colateral ligament and a varying degree of damage to the arcuate ligament.

The abnormal posterior motion of the lateral plateau may be difficult to detect clinically. We have found it useful to tape a radio marker (a paper clip) to the inner aspect of the knee and take lateral X-rays with the tibia pushed back and pulled forwards, being free to rotate as it wants. The relative excursion of the fibular styloid and its direction compared with the medial radio marker can be measured and a more accurate idea of the degree of laxity obtained (Fig. 11.1). In addition there is usually some degree of hyperextension with slight external rotation of the tibia when the lower limb is supported by the big toe.

11.3 Interpretation of clinical signs

The physical signs have been described at some length as they represent the current 'language' in this field. It remains tempting to allocate to each a specific anatomical lapse. This course has, however, led to so much confusion in the past that I shall merely describe how I correct the abnormal motion that I believe to be the cause of the symptoms.

The 'pure' anterior drawer sign of any size means that both sides of the tibia are coming forwards and correction must be directed to holding back both sides of the joint. The same situation may be described by a positive Slocum–Larsen plus 'pivot shift' – in other words, both sides move forwards. An isolated pivot shift with minimal anterior drawer sign and minimal or absent 'Slocum–Larsen' directs my attention in isolation to the lateral side.

A minimal anterior drawer sign, minimal 'Slocum–Larsen' and mimimal valgus laxity directs one's attention to the posteromedial corner. This is almost without exception an acute lesion. Secondary stretching somewhere else will have occurred in the chronic lesion.

Thus, the crucial decision to make (and for which reason all these tests are done) is whether surgery to one side of the joint alone is adequate and if so which side. On the whole now I operate most frequently in isolation on the lateral side, sometimes combining it with the inner side and 'never' on the inner side in isolation. Whether an intra-articular repair needs to be added still awaits confirmation. X-ray examination is essential, as is arthroscopy, as there is growing evidence that radiological or arthroscopically confirmed degenerative changes will reduce the quality of the result of any type of reconstruction.

11.4 Operative correction

Once the decision has been made to operate on the medial, lateral or both sides of the joint there is a large choice of operations.

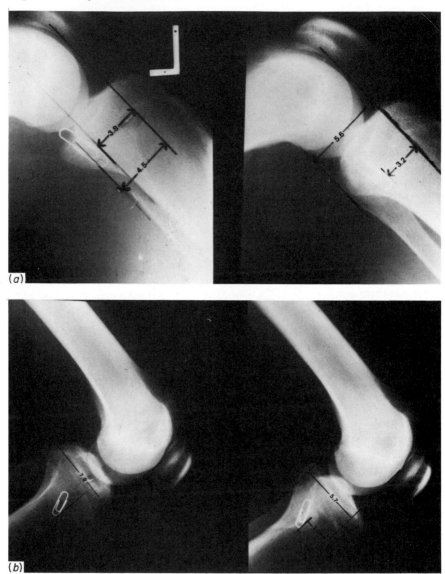

Fig. 11.1 (*a*) Shows the vastly increased posterior excursion of the fibula; (*b*) as opposed to the radio marker (paper clip) on the medial side of the knee when the tibia is stressed posteriorly.

11.4.1 MEDIAL SIDE: POSTERIOR PART

Slocum, Larsen and James (1974) describe a procedure to reef the posteromedial capsule. Through a longitudinal medial incision

214

sufficiently distal and curved so as to inspect the tibial insertion of the medial collateral ligament, the area of insertion of semimembranosus is explored. The tendon sheath is opened and that part of the tendon contributing to the oblique popliteal ligament freed. The medial head of gastrocnemius is separated from the posterior capsule and an incision made into this latter structure. This incision is basically vertical, being parallel to and just behind the posterior fibres of the medial collateral ligament. Using the space made by mobilizing the head of gastrocnemius the capsule is elevated from the tibia a short distance anteriorly and posteriorly.

Slocum states that on the whole this can be done without having to remove the medial meniscus, especially if the main component of laxity is meniscofemoral. In severe laxity the capsule is elevated with an osteotome to provide a fresh surface for attachment. Such extensive dissection is unnecessary with lesser laxity.

Repair, performed with the knee in flexion, commences with a suture in the distal part of the anterior flap pulling it down onto the insertion of semimembranosus (or onto the bone if that is inadequate). The posterior flap is then pulled over the anterior and sutured to it. This repair is reinforced by bringing up the distal part of the semimembranosus, leaving it attached to its normal bone site distally and suturing the distal 2 cm along the repair line. There should be resistance to further extension at about 10–15° when this has been correctly tensioned.

I have for a number of years been doing a modification of this technique in that the capsular incision is oblique downwards and forwards, stopping within the peripheral substance of the meniscus if still present. The two flaps are overlapped with the knee flexed and, if the operation is done in isolation, in internal rotation. Overlapping sutures are laid with a 'fishhook' needle and left long. The ends of the stitches are rethreaded and passed through the distal 2cm of semimembranosus. As these stitches are tied on top of semimembranosus it is brought up onto the capsular incision. This produces support from the tendon in a downwards and forwards direction and in addition has a longitudinal capsular scar in the line best capable of resisting stretching.

The idea is that this should duplicate the line of fibres in the posterior oblique ligament which is the posteromedial capsule, reinforced by downwards and forwards running fibres from the normal (and complex) insertion of semimembranosus. As the idea is to stop the tibia moving forwards, various addition fascial sutures which have been described in this context but pass downwards and posteriorly, thus seem to me to have little value as they would be passively shortened as the plateau advanced! However, I am sure that Slocum is correct in implying that some have too much capsular damage to be amenable to this operation in

215

isolation. In these cases it is my preference to support the reefing with a downwards and forwards darn of carbon fibre.

The addition, described by Slocum, of adding an Elmslie-Trillat type of medial transposition of the tibial tuberosity to this procedure is no longer needed with such a reinforcement. As an alternative to transposing the tibial tuberosity Slocum describes a medial transfer of the medial portion of the patellar ligament. The same criticism applies as in the previous paragraph.

The inadequacy of such a repair (without some reinforcement) in isolation in the presence of several injured tissues is rather reinforced by the operation described by Nicholas (1973) and described as the five-in-one.

He makes the point that abnormal anterior motion of the tibial plateau is mainly caused by weakness of the posteromedial capsule and not necessarily associated with anterior cruciate loss (but reports that at operation none had a functional anterior cruciate ligament). The emphasis on associated pure valgus laxity as part of the injury complex may be overstated.

Through an S-shaped medial incision the medial structures are indentified and exposed, the distal part of the medial collateral ligament being seen by rolling the distal part of the pes anserinus proximally after partial anterior freeing. The proximal part of the medial ligament (if there is no damage distally as usual) is elevated from the femur and anterior and posterior longitudinal incisions developed to leave it as a strip attached solely to the tibia. The capsule is then opened by a downwards and forwards incision which may extend as far anteriorly at the patella ligament as the collateral has been elevated and allows fully exploration of the joint.

Nicholas feels that adequate mobilization of the posterior part of the capsule cannot be done with any portion of the meniscus present and insists on total meniscectomy (part one of five). The proximal end of the medial ligament is now pulled proximally and posteriorly and reattached to a freshened bone surface with a staple or screw (part two). The posterior flap of capsule containing semimembranosus proximal to its insertion is pulled forwards and distally across the medial ligament and securely sutured to its anterior border (part three).

These last two manoeuvres produce the downwards and forwards running reinforcement as described above.

Part four consists of advancement of the distal part of the vastus medialis muscle in an anterior direction so that it can be sutured to the proximal half of the repositioned medial ligament and overlying advanced capsule. In practical terms the majority of this advancement ends up on the medial patellar retinaculum! The fifth and final part is a pes plasty (see below).

216

Despite such extensive surgery only half of Nicholas' patients could return to sport without a brace. This may be a reflection of the difficulties of the multiply operated patient (more than half had had previous operations of which less than half had been meniscectomies). This supports my own experience that a relatively small repair of the posteromedial corner, associated with carbon fibre reinforcement in the presence of very poor tissue, is perfectly capable of alleviating abnormal anterior motion of the medial tibial plateau.

11.4.2 MEDIAL SIDE: ANTERIOR PART

The other operation performed on the medial side to any great extent has been the Slocum–Larsen (1968) operation of pes anserinus transplantation (the pes plasty).

Through a longitudinal curved medial incision the insertion of semitendinosus, sartorius and gracilis into the medial aspect of the tibia is identified. The line of insertion of these three tendons is vertical, well anterior on the tibia and the tendons are somewhat merged at this point.

The distal half of this insertion (mainly semitendinosus) is elevated and rolled up over itself so that semitendinosus can be reinserted onto the tibia more proximally and even more anteriorly. Because it now has to negotiate the greater radius of the proximal tibial flare in flexion it is a more efficient internal rotator and in extension it is tightened and gives added medial support to the joint. From reports and papers (plus personal experience) the performance of this operation has diminished significantly over the last few years.

Without a doubt the results in the first reported series are good. However, in the 45 (80%) done for chronic ligamentous laxity 100% has associated meniscectomy. If a meniscus is torn to the extent that it needs to be removed, it is a potent cause of giving way, especially on twisting! My own experience is that about 20% of patients after meniscectomy and hamstring exercises come back to surgery despite proven anteromedial laxity, at follow-up of 5 years.

11.4.3 THE LATERAL SIDE

Although on the outer side of the knee reconstruction is now quite frequent posteriorly as well as anteriorly, the posterior repair is never done in isolation and thus both will be described together.

There are two basic approaches to the abnormal anterior motion of the lateral tibial plateau, namely static and dynamic. The dynamic approach is represented by the Ellison (1979) procedure. Through a longitudinal lateral incision somewhat curved posteriorly, the iliotibial tract is exposed and the tubercle of Gerdy identified. A piece of bone is elevated from Gerdy's tubercle bearing about 1.25 cm of iliotibial tract and anterior and posterior incisions made in the line of the fascia leaving a 15 cm pedicle, wider at its base than its apex which is the piece of bone.

The fibular collateral ligament is identified by sharp dissection and carefully freed from the underlying synovium. The capsular incisions anterior and posterior to the lateral ligament are approximated and sutured deep to the ligament to provide the deep wall of a tunnel bounded superficially by the fibular ligament.

Through the tunnel from above to below is passed the piece of bone carrying the strip of iliotibial tract with it. The bone is reinserted anteriorly to its original site on a freshened bone surface. The tract is carefully closed over the band to prolong the tunnel proximally. The idea is that the iliotibial tract is held posteriorly by the fibular ligament, remaining behind the centre of rotation even in extension and pulling back the lateral plateau. The tunnel created allows the tensor fascia lata to continue to exert a pull on the insertion of the iliotibial tract onto the tibia.

Kennedy *et al.* (1978) criticize this technique for allowing the rerouted band to advance too much and they insist that the tunnel should be developed only deep to the distal half of the fibular ligament. They claim that if the piece of bone of Gerdy's tubercle can be advanced more than 1 cm with the knee flexed to 70° the rerouting is not posterior enough. They state that repair of the defect in the fascia prevents resultant one-plane varus laxity.

The concept of dynamic stabilization is tempting, particularly in the face of reports of stretching of static support mechanisms with time. However, in no paper has a dynamic component to this procedure been proven and its results are better in those cases where the pivot shift has been lost (that is, it is acting as a static or passive stabilizer).

Other attempts at dynamic stabilization are being made by altering the mechanics of insertion of the biceps tendon. Slocum is attributed a biceps plasty, in Campbell (1980). Torg (personal communication) is completing an evaluation of biceps advancement and one must await their reports before further comment.

The static stabilization procedures began with the description by Galway, Beaupre and MacIntosh (1972) of a tenodesis operation utilizing a band of iliotibial tract which remains attached distally at Gerdy's tubercle. The precise routing and fixation of the strip of fascia have varied considerably since then, although the majority still seem to be described under the generic term 'MacIntosh' operation. Without further description this name now has come to mean a tenodesis procedure on the outside of the knee to stop abnormal anterior motion.

In the original operation the iliotibial tract was exposed in a longitudinal incision some 20 cm long, based distally at Gerdy's tubercle. A 1.25 cm strip of fascia was elevated in the length of the incision, being free proximally and attached distally. The lateral intermuscular septum was identified and freed with attention to the vessels in its deep distal portion. The fibular collateral ligament was freed and the fascia strip was threaded underneath it and the proximal end woven into the inter- muscular septum with the knee flexed to about 60° and the foot maximally externally rotated.

Because of some early stretching possibly allowed by this type of fixation, it was recommended that bone be exposed deep to the proximal part of the fibular ligament to provide secure fixation. I found it easier to wrap the fascial strip completely around the fibular ligament and suture through both. Once more secure fixation of the strip was achieved at the fibular ligament the necessity to use the proximal part in a weave in the the intermuscular septum no longer existed.

Campbell (1980) attributes to MacIntosh a rerouting of the proximal strip through the septum, then back under the lateral ligament at its distal part, and finally into the soft tissues near Gerdy's tubercle.

More complex procedures are also described. In Losee *et al.*'s (1978) reef and sling operation a strip of fascia is developed as for the MacIntosh procedure described above. However, the skin incision is a lazy S with the proximal part posterior so as to give more access to the posterior capsular structures. The fascial strip is passed through a bone tunnel from front to back made just above the insertion of the fibular ligament in the femur. The precise positioning is a matter of trial and error by holding the strip at various points and assessing its looseness in flexion and extension. Occasionally excessive looseness in flexion necessitates its being threaded under the ligament. It is important not to damage the articular surface during creation of the tunnel.

Once the strip has been passed through the tunnel it is sutured to periosteum at entry and exit points. It is then passed through the proximal part of the lateral head of gastrocnemius grasping about one-third of its bulk, above the joint line. It is then passed downwards and forwards picking up the arcuate ligament and going into the lowest part of the fibular ligament below the level of the joint.

When it is pulled hard the lateral gastrocnemius and posterior capsule will reach the fibular ligament to the back of which they are sutured. The final part of the fascial strip is imbricated into the fibular ligament and anteriorly towards the tubercle of Gerdy. As is obvious the strip needs to be longer than that for a 'simple' MacIntosh procedure. The repair is made in mid-flexion of the knee and external rotation of the foot. The operation produces a double downwards and forwards passive resistant mechanism. Its only potential disadvantage is of stretching of the collagen of the repair material.

I have been using a similar modification of the 'simple' MacIntosh procedure. A long strip of fascia is developed as above. It is passed behind and around the fibular ligament close to its proximal end and sutured there. It is then threaded once through the intermuscular septum and passed into the lateral head of gastrocnemius *below* the joint line. It is then passed into the periosteum (at its junction with posterior capsule) on the back of the tibia and backed through the lateral head of gastrocnemius. There is not usually enough strip to do anything more than suture it there.

The idea of this is to produce a short posterior tenodesis with gastrocnemius tendon attached firmly to both sides of the joint so that the back of the tibia cannot move away from the tensed gastrocnemius muscle. As only the lateral third is caught in sutures it probably does not cause interruption of the blood supply and does not seem to stretch out. The descending posterior band from the intermuscular septum also tends to hold the lateral tibia posteriorly.

Since the advent of carbon fibre I have been using a degradably coated carbon fibre suture instead of the fascial strip. It is threaded in exactly the same way as the fascial strip except that it can be continued forwards from gastrocnemius and passed through the distal fibular ligament before being reattached at Gerdy's tubercle. It can safely be anchored by using it to close the incision on the fascia lata (Figs. 11.2, 11.3, 11.4, 11.5, 11.6 and 11.7).

In a direct comparison between the fascial and carbon fibre reconstructions, the results show better clinical results using carbon fibre but there is debris within the joint.

11.4.4 COMBINED

On occasions both tibial plateaux come forward abnormally. While there may be an indication here for intra-articular reconstruction in isolation or combined with peripheral reconstructions, I shall simply mention peripheral procedures.

When the patient recognizes a laxity as instability and there is a big anterior motion on the other side it seems logical to repair both sides. A unilateral repair will alter the pivot point significantly and may make the symptoms (or articular damage) from the other side greater.

A combination of a medial and lateral reconstruction from those already described is used. I prefer the small posteromedial repair plus the

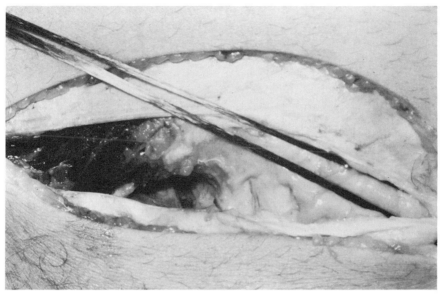

Fig. 11.2 Carbon fibre traversing tubercle of Gerdy.

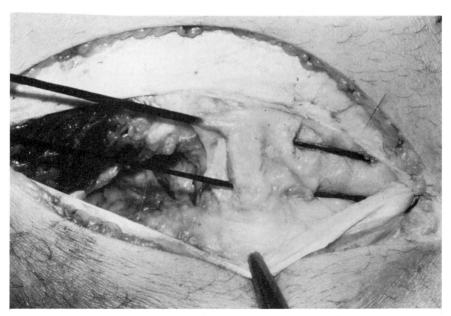

Fig. 11.3 Fibre underneath fibular collateral ligament including a piece of mid one-third capsular ligament.

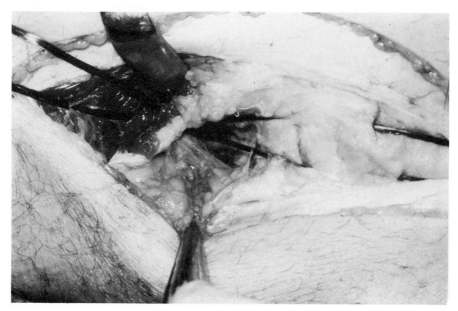

Fig. 11.4 Fibres through lateral intermuscular septum.

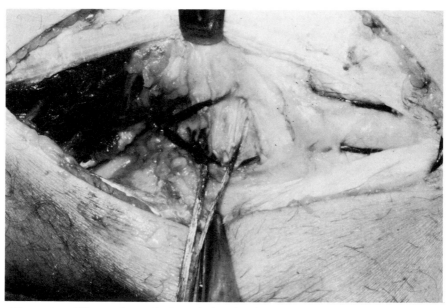

Fig. 11.5 Fibres through lateral head of gastrocnemius and underlying periosteum.

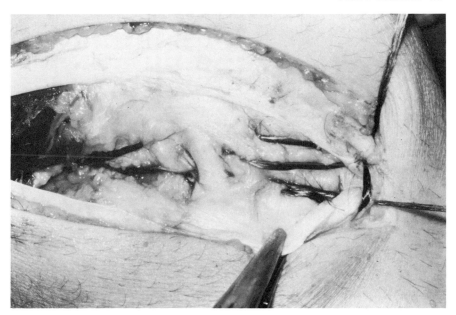

Fig. 11.6 Fibre returning under fibular collateral ligament to tubercle of Gerdy.

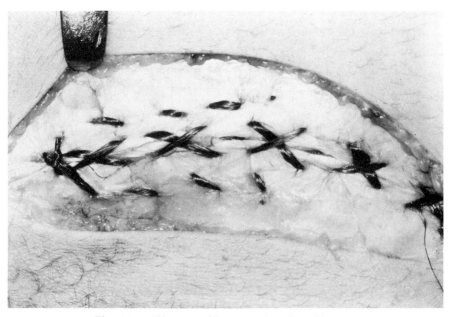

Fig. 11.7 Closure of fascia with carbon fibre.

lateral reconstruction noted above. The main problem is in deciding in what position to hold the knee. When doing one side alone, maximal advantage is given to the repair by turning the foot to that side. In these cases neutral rotation has to be used.

11.5 Postoperative management

There is general agreement that the knee should be immobilized in flexion (about 30°) and for unilateral repairs, in tibial rotation to that side. Because tibial rotation is important the foot has to be incorporated. The length of time in plaster, the necessity for bracing afterwards and the type of (or even the need for) physiotherapy remain debated. From a purely pragmatic point of view it is probably safest to stick to the programme used and understood in a particular unit.

My own regime is to plaster as above and start isometric knee and ankle exercises as soon as postoperative pain allows, plus range-of-motion hip exercises. The patient is non-weight-bearing on crutches.

At 4 weeks the cast is removed and stitches taken out. There is immediate fitting of a modified cast brace with thigh and leg pieces plus a free ankle hinge and lockable knee hinge. The knee hinge is locked so as to allow a range-of-motion of 20–70°. The patient is encouraged to work hamstrings and quadriceps within this range and may weight-bear when good quadriceps control is achieved.

After a further 4 weeks the locks are changed to 5–90° and more intensive work done within the allowed range. At 12 weeks postsurgery all bracing is removed and range-of-motion plus strengthening exercises done, with emphasis on the hamstrings. Analgesics may be allowed but only in the absence of local reaction expressed as heat, swelling or effusion, as they may otherwise allow damage to be done. Some patellar pain is not unusual and may be treated.

Wobble board exercises (a wobble chair is being evaluated) are important to re-educate proprioception so as to allow protection by muscle of the repair. Graduated activities through jogging, running and cutting are encouraged, the next step being allowed when the previous activity is 100%.

No return to sport is allowed until there is full range of motion, good muscle bulk and an ability to run fast backwards in a figure-of-eight.

References

Campbell, (1980), *Campbells Operative Orthopaedics* 6th edn C. V. Mosby, St Louis, p. 967.

Deacon, O. (1981), *Sicot Proceedings*, 480.

Ellison, A. E. (1979). *J. Bone. Joint Surg.*, **61A**, 330.

Erikson, E. (1976), *Orthop. Clin. N. Am.*, **7**, 167.

Freeman, M. A. R. (1965), *J. Bone Joint Surg.*, **47B**, 661.

Galway, R. D., Beaupre, A. and MacIntosh, D. L. (1972), *J. Bone Joint Surg.*, **54B**, 763.

Hughston, J. C. *et al.* (1976), *J. Bone Joint Surg.*, **58A**, 159.

Jones, K. G. (1963), *J. Bone Joint Surg.*, **45A**, 925.

Kennedy, J. C. *et al.* (1978), *J Bone Joint Surg.*, **60A**, 1031.

Losee, R. E. *et al.* (1978), *J. Bone Joint Surg.*, **60A**, 1015.

Nicholas, J. A. (1973), *J. Bone Joint Surg.*, **55A**, 899.

Slocum, D. B. and Larsen, R. L. (1968), *J. Bone Joint Surg.*, **50A**, 211, 226.

Slocum, D. B., Larsen, R. L. and James, S. L. (1974), *Clin. Orthop.*, **100**, 23.

PART THREE
The Use of Graft Materials

Introduction

The five chapters which follow comment on grafting materials that are in current use. I have not included experimental materials, or materials that have not reached the human implantation stage. Carbon fibre is dealt with at some length, and the bovine xenograft is commented on by McMaster and Jaffe (Chapter 16), and certainly shows promise.

In the chapters on carbon fibre implantation, those by myself and Neugebauer and Claes (Chapters 12 and 13) deal with our own experience in the use of carbon fibre as a primary ligament replacement material. Chapter 14 by Strover lists his own contribution to the improved operative techniques and instrumentation in the use of carbon fibre. Chapter 15 by Lemaire uses carbon fibre in a somewhat different manner to those demonstrated by myself, Neugebauer and Strover. Lemaire prefers to use the carbon as a ligament reinforcement agent rather than as a primary repairing material. It is interesting that the results of either of the two methods are similar, in that new collagen is encouraged to be laid down by fibroblast activity, leading to new ligament-like tissue to be formed, both in and around the carbon fibre matrix. Worldwide, there are at this time over 10 000 carbon implants functioning in humans, and the longest implant is in a man from Cardiff, South Wales, who was implanted late in 1975. There has been no evidence or suggestion of a neoplastic response to carbon, and it is now generally accepted that this is a safe material for human use. While the material is approved for use in Britain, most European countries and South Africa, it is anticipated that FDA approval in the United States may be achieved within the year 1985.

D.H.R.J.

12   *Carbon fibre I*

DAVID H. R. JENKINS

12.1   Introduction

It has been my particular experience that the conventional methods of ligament replacement and ligament reinforcement are somewhat lacking. It is true that there are certainly excellent results which can be achieved by certain surgeons, but at fault has been the major absence of any one material which can possibly encourage ligament-like material to grow.

Our initial experiments with carbon fibre began in 1970, when we had an interest in not only the filamentous form of carbon, but also the rigid forms of carbon. At that time there were three types of carbon implant available (Fig. 12.1).

The first was pure carbon reinforced carbon. This is a type of carbon in which the molecules are arranged in three dimensions, providing a light, strong, yet somewhat brittle type of material. It has the theoretical advantage of being biologically acceptable in that the material is pure carbon, but it also has the practical disadvantage of not only being expensive to manufacture, but also having a high Young's modulus such that its brittleness proved awkward in the management of bone fixation.

The second type of carbon in which we developed an interest was epoxy-based carbon. This material can be thought of as similar to reinforced concrete – the concrete is the epoxy, and the reinforcing bars are the individual carbon filaments. This is the material from which fishing rods, helicopter blades, and now car springs, are made. It has the major advantage of a moderate degree of biological acceptability and compatability. It is cheap to manufacture and Young's modulus can be altered by the proportion of carbon to epoxy. Its major disadvantage, however, is that it cannot be formed in the way metal can be formed, and at the moment experiments are still in progress with this material.

Our major interest, however, has been in the filamentous type of carbon. We have been using Courtaulds' Grafil A.S. and have developed a method in which 4× 10 000 individual filaments are loosely plaited, so

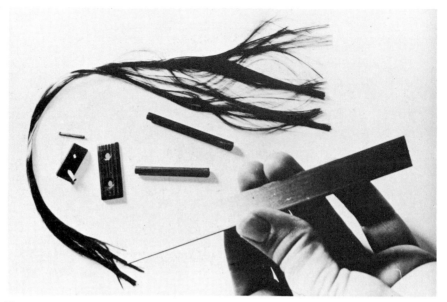

Fig. 12.1 *Top left*: Filamentous carbon fibre. *Centre*: Carbon reinforced carbon. *Lower right*: Epoxy based commercial carbon fibre.

that they form a ligamentous-like structure, roughly the size of a shoe lace. For large joints such as the knee we have found this suitable, but for smaller joints such as the carpometacarpal and interphalangeal joints, we have used half or a quarter of this quantity. Each carbon filament is approximately 9 μ in diameter (Fig. 12.2).

In our initial experiments in tissue culture, we were able to demonstrate that carbon filaments appear to have a special affinity for living tissue, in that the latter could be persuaded to grow around the filaments. In the scanning electron micrograph presented (Fig. 12.3) fibroblasts can be seen to be growing around and along the individual carbon filaments, rather as if the carbon filaments are railway lines, and the carbon is growing along those particular lines. We were encouraged by these findings to experiment in animals. In our initial experiments in sheep, we replaced the tendo-achilles, using four strands, each of 10 000 individual filaments, in such a manner that the tendo-achilles was totally replaced from its musculotendinous junction to the oscalcis (Fig. 12.4). Experiments were carried out on 50 sheep, and no immobilization was used. Figure 11.5 shows the typical appearance of the neotendon induced in response to the presence of the carbon fibre, at 1 year postimplantation. Attention is drawn not only to the physiological function of the tendon, but also to the anatomical shape of the neotendon. As a result of the

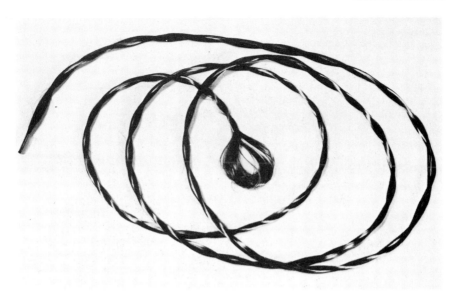

Fig. 12.2 The Jenkins Ligament. A double helical loose weave of approximately 140 000 individual carbon fibre units.

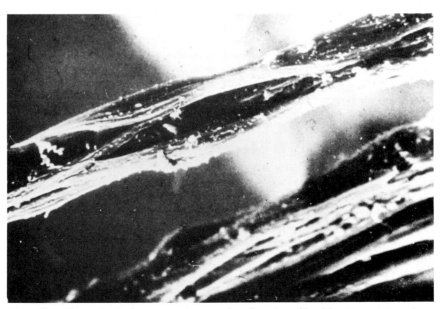

Fig. 12.3 Scanning electron micrograph, showing fibroblastic activity along individual carbon fibre filaments. (Courtesy of A. Goodship, Bristol University.)

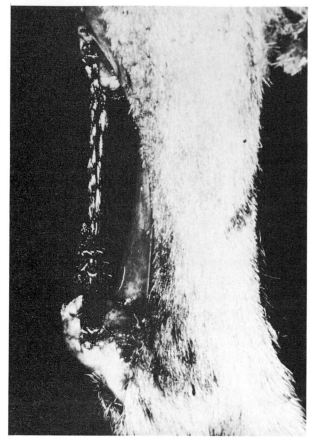

Fig. 12.4   Replacement of the tendo-achilles in the sheep.

implantation of the carbon, collagen has been laid down by fibroblasts which have grown along the individual carbon filaments, pushing aside the filaments as the collagen has been laid down. In this way, the bulk of the tendon has been increased as it has formed. Experiments in lower animals, such as rabbits, have shown that approximately 16 times the bulk of the initial carbon implant can be achieved by collagen infiltration. In higher animals, such as sheep, the increase in size of the tendon is approximately four-fold, and in humans it is between two- and three-fold. We were able to demonstrate that the neotendon did not break, stretch, or in any way lose its functional ability to act as a tendon. In fact, as months went by, the neotendon appeared to increase in both size and strength. Once a physiological state had been reached, there was a balance between the increase in size and the physiological function.

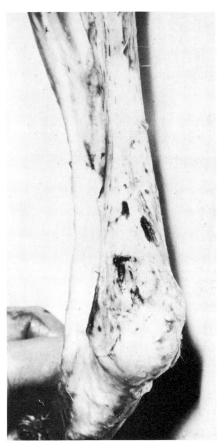

Fig. 12.5 The appearance of the tendo-Achilles following implantation of approximately one year.

Examination of the perilymphatic tissue in the regional nodes (Fig. 12.6) showed that there was some carbon infiltration into that particular tissue. This led us to question whether the carbon could be breaking down biologically or mechanically. We came to the conclusion that it was impossible for carbon to be broken down biologically, since by its very nature it is an inert material, and that the partial breakdown was occurring because of mechanical fragmentation of the carbon. Initially we were enthusiastic because there was an indication that the carbon might be inducing a neotendon to form, and then, because of mechanical breakdown it would be leaving the site of implantation and travelling to the regional lymph nodes. In fact, only a small proportion of the carbon fragments appears in the regional nodes. We then turned our attention to

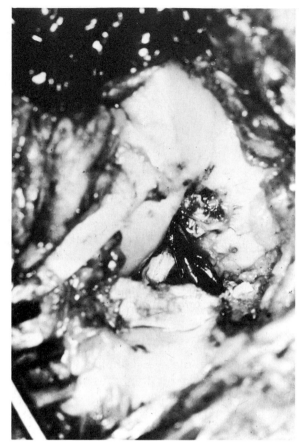

Fig. 12.8 The anterior cruciate has been replaced in the knee of the sheep. The posterior cruciate is intact.

there was no evidence of neoplasia, and because in different animals it appeared that the response to the carbon fibre implantation was similar, we concluded that it would be reasonable to attempt to repair old late chronic, severe, unstable joints in humans.

12.2 Ankles

There are well-established surgical procedures for the reinforcement or replacement of the lateral ligament complex of the ankle. To my mind the disadvantage of the Watson Jones procedure is that the peroneal tendons are not long enough, and the disadvantage of the Evans procedure is that

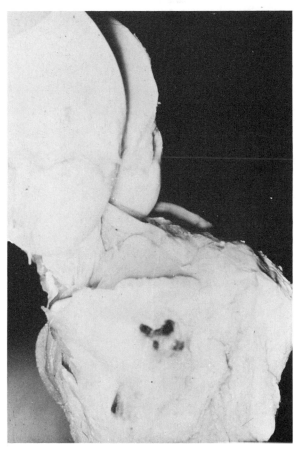

Fig. 12.9 A lateral view of a similar knee to that in Fig. 12.8 but 6 months after implantation of carbon fibre. The neo-anterior cruciate can be clearly seen. It is similar in shape, size and anatomical form to the posterior cruciate.

one is only replacing one particular aspect of the complex nature of the instability. By the use of carbon fibre, one can actually replace the particular ligament component which has been damaged. For example, if the anterior part of the ligament only is damaged, this only can be replaced; if the fibulocalcaneal part of the ligament is damaged this can be replaced. A major advantage, however, is that if the subtalar joint is not compromised in any way, then the fibulotalar part of the ligament can be replaced, without any compromising of the subtalar joint. Figure 12.11 shows an ice skater with a gross degree of varus instability. All components of the particular ligament complex have been damaged, but it is noteworthy that the subtalar joint remains stable and intact. The method

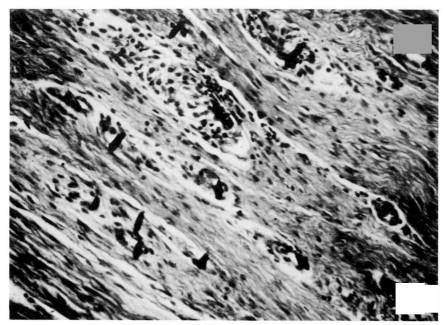

Fig. 12.10   A cross section from the induced anterior cruciate, at 6 months.

used on this particular occasion was that as shown in Fig. 12.12, in which a double strand of carbon is led through a drill hole in the distal fibula, and then across the lateral aspect of the ankle joint, to pass through the talus. The anchorage on the medial side is either by the use of one of the cyanoacrylate glues, or by suture. It is important to emphasize that the carbon should fit snugly and tightly in the bone tunnels, otherwise there will not be adequate fixation. Figure 12.13 shows a clinical example, similar to that shown in Fig. 12.12.

It has been our practice to immobilize individuals with this form of implant in a below-knee plaster for at least 6 weeks, and active sporting activity is then discouraged for at least 3–6 months.

Eight medial ligaments have been replaced, and all have been successful; 30 lateral ligament complexes have been repaired or replaced, and 28 have been successful (Table 12.1). The two failures occurred early in the series, because of erosion of the skin over the carbon implant; this occurred where the edge of the shoe impinges on the skin just below the ankle. This led us to the conclusion that carbon must be deeply placed. If it is too superficially placed because of its slightly bulky nature, it is possible that the skin will be eroded. Should that happen marsupialization of the carbon will occur, leading to infection and the inevitable

238

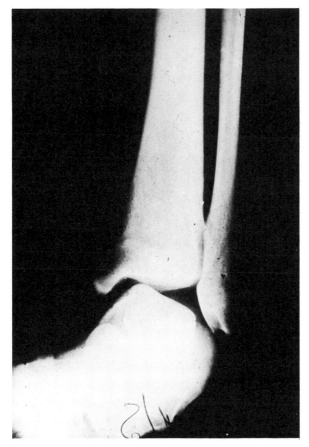

Fig. 12.11 Gross lateral instability in a human ankle.

removal of the material. In the two failures, both became infected and both had to be removed. There has been one subsequent early failure, in which the patient appeared to develop a reaction to the presence of the carbon fibre, and while the ankle was totally stable, there was sufficient pain to merit removal of the carbon implant. In all patients, the integrity of the subtalar joint has been maintained, and in all our successful patients, both full mobility and full stability has been achieved.

12.3 Knees

In the knee it is my view that it is important to recognize the complex nature of the instability. Examination will often suggest that only one

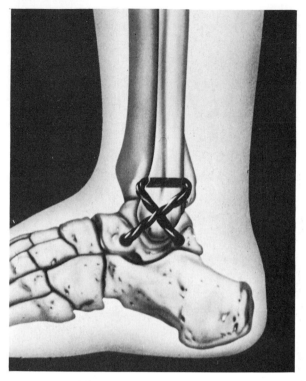

Fig. 12.12 The diagramatic representation of the method used to repair the instability demonstrated in Fig. 12.11.

ligament is damaged. Classical tests to delineate the anterior or posterior parts of the distorted anterior cruciate will suggest that only that ligament is damaged. However, for there to be an adequate degree of instability, to demonstrate, for example, the drawer sign, it is my view that there must be a degree of lateral and medial ligament or capsular disruption. If the anterior cruciate alone is cut, in an otherwise normal knee, it is unusual for one to be able to demonstrate a true anterior cruciate instability. When there is a marked degree of anterior cruciate instability, it is unlikely that a single surgical procedure designed to replace the anterior cruciate alone will be adequate to bring enough stability to an otherwise unstable knee. Similarly, when there is good clinical evidence of medial ligament disruption, it is important to look for signs of cruciate ligament instability as well. That being the case, it seems logical to try and attempt to repair all aspects of the particular patient's instability. Where one is using an artificial material, there is no limitation on the length of material which can be used. Thus, in the grossly unstable knee, one can replace not only

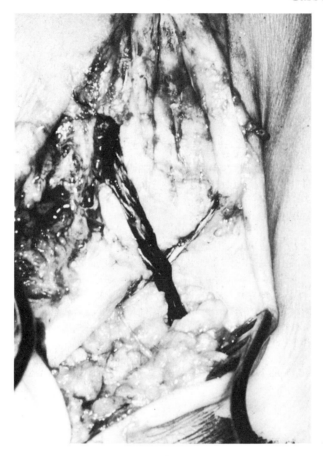

Fig. 12.13 An actual clinical photograph of the mode of implantation of the carbon fibre in the human ankle, for lateral collateral ligament instability.

Table 12.1 Success and failure rates in ankle ligament complex repairs

Medial ligaments	Eight successful
Lateral ligaments	28 successful,
	Two failures

the anterior but posterior cruciate, and the medial and lateral ligament complexes. One can overcome anterolateral instability demonstrated by the jerk test, by placement of the carbon in such a manner that as the knee

241

fully extends, the lateral tibial plateau is pulled backwards, so that the pivot shift or jerk sign cannot exist.

The method of replacement of the medial and lateral collateral ligaments can be simple, and can be carried out by percutaneous means. Figure 12.14 demonstrates an individual in whom the lateral collateral ligament of knee has been replaced by percutaneous stab incisions, and the carbon fed beneath the skin. Figure 12.15 shows a patient who has had multiple previous procedures. The medial and lateral collateral ligaments have been replaced by stab incisions, and the anterior cruciate ligament has been replaced by arthrotomy. It can be clearly seen that there has been a hypertrophy of the medial and lateral collateral ligaments, which has occurred in response to the presence of the carbon fibre, and has contributed to the stability of the knee. Various methods have been described elsewhere in this book (Strover, chapter 14), and details have been provided about the positioning and placement of the anterior cruciate. It has been my habit to pass the carbon fibre through a drill hole low down and far back on the lateral wall of the intercondylar notch. The drill is passed through bone, and the carbon anchored by a single knot on the lateral aspect of the femur, deep to the vastus lateralis. The carbon is then fed across the joint, and follows the anatomical path of the original anterior cruciate ligament. It is then brought out through a drill hole on the anterior aspect of the tibia. Where there is an attenuated, but not divided anterior cruciate ligament, that ligament is split longitudinally and wrapped around the carbon so that the carbon is buried.

Where the anterior cruciate ligament has been removed by other surgeons, or where the ligament is totally disrupted, it is now my practice to turn down a medial slip of patella tendon, pass this through a drill hole in the tibia up into the knee, and then pass that slip of patella tendon out through the same drill hole as the carbon occupies on the lateral aspect of the femur. The carbon is then wrapped inside that particular strip of tendon, and this way the carbon is buried within tendon within the joint. Earlier experience, in which naked carbon was left in the joint, showed heavy carbon staining of the synovium and led to a fairly marked degree of inflammation within the joint. The inflammation invariably settled after 2–3 months, but caused pain in patients over that period. Since starting the practice of burying the carbon within either the original anterior cruciate or a substituted piece of tendon, we have seen a marked reduction in inflammation, and practically no carbon staining when patients have had arthroscopy postoperatively.

Figure 12.16 demonstrates the implantation of carbon fibre in the replacement of the anterior cruciate ligament. In this particular figure, the anterior cruciate has not yet been wrapped around the carbon. The

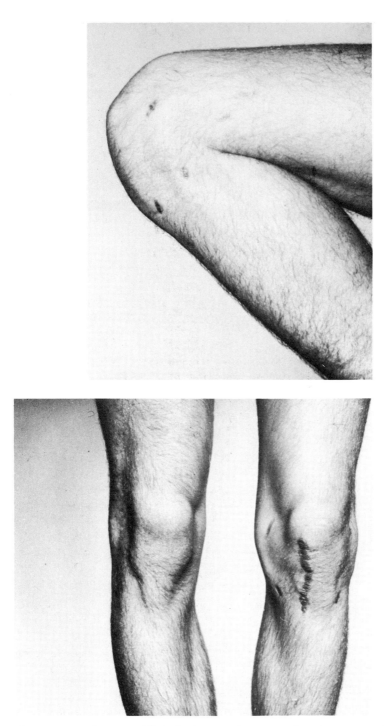

Figs. 12.14 and 12.15 Clinical pictures demonstrating the range of movement and stability in the human knee, following carbon fibre implantation.

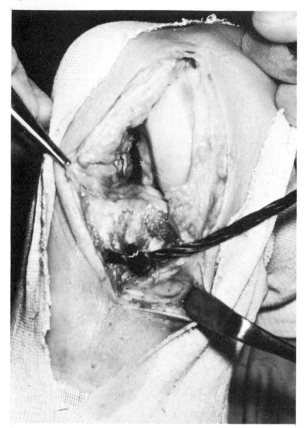

Fig. 12.16 A clinical picture showing the actual implantation of the carbon fibre in the replacement of the anterior cruciate.

carbon has been led out through a drill hole on the tibia, and has been continued around the knee, to replace the medial and lateral collateral ligaments in one continuous loop.

Our findings in the human have been similar to those in the animal. In other words, that provided that there is an adequate matrix of collagen tissue associated with the carbon, a neoligament will form in response to the presence of the carbon fibre. This statement is true whether the carbon is placed within or outside the knee. Figure 12.17 demonstrates a medial collateral ligament which was replaced in a man aged 60, 7 years prior to this photograph, and shows that there has been ingrowth of fibroblasts, with the subsequent laying down of collagen, such that a ligamentous-like structure has formed in response to the presence of the carbon fibre.

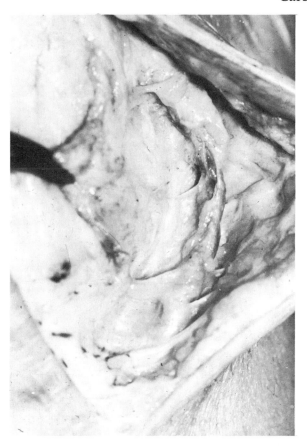

Fig. 12.17 Collateral ligament in a knee. This photograph was taken 7 years following implantation, and demonstrates the development of the neo-ligament.

12.4   Fixation

We have experimented with autofixation, and with screws and nails, in an attempt to fix the carbon on to bone. Strover (Chapter 14) in South Africa has developed a system of bollards and toggles (Table 12.2). There is no criticism of that particular system, but is the author's view that a word of caution is required in the use of metal implants associated with carbon fibre. Figure 12.18 shows a Steinman pin which was inadvertently inserted through the oscalcis, in a lady in whom carbon fibre had been implanted in the repair of the lateral ligament complex 6 years earlier. The Steinman pin was inserted in the management of a subsequent ankle fracture; at 6 weeks the pin collapsed, and its removal demonstrated gross

245

Table 12.2 Types of fixation

1. Bollards and toggles
2. Autofixation – friction ± glue
3. Screws and nails

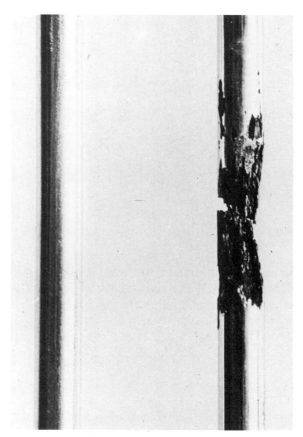

Fig. 12.18 The Steinman Pin on the left is a normal pin. That on the right shows a pin passed through a carbon fibre implant inadvertently, and demonstrates the corrosion which may occasionally be seen.

corrosion. We have formed the view that corrosion is a real risk when metallic implants are used next to carbon, and therefore we would caution against this particular method of fixation.

Autofixation consists of the carbon itself becoming incorporated into the bone. Provided that the carbon fits snugly and tightly within drill holes, and that the patient is immobilized in plaster for at least 6 weeks, it

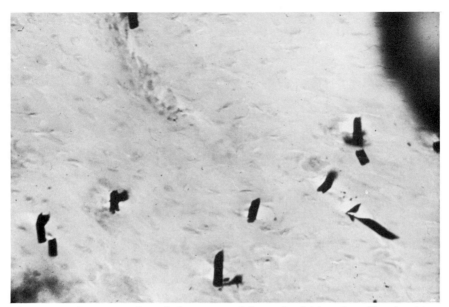

Fig. 12.19 A cross section of a bone tunnel through which carbon fibre has been passed. This demonstrates new bone ingrowth with firm anchoring of the carbon fibre.

has been our experience that in the majority, bone growth into the interstices of the carbon will occur, thus leading to adequate fixation. We initially reinforce the carbon within the bone with cyanoacrylate glue. The glue is designed not to hold the carbon for any long particular period of time, but is designed instead to hold the carbon in its correct position until the plaster of paris can be applied. In this way, the correct degree of tension of the carbon ligament can be applied and held, until external immobilization can be achieved. Figure 12.19 demonstrates a cross section from a carbon implant, where it passed through a hole in the bone, and shows that true bone ingrowth into the interstices of the carbon can occur, thus lending truth to the claim that autofixation really does occur.

12.5 Results

The successes and failures in ankle replacements have been dealt with above (pp. 236–239).

At the time of writing, 510 implants in human knees have taken place. Because it has been our practice to treat chronic severe instability by multiple ligament replacements, the majority have been implants of more

Ligament Injuries and their Treatment

than one ligament. We have found that provided that the postoperative routine of the application of plaster of paris for 6 weeks, a stick for 4 weeks, jogging at 4 months and sports not earlier than 6 months, is followed (Table 12.3) we achieve satisfaction in 80% of patients (Table 12.4). Satisfaction is measured in terms of an alternative surgeon describing the procedure as satisfactory, and the patient himself/herself stating that he/she has achieved what he/she wished to achieve from the implants. This means that in patients with poliomyelitis, the treatment of recurvatum deformities has overcome the recurvatum deformity, but does not of course make them walk normally. On the other hand, high-class sportsmen, who have slipped to the level at which ordinary mortals function, have regained some degree of their sporting prowess. Ordinary individuals who cannot, for example, climb in and out of a car without the knee collapsing, can now achieve that as a result of their carbon implantation.

Table 12.3 Anterior cruciate replacement, all knee ligament replacements: postoperative routine

1. Plaster of paris with knee at 20° for 6 weeks – no weight bearing on crutches
2. Stick for 4 weeks – full weight bearing
3. Jogging only at 4 months
4. Sports at 6 months

Table 12.4 Outcome of 380 knee implants (Jenkins, Cardiff)

380 Knee implants
  Satisfaction in 80%
  Follow-up 1–7 years

We have been impressed by the fact any failures which occurred did so early following implantation. This is usually because the carbon implant has broken due to insufficient time having elapsed to allow tissue ingrowth to occur (Tables 12.5 and 12.6). Provided that the patient has

Table 12.5 Success and failure in knee implants

	Success	
	Patient (%)	Surgeon (%)
Extra-articular	90	80
Intra-articular	70	60

Table 12.6 Failures in anterior cruciate replacement (Jenkins, Cardiff)

Cardiff: Four certain failures in 120
     : Three in first 6 months

patience, and that there is adequate supervision in the post-plaster period, it has been our experience that the ligament will grow stronger rather than weaker, as its bulk increases. This inevitably leads to some slight loss of extremes of flexion in the knee, and can occasionally rather overstabilize an ankle, but that is a small price to pay for stability.

Table 12.7 shows the range of places in which carbon fibre has been used in the human, and demonstrates the success rate of approximately 80% in all implants.

Table 12.7 Range of places and success rate of carbon fibre in humans (Jenkins, Cardiff)

	Number	Success
Knee implants	380	310
Ankles	40	38
Anterior cruciate joint	32	28
Metacarpophalangeal joint, thumb	6	4
Radio ulna joint	4	4
Unstable shoulder	8	6
Tendo-achilles	8	7
Patella tendon	8	6
Poliomyelitis knees (genu recurvatum)	8	6
Sternoclavicular joint	6	6

Percentage succcess rate about 80%

In conclusion (Table 12.8) it is my view that carbon fibre is ideal in ankle instability. It has the merit of replacing the part of the unstable joint complex, which needs to be replaced, and does not compromise other parts of the ankle joint complex and its movements. It is excellent in extra-articular situations, although we have some doubt about its intra-articular use when it is buried in the knee in a naked position. Provided that it is covered with tendon or ligament, synovitis is reduced and the results are adequate. Still the question remains: 'should we restrict ourselves to its extra-articular use'. It is my belief that the material has a place both within and outside joints. It is not the universal panacea for all ligament

Ligament Injuries and their Treatment

Table 12.8 The place of carbon fibre

---

1. Ideal in ankles
2. Excellent in extra-articular situations
     Ease of method
     Speed of operation
     Standard results in many centres
3. Some doubt about intra-articular situations
     Synovitis 3–4 months
     Failures
         possibly related to postoperative regime
         possibly the claims by Jenkins and Strover are incorrect
4. Should we restrict ourselves to extra-articular use only?

---

instability, but it certainly has a place in the surgeon's armamentarium, especially in complex problems.

References

Alexander, H. *et al.* (1979a), An absorbable polymer-filamentous carbon scaffold for ligament and tendon replacement. *Proceedings 7th New England Bioeng. Conf.*, pp. 400–03.

Alexander, H. *et al.* (1979b), Ligament and tendon replacement with absorbable polymer-filamentous carbon tissue scaffolds. *Transactions of the 11th International Biomaterials Symposium in conjunction with the Fifth Annual Meeting of the Society for Biomaterials, Clemson, South Carolina*, **III**, 72, (28 April–1 May).

Alexander, H. *et al.* (1981), A filamentous carbon-absorbable polymer medial collateral ligament replacement. *Transactions of the 7th Annual Meeting of the Society for Biomaterials in conjunction with the 13th International Biomaterials Symposium, Rensellaer Polytechnic Inst. Troy, New York*, **4**, 129, 28–31 May.

Alexander, H. *et al.* (1982), Anterior cruciate ligament replacement with filamentous carbon. *28th Annual ORS, New Orleans, Louisiana*, **19–21**, 45.

Amis, A. A. *et al.* (1980), Filamentous implant construction of tendon defects. *British Orthopaedic Society Meeting at Princess Margaret Rose Orthopaedic Hospital, Edinburgh (14 November)*.

Amis, A. A. *et al.* (1981), Filamentous implant reconstruction of tendon defects. *J. Bone Joint Surg.*, **63B**, 296.

Aragona, J. *et al.* (1981a), Attachment of a partially absorbable tendon and ligament to soft tissue. *Proceedings of the 9th Northeast Conference, Rutgers University, New Brunswick, New Jersey*, **25–28**, 19–20 March.

Aragona, J. *et al.* (1981b), Soft tissue attachment of a filamentous carbon-absorbable polymer tendon and ligament replacement. *Clin. Orthop. Rel. Res.*, **160**, 268–78.

Beacon, J. P. and Aichroth, P. M. (1980), A method of reconstruction of the goat knee joint using carbon fibre. *J. Bone Joint Surg.*, **62B**, 534–5.

Beacon, J. P. *et al.* (1980), A mechanical investigation of the human anterior

250

cruciate ligament. *Programme, British Orthopaedic Society Meeting at Princess Margaret Rose Orthopaedic Hospital, Edinburgh*, 14 November.

Beacon, J. P. *et al.* (1981), A mechanical investigation of the human anterior cruciate ligament. *J. Bone Joint Surg.*, **63B**, 299.

Bejui, J. *et al.* (1980), Experimental study of the prosthetic replacement of the anterior cruciate ligament in the dog's knee with a carbon fibre joint. *First World Biomaterials Congress, Austria, Final Programme, Book of Abstracts, 4.7.6*, 8–12 April.

Bejui, J. *et al.* (1983), Carbon fibre reconstruction of anterior cruciate ligament. *Book of Abstracts 4th European Conference on Biomaterials, Leuven, Belgium*, 31 August–2 September, **113**.

Blobel, K. *et al.* (1983), Die perdutane Intratendinale carbonfaserimplantation beim Pferd. *Vet. Bull.* **53**, 716 (abstract).

Bokros, J. C., Artificial tendon prostheses, United States Patent 4 149 277.

Bokros, J. C. Artificial tendon or ligament prostheses. GB Patent 1 593 700.

Burri, C. and Claes, L. (eds) (1983), Alloplastic ligament replacement. *Aktuelle Probleme in Chirurgie und Orthop.*, **26**, Hans Huber, Bern.

Burri, C. (1980), Grundlagen des Kniebandersatzes durch Kohlenstoff. *Unfallheilkunde*, **83**, 208–13.

Burri, C. and Neugebauer, R. (1981), Technik des alloplastischen Bandersatzes mit Kohlefasern. *Unfallchirurgie*, **7**, 289–97.

Claes, L. *et al.* (1978), Physical and biological aspects of carbon fibres in the ligament prosthesis. *BES 71st Scientific Meeting, 3rd Conference on Materials for Use in Medicine and Biology, Mechanical Properties of Biomaterials and Bioceramics Symposium, University of Keele, 13–16 September*.

Claes, L. *et al.* (1983), The ligament replacement with various alloplastic materials. *4th European Conference on Biomaterials, Leuven, Belgium, 31 August–2 September*, **112**.

Coombs, R. R. H. *et al.* (1980), Collagen typing in carbon fibre induced tendon. *Programme, British Orthopaedic Society Meeting at Princess Margaret Rose Orthopaedic Hospital, Edinburgh, 14 November*.

Coombs, R. R. H. *et al.* (1981), Collagen typing in carbon fibre-induced tendon. *J. Bone Joint Surg.*, **63B**, 196.

Dahhan, P. *et al.* (1981), Reparation du ligament croise anterieur par fibres de carbone. *J. Chir (Paris)*, **118**, 275–80.

Dandy, D. J. *et al.* (1982), Arthroscopy and the management of the ruptured anterior cruciate ligament. *Clin. Orthop. Rel. Res.*, **167**, 43–9.

Denny, H. R. and Goodship, A. E. (1980), Replacement of the anterior cruciate ligament with carbon fibre in the dog. *J. Small Anim. Pract.*, **21**, 279–86.

Fitzer, E. *et al.* (1977), Preparation of pyrocarbon-coated carbon fibres for use in ligament replacement. *Extended Abstracts and Program, 13th Biennial Conference on Carbon, Irvine, California*, 18–22 July, pp. 180–1.

Forster, I. W. (1976), A study of the mechanisms by which carbon fibre acts as a tendon prosthesis. *J. Bone Joint Surg.*, **58B**, 376.

Forster, I. W. *et al.* (1978), Biological reaction to carbon fibre implants: the formation and structure of a carbon-induced 'neotendon'. *Clin. Orthop. Rel. Res.*, **131**, 299–307.

Goodship, A. E. *et al.* (1978), Use of carbon fibre for tendon repair. *Vet. Rec.*, **102**, 322.

Ligament Injuries and their Treatment

Goodship, A. E. *et al.* (1980), An assessment of filamentous carbon fibre for the treatment of tendon injury in the horse. *Vet. Rec.*, **106**, 217–21.

Goutallier, A. *et al.* (1981), Prosthetic replacement of the anterior cruciate ligament with carbon fibre strands – fibre fragmentation and migration study. *Proceedings of the 2nd European Conference on Biomaterials, Interactions between Material and Tissue in Orthopaedic, Maxillofacial, Dental and Plastic Surgery. Review of Progress in Basic Understanding of the Interface, Gothenburg, Sweden*, **59–60**, 27–29 August.

Hutchins, D. R. and Rawlinson, R. J. (1981), Treatment of tendon injuries. *Conference Conducted by Postgraduate Committee in Vet. Sci., Univ. Sydney, Suite 93, Lincoln House, 280 Pitt St. Sydney. Proc. No. 54 'Soft Tissue Surgery'* pp. 229–236.

Jenkins, D. H. R. Improvements relating to replacements for ligaments and tendons. BP 1 602 834.

Jenkins, D. H. R. (1976), Carbon fibre as a prosthetic implant material in orthopaedics. *J. Bone Joint Surg.*, **58B**, 253.

Jenkins, D. H. R. (1977a), Experimental and clinical application of carbon fibre as an implant in orthopaedics. *J. Bone Joint Surg.*, **59B**, 501.

Jenkins, D. H. R. (1977b), Experimental and clinical application of carbon fibre as an implant in orthopaedics. *Extended Abstracts and Program, 13th Biennial Conference on Carbon, Irvine, California, 18–22 July*, pp. 178–9.

Jenkins, D. H. R. (1978a), Ligamentous induction of filamentous carbon fibre. *Surg. News*, **6**.

Jenkins, D. H. R. (1978b), The repair of cruciate ligaments with flexible carbon fibre: a longer-term study of the induction of new ligaments and of the fate of the implanted carbon. *J. Bone Joint Surg.*, **60B**, 520–2.

Jenkins, D. H. R. (1979a), The induction of a new anterior cruciate ligament in the sheep and the clinical use of filamentous carbon fibre in the human. *J. Bone Joint Surg.*, **61B**, 120.

Jenkins, D. H. R. (1979b), Carbon fibre in ligament and tendon repair. *Vet. Rec.*, **105**, 312.

Jenkins, D. H. R. and McKibbin, B. (1980), The role of flexible carbon-fibre implants as tendon and ligament substitutes in clinical practice. *J. Bone Joint Surg.*, **62B**, 497–9.

Jenkins, D. H. R. and Parkington, R. (1978), The clinical use of flexible carbon fibre materials. *BES 71st Scientific Meeting, 3rd Conference on Materials for Use in Medicine and Biology, Mechanical Properties of Biomaterials and Bioceramics Symposium, University of Keele, 13–16 September*.

Jenkins, D. H. R. *et al.* (1976), Filamentous carbon fibre as an orthopaedic implant material. *BES 63rd Scientific Meeting. Second conference on Materials for Use in Medicine and Biology: Problems of Biocompatibility, Brunel University*.

Jenkins, D. H. R. *et al.* (1977), Induction of tendon and ligament formation by carbon implants. *J. Bone Joint Surg.*, **59B**, 53–7.

Johnson-Nurse, C. and Jenkins, D. H. R. (1980), The use of flexible carbon fibre in the repair of experimental large abdominal incisional hernias. *Br. J. Surg.*, **67**, 135–7.

Kennedy, J. C. (1983), Application of prosthetics to anterior cruciate ligament reconstruction and repair. *Clin. Orthop. Rel. Res.*, **172**, 125–8.

Kinzl, L. *et al.* (1979), Aspects of coated carbon fibres in the ligament-prostheses.

Transactions of the 11th International Biomaterials Symposium in conjunction with the Fifth Annual Meeting of the Society for Biomaterials, Clemson, South Carolina, **III**, 71, *28 April–1 May.*

Kramer, B. and King, R. E. (1983), The histological appearance of carbon fibre implants and neo-ligament in man. *SA Med. J.*, **63**, 113–15.

Leyshon, R. L. *et al.* (1983), Late flexible carbon-fibre for knee instability. *J. Bone Joint Surg.*, **65B**, 227.

Littlewood, H. F. (1979), Treatment of sprained tendons in horses with carbon fibre implants. *Vet. Rec.*, **105**, 223–4.

Merz, B. (1982), Try a carbon ribbon 'round the old hurt knee (and shoulder). *J. Am. Med. Assoc.*, **248**, 1681–2.

Minns, R. J. and Flynn, M. (1978), Intra-articular implant of filamentous carbon fibre in the experimental animal. *J. Bioeng.*, **2**, 279–86.

Minns, R. J. and Muckle, D. S. (1978), The use of filamentous carbon fibre for the repair of osteoarthritic articular cartilage. A preliminary investigation. *Programme, Br. Orthop. Res. Soc. Meet. Bradford*, RI 16 November.

Mockwitz, J. and Contzen, H. (1982), Die behandlung des veralteten Kniebandschadens mit alloplastischem Material. *Unfallchirurgie*, **8**, 176–9.

Murray, G. A. W. and Semple, J. C. (1979), A review of work on articicial tendons. *J. Biomed. Eng.*, **1**, 177–84.

Neugebauer, R. amd Burri, C. (1981), Ergebnisse nach alloplastischem Bandersatz mit Kohlenstoffasern. *Unfallchirurgie*, **7**, 198–304.

Neugebauer, R. *et al.* (1980a), The trap door, a possibility of fixation of carbon-fibre-strands into cancellous bone. *First World Biomaterials Congress, Austria, Final Programme, Book of Abstracts*, 4.7.5, 8–12 April.

Neugebauer, R. *et al.* (1980b), Kohlenstoffasern als Bandersatz am Kniegelenk, eine Biomechanische und Histologische Untersuchung. *Langenbecks Arch. Chir.*, **351** (Suppl.) 35–9.

Neugebauer, R. *et al.* (1982), Biocompatibility and biomechanics of carbon-fibre strands coated with a quick resorbable collagen. *Transactions of the 8th Annual Meeting of the Society for Biomaterials in conjunction with the 14th International Biomaterials Symposium.* **41**, 24–27 April.

Parsons, J. R. *et al.* (1981), Medial collateral ligament replacement with a partially absorbable tissue scaffold. *Proceedings of the 9th Northeast Conference, Rutgers University, New Brunswick, New Jersey*, **29–32**, 19–20 March.

Ralis, Z. A. and Forster, I. W. (1980), Choice of the implantation site and other factors influencing the carbon fibre tissue reaction. *Programme, British Orthopaedics Research Society Meeting at Princess Margaret Rose Orthopaedic Hospital, Edinburgh, 14 November.*

Ralis, Z. A. and Forster, I. W. (1981), Choice of the implantation site and other factors influencing the carbon fibre–tissue reaction. *J. Bone Joint Surg.*, **63B**, 294–5.

Rushton, N. *et al.* (1983), The clinical, arthroscopic and histological findings after replacement of the anterior cruciate ligament with carbon fibre. *J. Bone Joint Surg.*, **65B**, 308–9.

Saha, S. *et al.* (1982), Biomechanical evaluation of filamentous carbon fiber implant in patellar tendon replacement. *Transactions of the 8th Annual Meeting of the Society for Biomaterials in conjunction with the 14th International Biomaterials Symposium. 24–27 April*, **42**.

Ligament Injuries and their Treatment

Schweitzer, G. (1982), The current status of carbon fibre in knee ligament repair. *Ann. Chirurg. Gynaecolog.*, **71**, 308–11.

Strover, A. E. and Hunt, M. S. (1982), Carbon fibre reconstruction of knee ligaments. *Transactions of the 8th Annual Meeting of the Society for Biomaterials in conjunction with the 14th International Biomaterials Symposium*, **5**, 24–27 April.

Valdez, H. *et al.* (1980), Repair of digital flexor tendon lacerations in the horse using carbon fiber implants. *J. Am. Vet. Med. Assoc.*, **177**, 427–35.

Vaughan, L. C. (1979), Muscle and tendon injuries in dogs. *J. Small Anim. Pract.*, **20**, 711–36.

Vaughan, L. C., Tendon injuries in dogs. *California Vet.*, **1**, 15–19.

Vaughan, L. C. and Edwards, G. B. (1978), The use of carbon fibre (grafil) for tendon repair in animals. *Vet. Rec.*, **102**, 287–8.

Wolter, D. *et al.* (1977), Ligament replacement in the knee joint with carbon fibres coated with pyrolytic carbon. *3rd Annual Meeting of the Society for Biomaterials, 9th International Biomaterials Symposium, New Orleans, Louisiana, Hyatt Regency Hotel*, **119**.

Wolter, D. *et al.* (1978a), Der Alloplastische Ersatz des medialen Knieseitenbandes durch beschichtete Kohlenstoffasern. *Unfallheilkunde*, **81**, 390–7.

Wolter, D. *et al.* (1978b), Die Reaktion des Körpers auf Implantierte Kohlenstoff-mikropartikel. *Arch. Orthop. Traum. Surg.*, **91**, 19–29.

13 Carbon fibre II: Biomechanics

R. NEUGEBAUER AND L. CLAES

13.1 Introduction

Knowledge of the biomechanical properties of human ligaments is an essential requirement for the development of an alloplastic ligament replacement. Therefore, it is most important to study the biomechanical behaviour of both the natural ligaments on cadaveric specimens and the alloplastic replacement *in vitro* and in animal trials. This chapter first gives details of human ligaments that are important for alloplastic replacement.

13.2 Properties of human knee ligaments

The various experimental procedures for the determination of the biomechanical properties of ligaments can be categorized into three groups.

(1) Ligamentous stress under nearly physiological conditions.

(2) The rupture strength as determined on individual ligaments isolated at the joint.

(3) Isolated ligaments used to determine specific ligamental properties such as the modulus of elasticity, extensibility and relaxation.

13.2.1 KNEE LIGAMENTS UNDER NEARLY PHYSIOLOGICAL CONDITIONS OF MOVEMENT AND STRESS

The motions of flexion, abduction, adduction and rotation which the knee joint is able to perform exert various amounts of tensile forces on the four main ligaments of this joint. A lack of homogeneity of the ligaments and the irregular ligamental cross-sections supported the assumption that there is no linear correlation between the tensile force and the extension of the ligaments.

In extension the forces and strains are most on the dorsal portion of the ligament, the least values are on the ventral part. As the range of flexion increased, the strains and tensile forces decreased dorsally and increased ventrally. Tensile forces are carried between 0° and 25° by the dorsal ligament portions. These forces are at their minimum between 25° and 80°, then greatly increase in the ventral portion of the ligament to reach their maximum at 135°. Additional abductional moments increased the tensile forces in all portions of the ligament. The major portion of the load here is taken up by the ventral portion of the ligament. The lateral collateral ligament is affected by tensile forces in extension, and they diminish with increasing angle of flexion and approach 0 at 40°. An adduction moment also results in a great increase in tensile forces on the ligament with a maximum at around 70°. The strains are not proportional to the forces. Under pure flexion the highest strains are at around 5%. Under abductional and adductional moments these values increase.

The results of strain measurements by various authors diverge greatly (Chaes *et al.*, 1978; Edward, Lafferty and Lange, 1970; Wang, Walker and Wolf, 1973). This is partly due to the fact that measurements were performed on different portions of the ligament. Wirth (1981) and Claes and Mutschler (1981) agree in the measurements on the medial collateral ligament and show that the strains on the ventral and dorsal portion behave in opposite ways. The dorsal portion of the medial collateral ligament and of the lateral collateral ligament have their greatest strains in extension (Claes and Mutschler, 1981; Edward, Lafferty and Lange, 1970; Wirth, 1981). The strains are cited as 5% (Claes and Mutschler, 1981) up to over 20% (Edward, Lafferty Lange, 1970). There are still conflicting statements concerning the load on the cruciate ligaments (Edward, Lafferty and Lange, 1970; Wang, Walter and Wolf, 1973) so that nothing definite can be said about the actual conditions.

13.2.2 STRENGTH AND EXTENSIBILITY OF THE LIGAMENTS

Tests for rupture strength are in most cases not performed on the isolated ligament, but instead on the ligament with its bony attachment. Rupture strength is determined by a test for tensile strength in which a force–strain diagram is graphed. The force at the linear limit indicates the load at which stress is reversible without doing damage to the ligament. Higher loads lead to the rupture of individual ligament structures without causing a total rupture. Corresponding to these two forces, the strains at the linear limit and the rupture strain provide a measure for the extensibility of the ligaments. Despite the considerable differences in the results by the various authors, it is recognized that there are distinct differences in the rupture strength of the different ligaments.

On the average, the highest values are cited for the posterior cruciate ligament, for which values between 571–1745 N have been published (Kennedy *et al.*, 1976; Piziali *et al.*, 1980; Trent, Walker and Wolf, 1976). For the anterior cruciate ligament, the rupture forces are in the range of 350–734 N. Higher average values are reported only for young ligaments, for which Noyes and Grood (1976) found an average value of 1730 N. These values are distinctly higher than the strength of old ligaments, which averaged 734 N in the same study.

The measurement results on the medial collateral ligaments varied much less than those on the cruciate ligaments. The average values stated are between 477 and 654 N and are thus approximately in the range of the strength of the anterior cruciate ligaments. The weakest ligament of the knee was definitely the lateral collateral ligament, here the average values of the different authors range from 354 to 384 N (Kennedy *et al.*, 1976; Neugebauer *et al.*, 1981; Trent, Walker and Wolf, 1976).

The rupture strain show no distinct differences in relation to the ligament type. The published values average between 18.1% and 30.8%. However, Noyes also stated an average of 44.3% for young anterior cruciate ligaments. The force at the linear limit averaged about 80% of the rupture force, and the strain at the linear limit is about 65% of the rupture strain of the ligaments (Claes and Mutschler, 1981; Kennedy *et al.*, 1976; Noyes, 1977; Noyes and Grood, 1976; Tremblay, Laurin and Drovin, 1980).

13.2.3 VISCOELASTIC PROPERTIES OF THE LIGAMENTS

Like all biopolymers, collagenous structures such as ligaments exhibit viscoelastic behaviour. This behaviour is characterized by the dependence of the material properties on both time and on load velocity. An increase in load velocity for ligaments leads to an increase of stiffness, the modulus of elasticity and the rupture strength as well as a reduction of strains (Hartung, 1975). Experiments have shown that the essential changes of relaxation and force recovery take place within the first minute.

The results of the relaxations and force recoveries after 1 min are presented in Table 13.1 as averages with their respective standard deviations for the different ligaments of the knee joint. The medial collateral ligament shows the highest values, but the differences between the various ligaments are not evident. Statements are given about the differences between the various ligaments only. The absolute values for relaxation and force recovery are of qualified significance only, because they are considerably influenced by the load velocity and the level of the initial load (Hartung, 1975).

However, human ligaments have pronounced viscoelastic properties.

Table 13.1 Viscoelastic properties of human knee ligaments

Ligament	Relaxation (%)	Recovery (%)
Medial collateral	19.6 ± 3.0	5.1 ± 0.8
Lateral collateral	14.1 ± 2.5	4.3 ± 0.8
Anterior cruciate	17.0 ± 3.1	3.7 ± 0.8
Posterior cruciate	18.9 ± 2.0	3.7 ± 0.6

Due to these properties, the ligaments can store deformation energy under dynamic load and release it in phases of relief. The ligaments are thus in a position to reduce peak loads and absorb impacts to the knee joint.

13.3 Properties of the ligament replacement by an alloplastic material (carbon fibres)

Ligament replacement materials should be fashioned in a way to ensure a function similar to a natural ligament under long-term *in vivo* conditions. In order to evaluate the suitability of a ligament replacement with carbon fibres, one therefore needs to know not only the mechanical properties of the carbon fibres, but also the biomechanical properties of the entire ligament replacement. These are essentially determined by the following factors:

(1) Mechanical properties of the fibres
(2) Structure of the carbon fibre prosthesis
(3) Anchorage of the prosthesis at the joint
(4) Behaviour under *in vivo* conditions.

For the determination of these properties a large number of materials studies, animal experiments and biomechanical investigations were performed.

13.3.1 MECHANICAL PROPERTIES OF FIBRES

A carbon fibre consists of pure carbon in a graphite structure (Böder *et al.*, 1981). The fibres have a diameter of 7–8 μm and are thinner than a hair. Carbon fibres can be produced with various material properties (Table 13.2) and are offered by various manufacturers. The high-modulus fibre type and the high-strength type are comparable in their modulus of

Table 13.2 Mechanical properties of carbon fibres

Properties/Type	High strength (HS)	High modulus (HM)	Isotropic (I)
Tensil strength (Pa–10—3)	2.5–3	2.0–2.5	0.9
Modulus of elasticity (Pa)	0.2–0.25	0.35–0.45	0.04

elasticity and their tensile strength to the properties of stainless steel (Fitzer *et al*, 1971).

Carbon fibres loaded up to the point of rupture only exhibit elastic deformation; there is no plastic deformation (Böder *et al.*, 1981). Fatigue loading does not produce creep, that is, the continuous increase in the length of the fibres. Under fatigue loading, values of fatigue strength constituting approximately 80% of the static strength were measured for the carbon fibres (Börder *et al.*, 1981). These values are higher than comparable values obtained for stainless steel.

Due to the anisotropic layer structure of the fibre, the shear strength perpendicular to the longitudinal axis of the fibre is slight. This means that high shear stresses occur when the fibres are bent over sharp edges, and that the fibres can break under these conditions.

13.3.2 STRUCTURE OF CARBON FIBRE PROSTHESES

If unidirectional strands of carbon fibre are used for ligament replacement, only very slight strains occur under tensile load due to the high modulus of elasticity (Wolter *et al.*, 1978). A bundle of carbon fibres (HS type) consisting of 96 000 fibres shows a strain of only 0.02% at 300 N load, whereas natural ligaments show strains of 10–20% at this load (Kennedy *et al.*, 1976). We therefore braided several tows of carbon fibres in order to obtain higher strain properties (Claes and Burri, 1981).

Seven ligaments with various numbers of tows, numbers of fibres per tow and various braiding angles were tested (Claes, Burri and Neugebauer, 1981; Claes *et al.*, 1979). The highest strains were achieved with a ligament consisting of 32 tows with 3000 filaments each braided at an angle of 43° (type A, Fig. 13.1). Whereas permanent changes in length occurred after the first tensile loads only reversible strains were registered after 15 load cycles had been applied. The permanent change of length following the first load was not due to fibre deformation, but to a shift of the fibres relative to each other.

The reversible, elastic extension of the type A ligament was 0.63% at 300 N (Fig. 13.2). It was therefore 31 times higher than the extensibility of

259

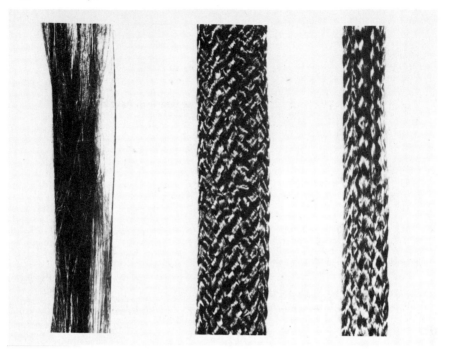

Fig. 13.1 Bundle with unidirectional carbon fibres, type U, left; braided carbon fibre ligaments with 3000 fibres per tow (type A, centre) and 1000 fibres per tow (type B, right).

a ligament with the same number of fibres worked in a unidirectional fashion (type U, see Figs 13.1 and 13.2). A further increase of ligament elasticity can be achieved by covering the fibres with an elastic or viscoelastic material. A layer of absorbable collagen 2–4 μm thick on all sides of the carbon fibres significantly ($p < 0.01$) increases the extensibility to 1.14% (see Fig. 13.2) and also increases the shearing strength of the carbon fibres.

Figure 13.2 depicts the differences between the three modifications by way of force–strain diagrams. This picture shows a progressive course of the graph due to the collagen layering in the region below 100 N tensile force, as it can also be observed for the natural ligaments (Neugebauer *et al.*, 1981; Trent, Walker and Wolf, 1976). Despite this significant improvement of ligament elasticity, the extensibility of the natural ligaments is not achieved. Elasticities corresponding to those of natural ligaments are only attained once the body's own connective tissue has grown into the carbon fibre ligament *in vivo* to form a compound.

The breaking stength of the ligament replacement is influenced by the

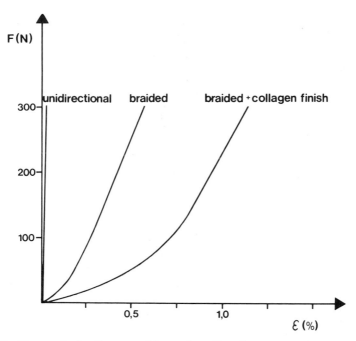

Fig. 13.2 Stress–strain diagram of the carbon fibre ligament replacement under traction.

strength of the ligament prosthesis and the anchorage of the ligament at the joint. The breaking strength of the alloplastic material depends on the number of fibres used and the braiding angle. The strength increases almost linearly with the number of fibres and decreases slightly with increasing braiding angle. The tensile rupture strength of the type A ligaments (32 tows, 3000 filaments/tow/43° braiding angle: see Fig. 13.1) was an average of 2461 ± 238 N. It was thus about three times higher than the breaking strength of natural ligaments of the knee joint. The smaller ligament type with 1000 filaments/tow for operations of the ankle joint (type B, see Fig. 13.1) achieved tensile strength of 996 ± 5 N.

13.3.3 ANCHORAGE OF THE PROSTHESIS AT THE JOINT

The anchorage of the alloplastic material to the joint is of greatest importance to the strength and stability of the ligament replacement. Even a ligament replacement of great strength will not permit a load on the joint if no sufficient anchorage to the joint is possible with the material. Various methods, such as suturing the carbon fibres to the periosteum or to the surrounding connective tissue (Alexander *et al.*,

Ligament Injuries and their Treatment

1981) as well as intraosseus anchorages (Burri, 1980; Burri and Neugebauer, 1981; Jenkins, 1978; Neugebauer, Burri and Claes, 1981; Neugebauer *et al.*, 1979, 1981; Wolter *et al.*, 1979) were tested clinically and experimentally. For the development of suitable intraosseus anchorage methods we performed investigations on cadaver knees as well as doing animal experiments. Three different types of anchorage were examined:

(1) Lateral anchorage of the prosthesis after drawing it through an intracondylar borehole (Fig. 13.3(a)).

(2) Medial anchorage of the prosthesis after drawing it through a V-shaped borehole (Fig. 13.3(b)).

(3) Medial anchorage of the prosthesis underneath a flake of bone (Fig. 13.3(c)).

In the case of the intracondylar (Fig. 13.3(a)) and V-shaped (Fig. 13.3(b)) borehole anchorages, the ends of the carbon fibre ligaments were fixed to the bone with screws and washers (Neugebauer *et al.*, 1981; Wolter *et al.*, 1979).

In the case of the anchorage shown in Fig. 13.3(c), the end of the carbon ligament was fixed by attaching the bone flake with a screw. We determined the intraoperatively obtainable anchorage strengths for 16 cadaver knees, fixing the carbon ligaments type A underneath a bone

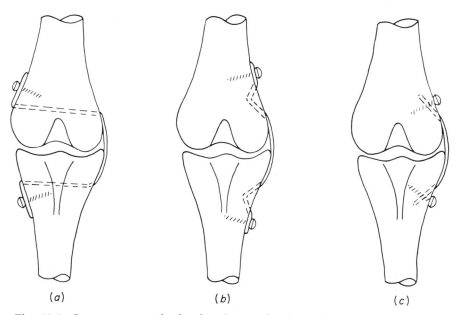

(a) (b) (c)

Fig. 13.3 Intraosseus methods of anchorage for the replacement of the medial collateral ligament of the knee in an animal experiment.

flake (Fig. 13.3(c)) in eight knees and drawing them through a V-shaped borehole (Fig. 13.3(b)) in the remaining eight knees.

The test for tensile strength (strain rate 10 mm/min) established an average breaking force of 434.3 ± 122.0 N for the flake anchorage. The natural medial collateral ligaments of the same knees tested for comparison exhibited a rupture strength of 650 ± 154 N. The intraoperative anchorage forces therefore achieved 66–89% of the strength of natural ligaments and permit an early functional exercise treatment of the ligament repair.

13.3.4 BEHAVIOUR UNDER *IN VIVO* CONDITIONS

We replaced the medial collateral ligament of the knee with a type A (see Fig. 13.1) carbon fibre ligament in 30 sheep. The anchorage of the ligament replacement was done according to the three methods described (Fig. 13 (a), (b) and (c)) in sets of ten sheep each.

After the knees were explanted 12 weeks postoperatively, all knee ligaments with the exception of the medial carbon fibre ligament were resected and the isolated medial ligament was subjected to a tensile test. Figure 13.4 shows the results of the tensile test for the three different anchorages in comparison to the natural medial collateral ligament. The rupture strength, which is indicated by the maximum of the graph, is higher for the intracondylar anchorage (625 ± 278 N) than it is for the natural ligaments (590 ± 204 N).

The two other types of anchorage achieved 50% of the natural ligament values with 291 ± 57 N (flake) and 291 ± 142 N (borehole) after an implantation time of 12 weeks. A further increase of these values is to be expected as the time of implantation increases.

The extensibility and elasticity of the ligament replacement increased greatly after implantation in comparison to *in vitro* values and reaches nearly physiological values. The reason for this is the growth of connective tissue in between the carbon fibres of the free ligament portion as well as the elastic fixation of the carbon fibre ligament in the intraosseus anchorage.

The connective tissue growth in between the braided carbon fibres constitutes a viscoelastic element. When tensile load is exerted on the braided carbon fibre ligament replacement, the connective tissue portions are compressed, as the model in Fig. 13.5 shows. After the load is released from the ligament replacement, the connective tissue pushes the fibres back into their original position like a spring (see Fig. 13.5). In this way, the complex of carbon fibres and connective tissue achieved an elasticity behaviour similar to that of a natural ligament. The same effect could be

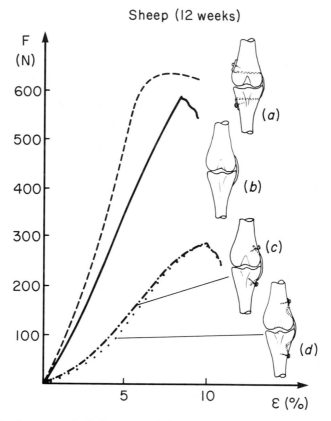

Sheep (12 weeks)

Fig. 13.4 Stress–strain behaviour of the replacement of the medial collateral knee ligament in sheep 12 weeks after the operation: (*a*) intracondylar anchorage; (*b*) normal medial collateral ligament compared with the flake anchorage medial (*c*); (*d*) borehole anchorage medial.

observed *in vitro* for the collagen-covered carbon fibre ligaments (see Fig. 13.2).

The influence of the anchorage on the elasticity of the ligament replacement is considerable at the onset of implantation, as Fig. 13.4 shows. However, this influence should diminish with prolonged implantation time as connective tissue fixation of the carbon fibre ligament to the bone is replaced by a bony fixation.

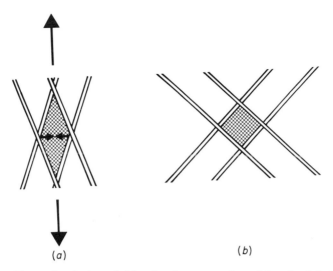

(a)   *(b)*

Fig. 13.5 Biomechanical model for the demonstration of the elastic behaviour of the ligament replacement with carbon fibres and connective tissue: (*a*) ligament replacement under tensile load; (*b*) ligament replacement after load removal.

13.9 Conclusion

Alloplastic materials which are suitable for a ligament replacement should offer a high biocompatibility and excellent biomechanical properties. In our opinion the materials should consist of a multifilament braided material, which allows natural tissue like collagen to grow in between the fibres. This will ensure a normal function in case of failure of the alloplastic fibres. In our experiments carbon fibres are most suitable for ligament replacements in respect of both biocompatibility and biomechanics. Therefore we can say in conclusion:

1. The tensile strength and modulus of elasticity of carbon fibres are comparable to those of stainless steel.

2. The small diameter (7–8 µm) produces high fibre flexibility, permitting braiding and weaving of this material.

3. The strength of braided ligament prostheses is about two to three times higher than the rupture strength of natural knee ligaments.

4. The elasticity and extensibility of a ligament prosthesis made of braided carbon fibres are higher than when the arrangement is unidirectional.

5. The growth of connective tissue in between the braided carbon fibres increases the elasticity and extensibility of the ligament replacement *in*

265

Ligament Injuries and their Treatment

vivo, so that 50–110% of the values for natural ligaments can be achieved.

6. The low shearing strength of the carbon fibres can be increased by a layer of collagen.

7. Intraosseus anchorages of the carbon fibre ligaments after 12 weeks of implantation exhibit strengths corresponding to 49–107% of the rupture strength of natural ligaments.

References

Alexander, H., Aragona, J., Parson, J., Weiss, A., Strauchler, I. and Mayott, C. (1981), A filamentous carbon-absorbable polymer medial collateral ligament replacement. *Transaction of the 7th Annual Meeting of the Society of Biomaterials*, Vol. 4, p. 129.

Böder, H., Gölden, D., Rose, Ph. and H. Würmseher (1981) Kohlenstoffasern-Herstellung, Eigenschaften, Verwendung. *Z. Werkstofftech.*, **11**, 275–81.

Burri, C. (1980) Grundlagen des Kniebandersatzes durch Kohlenstoff. *Unfallheilkunde*, **83**, 208–13.

Burri, C. and Neugebauer, R. (1981), Technik des alloplastischen Bandersatzes mit Kohlefasern. *Unfallchirurgie*, **7**, 289–97.

Claes, L., Burri, C. and Neugebauer, R. (1981), Biomechanik des Bandersatzes mit Kohlenstoffasern, in *Kapselbandläsionen des Kniegelenkes* (eds. M. Jäger, M. H. Hackenbroch and Refior, H. J.), Georg Thieme, Stuttgart, New York, pp. 56–61.

Claes, L., Burri, C., Neugebauer, R., Wolter, D. and Rose, P. (1979), The elasticity of various carbon fibre ligament prostheses. *2nd Meeting of the European Society of Biomechanics*, Strasbourg.

Claes, L., Burri, C., Neugebauer, R. and Wolter, D. (1981), Biomechanische Untersuchungen zum alloplastischen Ersatz von Bändern mit elastischen Kohlenstoffaser-Bandprothesen, in *Biomaterialien, Chirurgische Implantate und künstliche Organe* (eds F. Unger and J. Hager), Verlag Erdmann-Brenger, Munich, M. 219–21.

Claes, L. and Mutschler, W. (1981) Elektrische Messung von Dehungen und Kräften an den Kollateralbändern des menschlichen Knies, in *Kapselbandläsionen des Kniegelenkes* (eds M. Jäger, M. H. Hackenbroch and M. J. Refior) Georg Thieme, Stuttgart, New York, pp. 34–9.

Claes, L., Burri, C., Mutschler, W. and Plank, E. (1978), Measurement of stress and strain on ligaments with strain gauge cells. *Conference Digest of the 1st International Conference on Mechanics in Medicine and Biology*, pp. 136–9.

Edward, R. G., Lafferty, Y. S. and Lange, K. O. (1970), Ligament strain in the human knee. *J. Basic Eng.*, **92**, 131–6.

Fitzer, E., Fiedler, A. and Müller, D. (1971), Die Herstellung von Kohlenstoffasern mit hohem Elastizitätsmodul und hoher Festigkeit. *Z. Chem. Ing. Tech.*, **43**, 923–32.

Hartung, C. H. (1975), Zur Biomechanik weicher Gewebe. *Fortschr. Ber. VDI-Z.*, **17**, VDI Verlag, Düsseldorf.

Jenkins, D. H. R. (1978), The repair of cruciate ligaments with flexible carbon fibre. *J. Bone Joint Surg.*, **60B**, 520–2.

Kennedy, J. C., Hawkins, R. J., Willis, R. B. and Danylchuk, K. D. (1976), Tension studies of human knee ligaments. *J. Bone Joint Surg.*, **58A**, 350–55.

Neugebauer, R., Burri, C. and Claes, L. (1981), Tierexperimentelle Untersuchungen mit Kohlenstoffbändern, in *Kapselbandläsionen des Kniegelenkes* (eds M. Jäger, M. H. Hackenbroch and H. J. Refior), Georg Thieme, Stuttgart, New York, pp. 51–4.

Neugebauer, R., Burri, C., Helbing, G. and Wolter, D. (1979), The anchorage of carbon fibre strands into bone, a biomechanical and biological evalution on knee joints. *Digest of the 2nd Meeting of European Society of Biomechanics*, Strasbourg.

Neugebauer, R., Burri, C., Claes, L. and Helbing, G. (1981), *In vitro-* und *in vivo-* Untersuchungen zur Fixation von Kohlenstoffasersträngen als Bandersatz am Kniegelenk, in *Biomaterialien, Chirurgische Implantate und Künstliche Organe* (eds F. Unger and J. Hager) Verlag Erdmann-Brenger, Munich, pp. 222–5.

Noyes, F. R. and Grood, E. S. (1976), The strength of the anterior cruciate ligament in humans and rhesus monkeys. *J. Bone Joint Surg.*, **58A**, 1074–82.

Noyes, F. R. (1977), Functional properties of knee ligaments and alterations induced by immobilization. *Clin. Orthop.*, **123**, 210–42.

Piziali, R. L., Rastegar, J., Nagel, D. A. and Schurman, D. J. (1980), The contribution of the cruciate ligaments to the load-displacement characteristics of the human knee joint. *J. Biomech. Eng.* **102**, 277–83.

Tremblay, G. R., Laurin, C. A. and Drovin, G. (1980), The challenge of prosthetic cruciate ligament replacement. *Clin. Orthop. Rel. Res.*, **147**, 88–92.

Trent, P. S., Walker, P. S. and Wolf, B. (1976), Ligament length patterns, strength and rotational axes of the knee joint. *Clin. Orthop. Rel. Res.*, **117**, 263–70.

Wang, C. J., Walker, P. S. and Wolf, B. (1973), The effects of flexion and rotation on the length pattern of the ligaments of the knee. *J. Biomech.*, **6**, 587–96.

Wirth, C. J. (1981), Biomechanik des Kapselbandapparates des Kniegelenkes, in *Kapselbandläsionen des Kniegelenkes* (ed. M. Jager, M. H. Hackenbroch and H. J. Refior), Georg Thieme, Stuttgart, New York, pp. 2–12.

Wolter, D., Burri, C., Fitzer, E., Helbing, G., Müller, A. and Rüter, A. (1978), Der alloplastische Ersatz des medialen Knieseitenbandes durch beschichtete Kohlenstoffasern. *Unfallheilkunde*, **81**, 390–7.

Wolter, D., Claes, L., Burri, C. and Neugebauer, R. (1979), Untersuchungen zur intraossären Verankerung von Kohlenstoffasern beim Schaf. *Langenbecks Archiv. Chir.*, **Suppl.**, 221–4.

14 Carbon fibre III: Operative techniques and instrumentation

A. STROVER

14.1 Introduction

This chapter deals with some of the technical aspects of the use of carbon fibre tow in the repair of knee ligaments and with the development of operative techniques and instruments specifically designed to utilize the advantages of the material and to minimize its disadvantages.

The novel contribution of carbon fibre in the surgical field is two fold; its biological encouragement of collagen tissue ingrowth into its interstices, and its excellent mechanical strength in tension.

The ability of carbon fibre to induce fibrous tissue to grow along its fibrils was discovered in experimental animals in whom tendons or ligaments were excised and replaced by carbon fibre tows (Jenkins *et al.*, 1977, Forster *et al.*, 1978). The prolific ingrowth of collagenous tissue into the carbon fibre tow is probably related to the presence of an active healing process in the area of the excised structure. When this experimental evidence is related to human practice, it is logical to assume that carbon fibre will work best in acute ligamentous tears and disruptions. In the chronic injury, where the local reaction has subsided, the fibrous tissue response is unlikely to be as lively, and I have therefore considered acute injuries of ligaments and tendons to be the prime indication for the use of carbon fibre. Its mechanical strength allows the material to restore primary stability to an unstable joint, and in this sense carbon fibre can act as an internal fixation in a broken ligament, to restore its anatomical configuration and hold it while the healing process goes on.

The techniques described here have been developed during a personal experience of approximately 200 cases over the past 3 years, most of which were acute cases, usually operated upon during the first 2 weeks and occasionally as long as 4 weeks after their injuries. At this stage the remnants of the original ligament are usually able to be clearly identified, and the aim of the operation is to recreate the original anatomy by primary repair reinforced with carbon fibre.

As an implantable material carbon fibre tow displays the following disadvantages:

(1) The uncoated material is hairy and, as the individual fibrils are extremely brittle, they tend to break off during surgical procedures, leaving an unsightly decidua in the operative field.

(2) Also due to the brittle nature, or mechanical stiffness of their fibrils, carbon tows are apt to break whenever they are flexed over an edge with a small radius (of less than approximately 0.8 mm). Breakage tends to occur, therefore, in the following situations:

    (a) on being handled with metallic instruments such as dissecting forceps, artery forceps, needle-holding forceps etc.;

    (b) on being pulled over the sharp edge of a hole drilled in bone;

    (c) on being used as a suture, threaded through any standard surgical sewing needle.

These properties have led to problems in the design and execution of operations for ligament repairs where the aim is to make full use of the mechanical and the biological properties of the material. The main problems in this respect have been firstly in combating the fragility and hairiness of the material, secondly in designing a system of anchorage of the carbon fibre to bone without the use of knots, and thirdly in designing a set of instruments for use with this material.

14.2 Disadvantages of carbon fibre

14.2.1 HAIRINESS OR FLUFFINESS

Fluffiness is reduced to some extent by wetting the carbon fibre with sterile saline or water, but even more effective has been to coat the carbon fibre tow with gelatine. The tow is sterilized by irradiation. During the past 2 years we have used gelatine-coated carbon fibre tows exclusively. The dry gelatine is hard and brittle, however, and it is necessary to soften it by soaking the tow in saline for a few minutes before use. I have used this manoeuvre as an opportunity to impregnate the material with antibiotics usually in the form of 80 mg gentamicin in 20 ml saline.

It is worth repeating that gentle handling of the material without the use of metallic instruments greatly reduces the fragmentation and deciduation of the carbon fibrils from the tow.

14.2.2 ANCHORAGE PROBLEMS

The mechanical stiffness of pure carbon fibre makes it difficult to anchor the material to the tissues and especially to bone, as it will not tolerate being knotted or being stapled. Fixation by a screw and washer may be feasible but it is not recommended due to the electrochemical activity between the carbon and metal (Jenkins and Grigson, 1979).

(a) The bollard

A system of anchorage was therefore designed in the form of a stud or rivet made of carbon/polysulphone composite around which the carbon fibre tow can be wound and trapped between the expanded head of the rivet and bone (Hunt, 1981).

The functional resemblance of this system to a bollard which is used to secure a boat to a quayside led to the use of the term 'bollard' for the polysulphone expanding rivet (Figs 14.1 (a) and 14.2).

The bollard in use at present has a head size of 13 mm diameter and a stem length of 22 mm. The diameter of the unexpanded stem is 5 mm and when the 3 mm central pin is driven home the end of the stem expands to about 7 mm, thus anchoring itself firmly into cancellous bone.

When used as an anchorage for carbon fibre to be attached to bone, the head and neck of the bollard fit into a radiused hole which is made by the bollard drill (Fig. 14.1(b)). This ensures that pressure is evenly distributed on the carbon fibre trapped beneath the bollard head. Having wound the carbon fibre tow around the stem of the bollard, it is introduced into the prepared hole, mounted on the punch tube (fig. 14.1 (c)) into which the central pin fits snugly.

Having adjusted the tension in the carbon fibre tow (see below, p. 274), the bollard is punched down firmly using the punch tube and mallet, and is expanded into place by advancing the central pin by use of the punch itself which fits into the punch tube.

In vitro testing showed that it is best to wind the tow only one-and-a-half times around the bollard to obtain satisfactory anchorage as long as the tow contains not more than 40 000 filaments. It is essential to drive in the bollard perpendicular to the surface of the bone, because tilting its stem away from the direction of the carbon fibre fragments the tow on the edge of the head of the bollard, while tilting it in the opposite direction reduces the frictional area between the tow, the bone and the bollard.

The bollard was found to be overfilled when more than 40 000 filaments were used in the tow to be anchored. In this situation the carbon fibre is not adequately trapped beneath the head of the bollard due to its relative bulkiness.

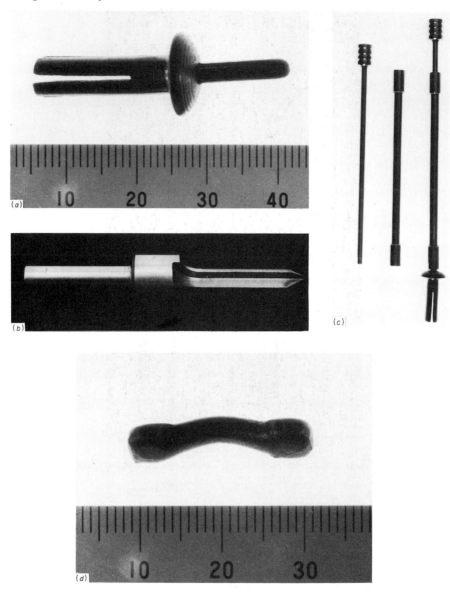

Fig. 14.1 (*a*) The bollard; (*b*) The bollard drill; (*c*) The bollard punch tube and punch; (*d*) The toggle.

(b) The toggle

The looped free end of the carbon fibre lends itself to an even more effective anchorage system than the bollard in the form of a carbon/

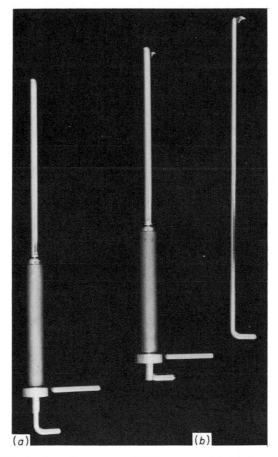

Fig. 14.2 (*a*) The back radius cutter; (*b*) The retractable blade of the back radius cutter.

polysulphone bar which has been called 'the toggle' for its functional resemblance to the duffle-coat toggle or wooden button (Fig. 14.1(d) and Fig. 14.3). When the tow is pulled through a hole in bone the toggle, which has been placed through the free looped end, jams itself transverely across the entrance of the hole resulting in a solid fixation.

(c)   Adjustment of tension

The system of bollard and toggle anchorage offers precise adjustment of tension in the carbon fibre prosthetic ligament and allows for the clinical testing of the stability of a repair on the operating table. Tension is adjusted after one end of the carbon fibre ligament has been anchored to bone. The bollard used for the second point of anchorage is introduced into its hole mounted on the bollard punch tube, with the carbon fibre tow wound a full turn around its stem. The slack is then taken up by pulling on the free end of the carbon fibre tow, and when the desired tension has been obtained the bollard is punched down and locked into place.

The correct tension in the carbon fibre should allow a full range of movement of the joint, but should restrict adequately any abnormal or unphysiological movements. Primary anatomical stability of the joint should be obtained after anchoring the carbon fibre to bone, so that the reconstructed ligament should be restored to its normal anatomical length during the phase of healing.

14.3   Instrumentation

14.3.1   RADIUS CUTTERS

Breakage of tows over the edges of drill holes in bones has largely been solved by rounding off the edges of the holes with radius cutters. Two instruments have been developed for this purpose. The bollard drill is used as a front radius cutter and rounds off the edges of holes accessible from the operative incision. It is made in the form of a self-counter-sinking drill bit (Fig. 14.1(b)).

The back radius cutter (Fig. 14.3(a)) is used on the far edge of a hole which is inaccessible to the front radius cutter. It is used, for example, on the edge of any hole emerging in the intercondylar area of the knee. The instrument is in essence a tube with a slot at one end through which a small retractable blade can be made to protrude (Fig. 14.3(b)).

It is introduced into a 4.8 mm drilled hole in bone with the blade in the retracted position. The functional end is pushed right through the hole and the blade is then made to protrude by a simple arrangement of levers. The handle is then gently pulled back and rotated by hand while the blade engages upon and carves off the edge of the drilled hole. Having completed this operation the blade is again retracted and the instrument removed.

14.3.2   THREADING INSTRUMENTS

Introduction or threading of carbon fibre tow through bony or soft tissue presents several additional problems. Metallic instruments applied directly to the carbon fibre tow and the use of wire or suture materials as railroading devices create the problem of fragmentation. The most practical development for threading carbon fibre tows through drilled holes has been the attachment of a piece of plastic coated steel wire onto one end of the carbon fibre tow (see Fig. 14.2). This introducing probe can be pushed

274

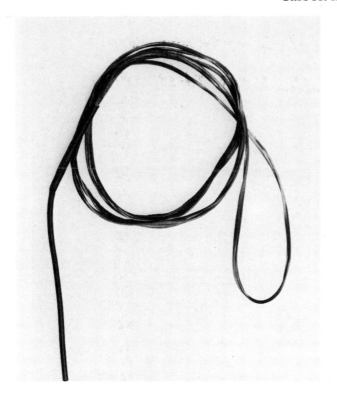

Fig. 14.3 The carbon fibre implant and its plastic-covered wire introducing probe.

into holes and can be handled with forceps. It can also be railroaded using wire or thread.

14.3.3 THE TUBULAR AND SEMITUBULAR GUIDES

In situations where the carbon fibre tow is to be threaded through the substance of tendons and ligaments, such as in the repairs of the collateral ligaments of the knee, tubular and semitubular guides have been found to be particularly useful (Fig. 14.4 (a) and (b)). These instruments are simply pushed through the tissues where they form tunnels through which the tow can be introduced. The straight semitubular guide can also be used in holes through bone where it prevents snagging of the carbon in sharp bony trabeculae.

Correct use of these instruments enables the surgeon to push the carbon through the remnants of the ligament in the direction which replaces the ligament into its original anatomical position.

275

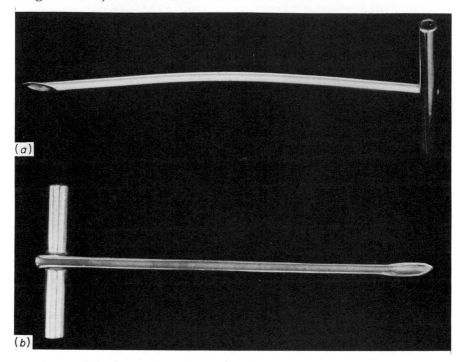

Fig. 14.4 (*a*) The tubular guide; (*b*) The semitubular guide.

14.3.4 THE DRILL JIG

The drill jig (Fig. 14.5 (a)) has been designed to place a hole through the proximal tibia for the anterior approach to the posterior cruciate ligament (see below, p. 287). It is used with a drill bush or sleeve and 4.8 mm drill and has a hole placed in its distal limb for the introduction of the railroading wire (Fig. 14.5 (b)).

Although originally designed for the posterior cruciate ligament, the same drill jig can be used for making the holes for any ligament reconstruction around the knee (see below, p. 282).

14.3.5 THE OVER-THE-TOP HOOK

This instrument (Fig. 14.6 (a) and (b)) has been designed to be introduced through the 'over-the-top' route of MacIntosh (MacIntosh, 1974), that is, to find its way around the posterolateral aspect of the lateral femoral condyle, appearing in the intercondylar notch of the femur. It serves a dual purpose, both as a dissector and as a threading device. In the latter context it is used with the railroading wire (see below, p. 282).

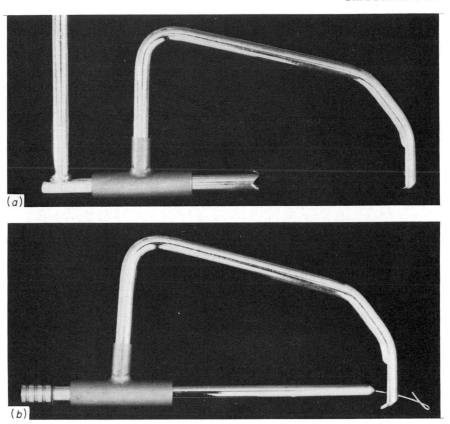

Fig. 14.5 (a) The drill jig; (b) The hole in the end of the drill jig is for the introduction of the lead-wire or railroading wire.

14.3.6 THE RAILROADING WIRE OR LEAD WIRE

This piece of stainless steel wire has a leading loop at the one end in the form of the Greek letter alpha (Fig. 14.7(a)) and a trailing loop in the form of the Greek letter omega (Fig. 14.7(b)). The leading loop has a protruding barb which allows it to be pushed through the hole in the end of the over-the-top hook/dissector and locks to prevent it from being pulled back through the hole (Fig. 14.7 (c)). It thus forms an immediate and powerful linkage when used in this way with the over-the-top hook and also with the hole in the posterior cruciate guide. The trailing end of the railroading wire can be clipped into the loop in the introducing probe (Fig. 14.7 (d)) of the carbon fibre tow and pulled through soft tissue without snagging. The railroading wire thus completes the linkage between the over-the-top

277

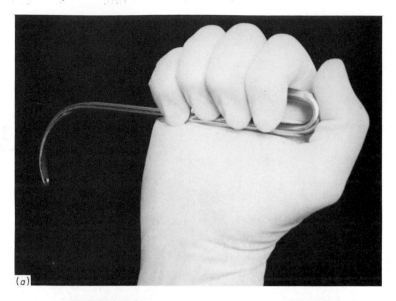

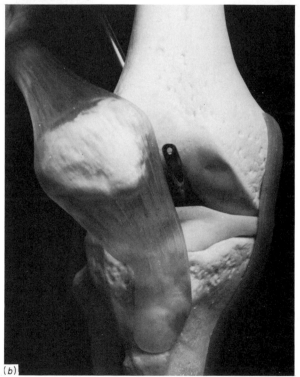

Fig. 14.6 (*a*) The over-the-top hook; (*b*) The over-the-top hook in position.

hook or the posterior cruciate threading device and the carbon fibre tow. It is used in both anterior and posterior cruciate repairs.

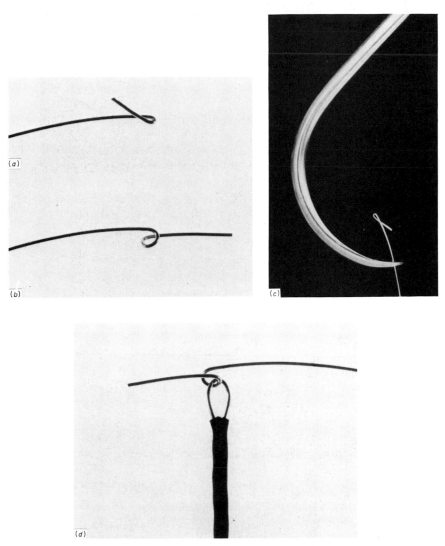

Fig. 14.7 (a) The alpha end of the railroading wire; (b) The omega end; (c) The railroading wire in the over-the-top hook; (d) The railroading wire linked to the introducing probe.

14.4   Indications for carbon fibre repairs of knee ligaments

The most practical time to repair a ruptured knee ligament is immediately after or within days of the injury. Delay leads to contracture of the torn ligament which obscures its normal anatomy and makes it difficult to find its exact bony attachments. Occasionally a torn ligament will reattach itself to the wrong anatomical site. On two occasions, for example, when both anterior and posterior cruciates have been found to be torn off from their femoral attachments, I have found that the posterior cruciate ligament has reattached itself to the origin of the anterior cruciate ligament on the lateral femoral condyle while the anterior cruciate ligament lay free in the intercondylar notch. Had this situation been allowed to persist a grossly unstable knee would have resulted.

Carbon fibre offers a method of regrowing an absent or badly mutilated ligament and if it fails it can be used again in a repeated attempt to restore the damaged anatomy without creating more damage.

14.5   Carbon fibre repair of acutely damaged knee ligaments

14.5.1   PREOPERATIVE EXAMINATION

Before beginning the operation, an examination under general anaesthetic is made with a careful assessment and comparison of the ligamentous laxity of both the affected and the unaffected knee. The aim of the operation is to achieve approximately physiological stability in the affected joint. This means that, if correctly anchored, the carbon fibre should allow a full and free range of movements in the joint and should achieve the same degree of stability as the unaffected joint.

It is a grave error to anchor the carbon fibre tow in an abnormally tight position because not only will the anchorage be put to excessive strain at the limits of the normal ranges of movement, risking failure of the carbon fibre fixation, but also a permanently limited range of movement may result from an abnormally shortened ligament. If any error is to be made, it is better to err on the side of allowing a little too much residual laxity in the carbon fibre.

14.5.2   STRESS RADIOGRAPHS

In my experience the best means of recording the extent and nature of the ligamentous damage in the acutely injured knee, is to take stress radiographs with the patient sedated or under anaesthetic immediately prior to the operation.

Cruciate views are obtained with the patient lying supine and his knee flexed to 90°. A lateral 'shoot through' is taken while the surgeon performs the drawer test anteriorly and posteriorly. Cruciate laxity is manifested by the amount of movement shown by the tibia in relation to the femoral condyles. The approximate centre of rotation of the femoral condyle lies towards its posterior aspect. A line joining the centres of each condyle gives the approximate axis of flexion and extension of the knee joint. A line drawn parallel to the posterior cortex and through the apex of the intercondylar eminence of the tibia should pass through or very close to the axis of flexion and extension.

The collateral ligaments are similarly assessed by anteroposterior radiographs taken while varus and valgus stress is applied with the knee just off full extension. Comparative films of the normal side should be taken whenever there is any doubt about the clinical significance of stress views.

Radiographic assessment of knee ligament injuries is more consistently accurate than clinical testing especially in swollen or fat knees.

14.5.3 POSITIONING OF THE LIMB

The operation is performed under a bloodless field with the knee flexed to 90° hanging freely over the end of the operating table.

14.6 Carbon fibre reinforced repair of the anterior cruciate ligament (ACL)

14.6.1 SURGICAL APPROACH

An anteromedial incision is made extending onto the proximal 4 cm of the tibia distally and allowing lateral dislocation of the patella if necessary.

14.6.2 OPERATIVE FINDINGS

All three compartments of the knee are examined under direct vision and a careful assessment of the joint surfaces, the menisci and the ligaments is made. Having discovered a torn anterior cruciate ligament it is important to determine whether it has been torn off from one of its bony attachments or whether it has been shredded within the body of the ligament. These considerations will influence the direction in which the carbon fibre tow will be introduced through the remnants of the ligament.

In chronic cases this consideration does not apply.

14.6.3 PROCEDURE

The following steps are then carried out in this order:

(1) Using a 4.8 mm drill a hole is made from the anteromedial surface of the tibia beginning about 2 cm distal to the joint surface and emerging within the tibial attachment of the anterior cruciate ligament in the intercondylar area of the tibial plateau. This exercise may be made more precise by using the drill guide (Fig. 14.8).

(2) The proximal and distal openings of the drill hole are radiused using the bollard drill and the back radius cutter. The hole is cleansed of bony debris using a saline rinse.

(3) Through a separate incision about 3 cm in length on the lateral aspect of the knee beginning just above the lateral epicondyle of the femur and extending proximally, a small triangular area of bone on the lateral femoral condyle is exposed deep to the iliotibial tract. The boundaries of this triangular area are precise and should be defined accurately. They consist of the following: anterosuperiorly, the inferior border of the vastus lateralis muscle; posteriorly, the attachments of the iliotibial tract to the supracondylar ridge of the femur; inferiorly the lateral epicondyle of the femur (Fig. 14.9). A bollard hole is placed in the middle of the supracondylar triangle.

(4) The over-the-top hook is now introduced into the supracondylar triangle and is passed around the posterior aspect of the lateral femoral condyle keeping close to the bone until its leading end appears in the intercondylar notch. (see Fig. 14.6 (b)). A little pressure in the direction of the long axis of the instrument and some additional flexion of the knee beyond 90° may be necessary to deliver the end of the hook to view. It is important to avoid entry into the posterior cruciate ligament on the medial side of the intercondylar notch. Some sharp dissection through the remnants of the anterior cruciate ligament may be required to visualize the end of the hook. The alpha end of a railroading wire is now introduced into the hole in the tip of the over-the-top hook and the hook and wire are withdrawn around the femoral condyle (see Fig. 14.7 (c)).

(5) The sequence of events from here on depends upon the operative findings:

(a) When the anterior cruciate ligament has been avulsed from its femoral attachment, the broken end of the ligament is pulled out of the intercondylar notch and two or three stay sutures are placed into it.

The introducing probe of the carbon fibre implant is now threaded through the hole in the tibia and through the substance of the remnant of the anterior cruciate ligament. The semitubular guide is used here to

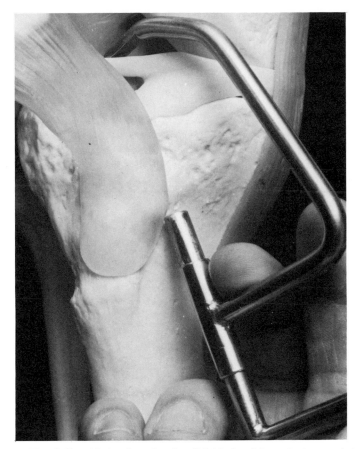

Fig. 14.8 The drill guide in place for the tibial hole of the anterior cruciate repair.

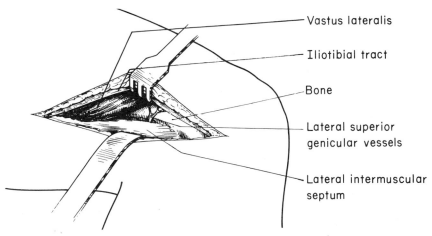

Vastus lateralis

Iliotibial tract

Bone

Lateral superior
genicular vessels

Lateral intermuscular
septum

Fig. 14.9 The lateral supracondylar triangle.

pierce the remnants of the ligament and to facilitate threading of the carbon fibre into its substance.

The stay sutures are passed through the wire loop in the end of the introducing probe which is then linked to the omega (trailing) loop of the railroading wire. Pulling the wire through the over-the-top route now brings the carbon implant and the stay sutures with it.

A toggle placed through the terminal loop of the carbon fibre anchors it at the tibial end.

At the femoral end, a bollard, with the tow wound one-and-a-half times around it, and mounted on the bollard punch tube, is introduced into the prepared bollard hole and held in place loosely by hand.

The tension in the carbon fibre is now adjusted and the bollard is seated down by tapping the punch tube with a small mallet. The tension in the tow is tested by performing the anterior drawer test and by putting the knee joint through as near a full range of movements as possible. When the correct degree of stability has been achieved the bollard is driven home and expanded as described earlier. The stay sutures are stitched into the iliotibial tract using a curved Mayo needle.

(b) When the ligament has been avulsed from its tibial end, the threading of the carbon fibre must go in the opposite direction, that is, it starts from the lateral femoral condyle, emerges through the inter-condylar notch, continues through the drill hole in the tibia, and ends on a bollard on the anterior surface of the tibia. For this purpose the alpha loop of the wire is bent around to resemble an omega (to prevent snagging on the tissue) and is attached to the introducing probe.

Anchorage on the lateral femoral condyle is secured by means of a bollard placed into the terminal loop of the implant. On the tibia it is best to bring the carbon fibre under the pes anserinus and anchor it to a bollard placed under the distal edge of the pes.

The stay sutures on the anterior cruciate ligament are brought through the hole in the tibia and sewn down to soft tissue on the front of the tibia.

(c) Where the ligament has torn in its middle or stretched within its substance, it is immaterial in which direction the carbon fibre is threaded.

(6) The carbon fibre tow is always cut off about 1.5 to 2 cm from a bollard and the free end is sutured down to periosteum or other soft tissue using interrupted sutures. This acts as an additional security to prevent unwinding of the tow around the bollard.

(7) The knee should now be gently flexed and extended to ensure that there is no restriction of movement which may indicate that the carbon has been secured in an excessively tight position. From this moment on

the knee is held in flexion while haemostasis is secured and the wound is closed in layers.

(8) Examination of the intercondylar area should now show that the carbon fibre tow has been placed retrosynovially and within the remnants of the ligament. If any of the tow remains uncovered it should be buried by closing soft tissue over it using fine interrupted sutures. It is desirable that the carbon should be buried towards the posterior part of the ligamentous tissue to allow the ingrown of neurovascular and fibrous elements to proceed from the retrosynovial tissues.

A well-padded plaster of paris splint is applied to keep the patient's knee between 20° and 30° of flexion, and this position is maintained in bed with elevation of the limb.

14.7 Postoperative management

During the postoperative phase load is transferred by stages from the carbon fibre to the newly formed ligament as the carbon fibre fragments and new collagen tissue is formed. The amount of protection needed during this phase depends upon the following combination of factors:

(1) the nature of the injury;
(2) the duration of symptoms, that is, acute or chronic;
(3) the operative findings;
(4) the mechanical adequacy of the carbon fibre support as judged on the operating table.

The personality of the patient also influences the surgeon to protect his repair for a relatively longer or shorter period of time. In my experience if the repair is going to fail it nearly always fails within the first 12 months after the operation. Three of my cases returned to active sport 3 months postoperatively and experienced a painful click during active exercise with subsequent demonstrable laxity of the ligament.

In the acute case where a single torn ligament has been repaired and in which an excellent fixation of the carbon fibre tow has given good primary stability on the operating table, the padded plaster of paris splint and dressings are removed after 5 days and gentle limited knee movements are allowed in a hinged cast-brace with the hinge blocked to allow movement only between 20° and 60°. The patient is allowed partial weight-bearing on crutches and after 6 weeks the cast-brace is removed and he is allowed to mobilize the knee walking only for at least 6 weeks. Full movement of the knee is not encouraged until after 3 months postoperatively.

Where extensive damage has occurred in the acute case but where excellent primary stability has been obtained at operation, a period of 4 weeks in a plaster cast may be followed by a hinged cast-brace with limited flexion and extension for 6 weeks and thereafter the patient should wear a knee brace of the Lennox-Hill type to protect the knee for 12 months

When the compliance of the patient is suspect for any reason a longer period in a plaster of paris cast may be necessary, but more than 6 weeks full immobilization is not recommended.

14.8 Carbon fibre reinforced repair of the posterior cruciate ligament (PCL)

14.8.1 APPROACH

The anterior approach to the posterior cruciate ligament (Strover, 1982) has been found to be practical and quick. The skin incision is identical to that used for the anterior cruciate ligament.

14.8.2 FINDINGS

The ligament may have been avulsed from either of its attachments or it may be shredded or stretched within its substance. These considerations once again decide the direction in which the carbon fibre should be introduced.

13.8.3 PROCEDURE

(1) If the synovium over the anterior part of the ligament is intact, this is incised and dissected off the ligament revealing the nature of the injury (Fig. 14.10 (a)).

(a) When the ligament has been avulsed from its posterior, or tibial, attachment the broken end is hooked forwards and delivered through the intercondylar notch. Two or three stay sutures of 2/0 absorbable thread are attached to the end of the ligament anteriorly.
(b) Where detachment has occurred from the anterior or femoral end, the synovium is usually also torn. Stay sutures on the free, anterior end now retract the ligament laterally.
(c) No stay sutures can be applied to the ligament shredded in its substance.

(2) The over-the-top hook is now introduced through the synovial defect in the intercondylar notch and a soft tissue track is dissected over the back of the tibial plateau to reach a point about 2 cm distal to its

posterior rim in the midline. This approximates the tibial attachment of the posterior cruciate ligament (Fig. 14.10 (b)).

(3) The drill jig is then introduced through the intercondylar area over the head of the tibia to reach the posterior aspect of the bone (Fig. 14.10 (c)).

When correctly positioned for the drill hole the connecting limb of the drill jig should run parallel to the tibial plateau.

(4) A 4.8 mm drill hole is made from front to back to reach about the middle of the tibial origin of the posterior cruciate ligament. A radiograph on the operating table may be used to confirm whether or not the drill hole has been correctly placed.

The drill bit and jig are removed and the drill hole is radiused front and back (Fig. 14.10 (d)).

(5) The wire-threading tube is now fitted into the jig and placed through the drill hole in the tibia. As the end of the tube touches the drill jig posteriorly a palpable click is felt. If there is soft tissue interposed between jig and tube this click is absent, and the soft tissue may be cleared by the use of the drill bit which is placed through the drill jig and turned by hand until metal upon metal is felt.

(6) With the threading tube in position the leading loop of the railroading wire is pushed down the tube and emerges through the hole in the drill guide. This loop locks automatically (Fig. 14.10 (e)) and the threading tube is removed leaving the wire *in situ*. On removal of the drill jig the wire is now drawn through the intercondylar region from posterior to anterior completing a full loop through the bone and over the head of the tibia (Fig. 14.10(f)).

(7) Using the drill jig a 4.8 mm hole is drilled through the medial femoral condyle to emerge in the middle of the femoral attachment of the posterior cruciate ligament. Having radiused the hole front and back, the pathway for threading the carbon fibre is now complete.

(a) If the ligament has been avulsed from its tibial attachment the threading begins through the medial femoral condyle. The leading loop of the railroading wire is bent to ensure that its free end trails through the soft tissues without snagging. It is attached to the introducing probe of the carbon fibre tow and threaded through the tibia.

(b) If the femoral attachment of the ligament has been avulsed or detached the threading will begin from the tibial side by linking the introducing probe onto the trailing end of the railroading wire. In either event the carbon fibre will be pulled in the direction which replaces the remnants of the ligament most closely into their anatomical position. The carbon fibre tow is anchored by a toggle in its looped end and by a bollard at its other end, having adjusted the tension.

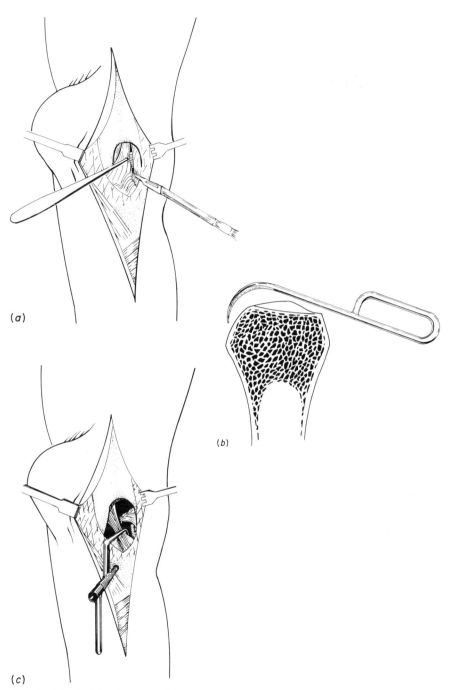

(a)

(b)

(c)

Fig. 14.10 (a) The intercondylar synovial curtain is incised and dissected off the posterior cruciate ligament; (b) The over-the-top hook dissects a track to reach the tibial attachment of the posterior cruciate ligament; (c) The drill jig in position for

288

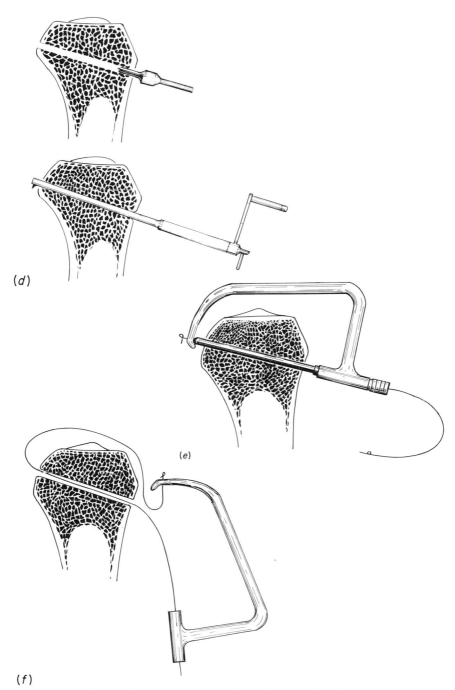

(d)

(e)

(f)

the P.C.L. drill hole (d) The drill hole is radiused front and back; (e) The railroading wire locks through the hole in the drill jig; (f) The railroading wire is pulled over the head of the tibia.

The excess of the tow is cut off and its free end is sutured down to soft tissues. The bollard and toggle are buried under deep fascia, and the synovial covering in the intercondylar notch is reattached by interrupted sutures.

14.8.4 CLOSURE

After irrigating the wound with saline and an antibiotic it is closed in layers with suction drainage.

Postoperative management is the same as for the anterior cruciate ligament. It should again be stressed that early stability may lead one to a false sense of achievement and full sporting activities should be delayed for 1 year.

14.9 Repair of the medial collateral ligament

14.9.1 APPROACH

This repair again begins with a standard medial arthrotomy and full examination of the joint. To gain access to the medial collateral ligament from this situation the skin incision is enlarged proximally and distally, turning posteriorly at both ends to expose the tendons of the pes anserinus distally and the distal muscle fibres of the vastus medialis proximally. A skin flap is raised to expose the medial epicondyle of the femur and both parts of the medial collateral ligament are carefully dissected out.

14.9.2 FINDINGS

An area of contusion indicates the site of pathology in acute cases. The femoral origin of the ligament may be avulsed and often takes a small flake of bone with it. The parallel part of the ligament (Brantigan and Voshell, 1945) may be torn in isolation and often detaches itself from its tibial origin under the tendons of the pes anserinus. The oblique part of the ligament may also be torn in isolation. It is found posterior to the parallel part with its tibial attachment much closer to the joint line. Commonly both elements of the ligament are torn or stretched and it is always worth stabilizing them as well as approximating the discontinuous pieces. Where it has been disrupted, the attachment of the medial collateral ligament to the meniscus should be restored.

The aim of the repair is to stabilize a broken ligament by burying carbon fibre tow into its substance and by attaching it to the tibial and femoral origins of the ligament.

Burying is achieved by the use of the tubular introducer (Fig. 14.11 (a)), or by splitting the ligament longitudinally and suturing it, using a round-bodied needle, over the carbon fibre tow.

Anchorage is gained by three bollards placed at the following three points:

(1) the medial epicondyle of the femur;
(2) the distal end of the parallel portion;
(3) the middle of the tibial attachment of the oblique portion of the ligament.

It is practical to start at the posterior tibial bollard passing upwards to the femoral bollard, round this once and down to the anterior tibial bollard which is placed at the distal margin of the pes anserinus.

The stability of the repaired ligament is tested in various degrees of flexion having ensured that none of the carbon remains superficial to the ligament.

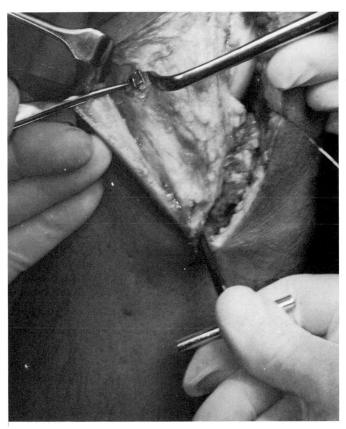

Fig. 14.11 Burying the carbon fibre is achieved by the use of the tubular guide.

14.9.3 CLOSURE

The wound is closed in layers as before and postoperative treatment is the same as for the cruciate ligament.

14.10 Repair of the lateral collateral ligament

Rupture of the lateral collateral ligament is frequently associated with rupture of other structures on the lateral side of the knee. A careful examination of the common peroneal nerve, the biceps tendon, the popliteus tendon, and the iliotibial tract is necessary both before and during the operation. It is also essential to examine the internal structures of the knee, and a medial arthrotomy or arthroscopy is a prerequisite to the repair of the lateral collateral ligament.

14.10.1 POSITIONING OF THE LIMB

Unlike the repairs of the cruciates and medial collateral ligament the repair of the lateral collateral ligament is most easily done with the knee nearly straight as the iliotibial tract tends to obscure the femoral origin of the ligament when the knee is flexed. The two structures – that is, the lateral collateral ligament and the iliotibial tract – move independently of one another and must be carefully identified during the surgical exposure.

14.10.2 APPROACH

A lateral approach is made beginning about 2 cm proximal to the origin of the ligament on the lateral epicondyle of the femur and extending 1 or 2 cm distal to the subcutaneous prominence of the fibular head. The following structures should be defined and positively identified:

(1) The posterior edge of the iliotibial tract in the anterior part of the incision.

(2) The biceps tendon towards the posterior part of the incision inserting in the head of the fibula.

(3) The tendon of popliteus on the lateral femoral condyle deep to the lateral collateral ligament.

(4) The common peroneal (lateral popliteal) nerve which lies deep and posterior to the biceps tendon; it is advisable to mark this important structure with a tape.

(5) The lateral patellar retinaculum of the vastus lateralis which may

292

appear in the proximal corner of the wound deep to the iliotibial tract.

(6) The remnants of the ruptured lateral collateral ligament which, in the acute case can be identified by an area of contusion which indicates the traumatized area. In the chronic case the lateral structures may be extensively scarred and adherent to one another. Any or all of them may have been involved in the original traumatic pathology and may have gained abnormal attachments. It is worth spending the time to sort out these scarified and malunited elements in order to reposition them in their correct plane.

14.10.3 PROCEDURE

(1) Having discovered the origin of the lateral collateral ligament on the lateral epicondyle of the femur, a bollard hole is drilled in this position at 90° to the surface of the bone.

(2) The neck of the fibula is cleared of soft tissue on its anterior surface for about 2 cm, and a 4.8 mm drill hole is made from anterior to posterior using the bollard drill and taking care to avoid the common peroneal nerve. The hole should traverse the junction of the head and neck of the fibula and the exit of the hole may require to be completed using the 4.8 mm drill bit.

(3) The posterior edge of the hole is rounded off using the back radius cutter.

(4) The remnants of the lateral collateral ligament are now pierced throughout their entire length by the tubular or semitubular guides in order to create a complete coverage for the carbon fibre.

(5) Carbon fibre tow is either introduced through the hole in the fibula and anchored by a toggle in its looped end or anchored by a bollard at this point. It is passed through the remnants of the ligament and fixed to a bollard on the lateral femoral condyle, with the required amount of tension. The direction in which it is threaded is determined by the pathology found. The movements of the knee are gently tested to ensure that the separate lateral structures move individually and that the carbon fibre tow has been positioned correctly.

14.10.4 CLOSURE AND POSTOPERATIVE CARE

The free ends of the carbon fibre tow are sutured down to soft tissue and all other exposed carbon is carefully buried in the tissue of the collateral ligament.

Other damaged lateral structures are repaired or reattached to their anatomical insertions where possible. Carbon fibre may be used in

Ligament Injuries and their Treatment

reinforcing the reattachment of the biceps tendon, the iliotibial tract and the popliteus tendon. These structures may be anchored to bone using bollards.

The wound is closed in layers, with suction drainage and the knee is immobilized in 20–30° of flexion.

Gentle movements are permitted in bed from the 5th to about the 10th postoperative day. If the repair was deemed to be well anchored and to have involved only the lateral collateral ligament, immobilization in a plaster cast is optional. I have treated several cases without any immobilization but the patient is encouraged to use non-weight-bearing crutches for 4–6 weeks.

If more than one ligament has been repaired the usual plaster cast is applied on the 11th day.

Postoperative stiffness is not a problem which I have encountered with this procedure when the ligament has been ruptured or avulsed in isolation, but when physiotherapy is used it must be stressed that total rehabilitation should not be aimed at too early.

14.11   Repair of combined ligamentous injuries

More often than not more than one ligament is involved in acute injuries to the knee and in these cases a single anchorage point may be placed in a convenient position to work for two or more ligaments. The following is a brief description of some typical combined repairs.

14.11.1   RUPTURED ANTERIOR CRUCIATE AND LATERAL COLLATERAL LIGAMENTS

In this case a bollard inserted at the lateral epicondyle of the femur may be shared by the lateral collateral and anterior cruciate ligaments.

14.11.2   COMBINED ANTERIOR CRUCIATE AND POSTERIOR CRUCIATE REPAIR

Only one bollard may be required on the tibia, depending on the direction in which the carbon has to be threaded. This situation arises when the anterior cruciate has been avulsed from its tibial origin and the posterior cruciate from its femoral origin, or conversely, when the anterior cruciate has been detached from its femoral origin and the posterior cruciate from its tibial origin. In other situations separate anchorage points are necessary for the individual ligaments.

A note of caution about the use of railroading wires is necessary here.

There is a danger of the carbon fibre tows being snagged and torn in the intercondylar notch when threading them past each other in combined anterior and posterior cruciate repairs. The use of nylon thread has been useful to avoid this danger.

14.11.3 COMBINED POSTERIOR CRUCIATE AND MEDIAL COLLATERAL REPAIR

Both ligaments may be approached by a long medial parapatellar incision extending rather more medially than one would normally do for a posterior cruciate repair alone. Drill holes are made and the railroading wire is positioned as described for the posterior cruciate repair, and the three bollard sites are positioned for the repair of the medial collateral ligament. The direction of the threading is planned according to the pathology found, and it is often possible to use a continuous carbon fibre tow, sharing the anchorage point at the distal border of the pes anserinus, and burying the carbon fibre under the pes by using the tubular introducer.

14.11.4 OTHER COMBINATIONS

Without going into details of the other combinations of ligament injuries that may occur around the knee joint, suffice it to say that the anchorage points and directions of threading of the carbon fibre can always be worked out by identifying the pathology and threading the carbon fibre accordingly. Where toggle fixation is possible it should be used as it is mechanically far more reliable than bollard fixation.

14.12 Concluding remarks

This chapter has dealt with our attempts to overcome the disadvantages of carbon fibre as a surgical material and to take full advantage of its mechanical properties. The tensile strength of carbon fibre is quite adequate for a tow containing 40 000 filaments to function as a prosthetic ligament independent of tissue ingrowth. The danger of fragmentation due to its mechanical stiffness is the main drawback in this context, however, and our efforts have been chiefly directed towards eliminating any situation which may result in falling short of the critical radius of 0.8 mm. To some extent we have been successful in this quest but the search for simpler and more effective techniques continues.

The solution to the problem of anchorage to bone is likewise an interim solution because, whereas the toggle appears to be completely satisfactory in its function, the bollard displays several dubious characteristics. Firstly, anchorage of the bollard in osteoporotic bone is tenuous. Secondly, the edge of the head of the bollard may be punched down onto the carbon tow if it is not placed perpendicular to the bone surface. This results in fragmentation of the tow. Thirdly, anchorage about the bollard depends upon friction and may be lost with any loosening or incomplete seating of the bollard. Attention to these technical details, therefore, is important if primary stability of the joint is to be achieved.

The question of whether primary stability using carbon fibre is either desirable or necessary has been asked. Burri and Neugebauer (1981) and Weiss and Alexander (personal communication, 1981) argue that collagen is significantly more elastic than carbon fibre and that bony anchorage of the tow may result in abnormally restricted joint movements. While it is conceded that it is possible to anchor the carbon fibre in an unphysiological position, which may result in a stiff joint, if the correct anatomical positioning of the carbon fibre is achieved, and if enough laxity allowed to permit full movements of the joint, unphysiological restriction of the movements cannot occur. The subsequent collagen ingrowth, furthermore, will be protected throughout the full range of movements of the joint.

The necessity of achieving primary stability can best be argued by considering the example of a ruptured anterior cruciate and lateral collateral ligament. The intact posterior cruciate ligament, pes anserinus muscles, popliteus muscle and quadriceps muscles now act both passively and actively in concert to shift the centre of rotation of the knee medially and to stretch the remaining lateral structures resulting in a chronic lateral pivot shift. It is almost impossible for any healing ligament on the lateral side of the knee to heal in its natural length unless actual mechanical opposition is brought to bear against the elastic deforming forces of the other intact ligaments.

In order to heal in its anatomical length, it is necessary, therefore, to appose the broken ends of the ligament and, until they are sufficiently healed, to protect the repair by restraining all the deforming forces.

A properly anchored carbon fibre repair constitutes the most plausible form of restraint in this context and should protect the damaged ligament during the early phases of healing.

Finally, the biological deposition of collagenous tissue into a carbon fibre scaffolding depends on the presence of actively proliferating fibroblasts. These in turn require an adequate blood supply and probably an intact nerve supply. We have observed that carbon fibre tow when placed intrasynovially does not gain an adequate ingrowth of fibrous tissue and it is for this reason as well as those outlined above that it is essential to place the carbon fibre tow retrosynovially in the intercondylar area.

References

Brantigan, O. C. and Voshell, A. F. (1943), The tibial collateral ligament: its function, its bursae, and its relation to the medial meniscus. *J. Bone Joint Surg.,* **25(1)**, 121–31.

Burri, C. and Neugebauer, R. (1981), Technik des alloplastischen Bandersatzes mit Kohlefasern. *Unfallchirurgie,* **7(6)**, 289–97.

Forster, I. W., Rális, Z. A., McKibbon, B. and Jenkins, D. H. R. (1978), Biological reaction to carbon fibre implants. The formation and structure of a carbon-induced 'neotendon'. *Clin. Orthop. Rel. Res.,* **131**, 299–00.

Hunt, M. S. (1951), An introduction to the use of carbon fibre reinforced composite materials for surgical implants. *CSIR Report ME 1689* Pretoria, South Africa.

Jenkins, G. H. and Grigson, C. J. (1979), The fabrication of artifacts out of glassy carbon and carbon fibre reinforced carbon for biomedical applications. *J. Biomed. Mater. Res.,* **13**, 371–94.

Jenkins, D. H. R., Forster, I. W., McKibbon, B. and Ralis, Z. A. (1977), Induction of tendon and ligament formation by carbon implants. *J. Bone Joint Surg.,* **59B**, 53–7.

MacIntosh, D. L. (1974), Acute tears of the anterior cruciate ligament. Over-the-top repair. *Presented at the Annual Meeting of the American Academy of Orthopaedic Surgeons, Dallas, Texas.*

Strover, A. E. (1982), The anterior approach to the posterior cruciate ligament. *A scientific display presented at the Autumn Meeting of the British Orthopaedic Association, Manchester, United Kingdom.*

15   *Carbon fibre IV: Ligamentous reconstruction*

M. LEMAIRE

15.1   Introduction

In the great majority of cases only two ligaments are involved in chronic instability of the knee: the anterior cruciate ligament (ACL) and the medial collateral ligament (MCL).

Since 1961, I have treated instability due to rupture of the anterior cruciate ligament by an anterolateral extra-articular plasty procedure, using a strip of facia lata (Lemaire, 1967). This does not replace the anterior cruciate ligament, since it does not follow its anatomical insertions, but its aim is merely to compensate the ligament for its essential functional role: internal rotation of the knee. I have performed this technique personally on more than 3000 occasions, making successive technical improvements. These improvements have made it possible to eliminate all need for postoperative immobilization. This has been my practice since 1973.

For the medial collateral ligament, classical techniques give results of poor immediate stability, and long immobilization in plaster cast is necessary. The example of plasty procedures for rupture of the anterior cruciate ligament clearly demonstrates the superiority of operations not followed by immobilization. By improving techniques of transfer of pes anserinus tendons, I have achieved more accurate anatomical results, an immediately stronger plasty, and it has been possible to eliminate progressively plaster cast immobilization. From 1968 to 1979, 315 plasty procedures were performed on the medial surface of the knee with, and then subsequently without, plaster cast immobilization. However, results remained variable, despite the precise nature of the technique. During reoperations, the failure was usually found to be due to degeneration of the transferred tendon which had become reduced to a simple cord, and with no functional value whatsoever.

In 1979, numerous experimental studies involving carbon fibres appeared to be quite conclusive. Under certain conditions and with certain reservations, these could be used without risk in human surgery. Thus strengthening of the transferred tendon by carbon fibres provided a solution to our principal problem for medial collateral ligament plasty procedures. In my department, 452 such procedures involving the medial collateral ligament have been carried out, including 297 by myself using two different techniques with pes anserinus tendons, strengthened with carbon fibres, and without any postoperative immobilization.

15.2 Palliative extra-articular technique for rupture of the anterior cruciate ligament

Since 1961, the technique of this procedure has been gradually improved, primarily in relation to its femoral fixation. However, the principle has remained the same: it is an extra-articular operation designed to stop excessive internal rotation of the knee, which is allowed by rupture of the anterior cruciate ligament. It is the abnormal amplitude of this internal rotation which causes instability, resulting from rupture of the ligament. Such problems are faithfully reproduced by the shift in internal rotation. This is the most reliable clinical sign of rupture of the anterior cruciate ligament. It is never present without rupture of the ligament, and no other lesion can cause it. I have been using this sign since 1964 and described it in 1967. Signs described, using the terms 'jerk test', 'pivot shift', etc. are later variants only.

The search for an extra-articular operation was justified, and is still justified, by repeated failures of intra-articular procedures designed to replace the anterior cruciate ligament. An operation placing a prosthetic ligament between the anatomical insertions of the ligament must have a very high percentage rate of success, and enable rapid recovery. Furthermore failure of such a prosthesis should not make the patient's condition worse in comparison with its preoperative state. It must always be remembered that the disability due to rupture of this ligament is relatively moderate. Only the eagerness to continue sporting activity without risk justifies surgical treatment. All intra-articular procedures suggested up to the present are far too major if instability due to rupture of the anterior cruciate ligament is put in its real place, and they involve a high risk of deterioration.

On the other hand, the complex structure of the anterior cruciate ligament must be borne in mind. It generally consists of two bands, each of which plays its own physiological role. There is no technique which makes it possible to reconstitute these two bands anatomically. This incompetence is proven by the fact that all intra-articular procedures are strengthened by an extra-articular anterolateral plasty. All the intra-articular procedures reconstruct only the anteromedial bundle of the anterior cruciate ligament. This controls the anterior drawer sign.

Our extra-articular technique does not pretend to replace the ligament. It seeks merely to control internal rotation which is no longer controlled by the ruptured anterior cruciate ligament. It avoids problems of instability, thereby preventing progressive degeneration of the joint. However, since it does not precisely reproduce the anatomy of the ligament, it decreases, but does not cause complete disappearance, of the anterior drawer sign, or the Lachman extension drawer sign. This abnormal anterior movement of the tibia is very well tolerated if its amplitude is low. If larger, the knee's instability demonstrates by virtue of a defect the anterior oblique ligament. It controls the anterior movement of the tibia in association with the anteromedial band of the anterior cruciate ligament. In fact, the choice between an intra-articular or an extra-articular procedure, is the choice of controlling the anterior movement of the tibia by reconstructing either the anteromedial band of the anterior cruciate ligament or the anterior oblique ligament (Lemaire and Miremad, 1983a).

The technique of the anterolateral operation to control the internal rotation is far from easy. It is very precise, with knee flexed between 45 and 60° and placed in complete external rotation, since it is internal rotation which must be controlled.

The principle of the operation is to stretch a strong band of fascia lata from its tibial attachment to Gerdy's tubercule to the upper insertion of the lateral collateral ligament. All the difficulty lies in the superior fixation to the femoral condyle. Only immaculate technique during this stage of the operation makes it possible to avoid postoperative immobilization, so potentially harmful for the joint (Lemaire and Combelles, 1980). The steps are as follows:

(1) The band used for the procedure is cut from the fascia lata, retaining its insertion into the tibia. It must be completely regular and cut following the direction of the fibres. It must measure at least 15 cm in length and 15 mm in width. All useless fatty tissue is carefully removed.

(2) The last 2 cm of the lateral collateral ligament, close to the femoral insertion, are freed, completely circling the ligament. After freeing the two edges, anterior and posterior, the underlying face is also freed, this being done very gently, in order to avoid damage to the synovial fold in contact with it.

(3) The fixation point of the plasty to the femur must then be prepared. The periosteum is separated from the bone using a rugine, taking great care not to risk the insertion of the lateral collateral ligament. It is necessary to remain posterior to its insertion. This periosteal separation,

starts immediately behind the ligament insertion, and must be continued for approximately 3 cm. This procedure is very difficult to do well without tearing the periosteum, but it is nevertheless highly important if the operation is to succeed.

(4) A bone tunnel is dug into the condyle, starting below and behind the insertion of the ligament, almost in contact with it. Superiorly, it reaches the end of the subperiosteal detachment. This tunnel cannot be made properly, and cleaned of small bone debris, without a special rasp for the digging and calibrating of tunnels in bone (Fig. 15.1).

(5) If the course has been well prepared, insertion of the plasty and stretching it presents no problem. The plasty is first passed below the upper part of the lateral collateral ligament (Fig. 15.2), then in the subperiosteal detachment (Fig. 15.3). It is then stretched, with the maximum tension possible, constantly confirming the position of the leg, which must remain in complete external rotation. A few sutures fix the plasty to the insertion of the ligament and to the detached periosteum. These are very strong tissues and, from this time onwards, there is no longer any risk of slackening of the plasty to the end of the operation.

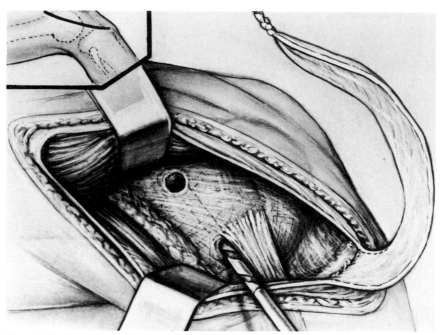

Fig. 15.1 Extra-articular procedure for rupture of the anterior cruciate ligament; the strip of the iliotibial band has been cut, and a bone tunnel is made into the lateral femoral condyle; it begins close behind the upper insertion of the lateral collateral ligament.

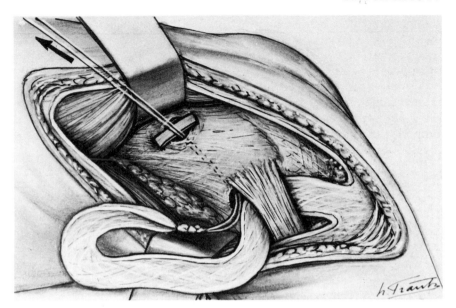

Fig. 15.2 Shows the strip which goes under the lateral collateral ligament; the periosteum has been released from the bone.

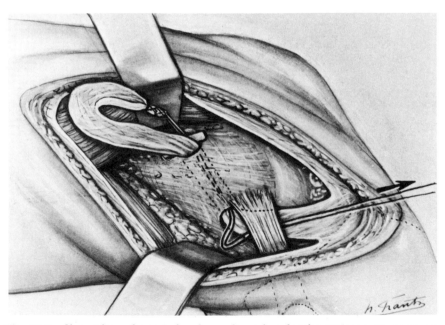

Fig. 15.3 Shows how the strip has been slipped under the periosteum, en route to the bone tunnel.

303

Ligament Injuries and their Treatment

(6) The plasty is then passed from above downwards, through the bone tunnel. It thus arrives behind the upper extremity of the ligament. It once again passes beneath the upper part of the ligament. It is then stretched very vigorously, in order to apply full tension of the intraosseous portion. It is then folded back on its initial portion, in order to provide a double layer. There it is very carefully sutured, since this suture, with those used for fixation to the lateral collateral ligament and to the periosteum, are the only means of attachment until fixation within the bone tunnel occurs, as a result of tissue growth (Fig. 15.4).

(7) Finally, the fascia lata is sutured. In order to oppose the edges well, it is useful to completely free the posterior one and to place the knee in extension which relaxes the aponeurosis.

No immobilization is necessary. However, the knee must be placed in complete extension as soon as operation has ended. The longer extension is delayed, the more difficult it is to obtain.

15.3 Techniques for the correction of medial laxity

Two techniques are used, one corresponding to correction of superior lesions, and the other to inferior lesions. Both of them are technically difficult.

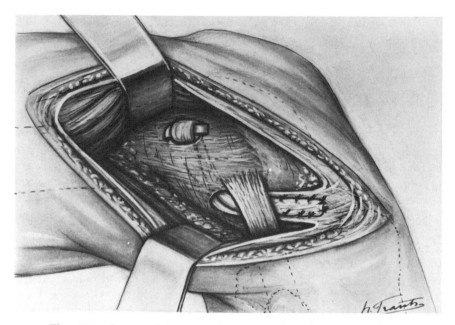

Fig. 15.4 Suture of the distal part of the strip to the proximal part.

15.3.1 COMMON PROBLEMS

Regardless of the technique, the two essential points are: absolute accuracy in the procedure and its immediate solidity (Lemaire and Miremad, 1983b).

(a) Accuracy of the technique

The course of the plasty must very precisely correspond to that of the normal medial collateral ligament. The lower part of the ligament is always clearly visible, since its edges stand out clearly against the surrounding tissues. Even if the scar of the initial tear is low, it is easy to identify the remains of the ligament above and below it. The same does not apply to the upper extremity; the insertion crest is always easily found, but it is not possible to place a marker in the middle of this insertion accurately, since both its anterior and posterior borders are poorly defined. In addition, the initial tear is most often located in the upper part of the ligament. It is thus later swamped in a mass of fibrous scar tissue, making precise location impossible, although this is essential. Only the use of a pair of compasses can provide the necessary accuracy (Fig. 15.5).

A marker is placed as low as possible in the middle of the medial collateral ligament, choosing the lowest area situated where the edges are clearly visible. The insertion crest may be easily located above by displacing vastus medialis. By trial and error and compass measurements, it is necessary to find on this crest the precise point remaining equidistant from the marker placed on the lower end, in mobilization of the knee from 0 through 90°.

This compass measurement is essential, otherwise the final result will be totally inaccurate.

(b) Identification of the initial lesion

In order to make a choice between the two techniques suggested, the initial lesion must be located with precision. Sometimes the scar is clearly visible, by dissection of the medial surface of the knee, underneath the aponeurosis of the sartorius muscle. However, very often, the haematoma following the accident leaves very diffuse fibrous tissue, and it is then impossible to localize accurately the precise site of the lesion. An incision must be made through the full thickness of the tissues from the upper insertion to the marker placed at the lower end. By examining the edges of this trench, the scar tissue zone may be easily found. At this time, the choice may be made between the two techniques described: one for lesions situated above the joint line and the other for those situated between the joint line and the lower insertion of the ligament.

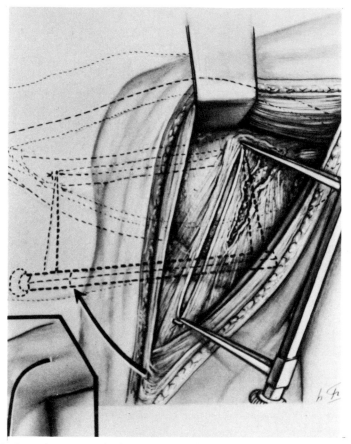

Fig. 15.5 Locating precisely the upper insertion of the medial collateral ligament by the use of dividers.

(c) *Immediate solidity of the procedure*

This is necessary in order to avoid the need for postoperative immobilization. There are two essential phases common to both procedures.

(i) Anchoring of the plasty in a bone tunnel
All other techniques are inadequate and do not definitely ensure solid fixation. However, this implies the need for a curved, intraosseous tunnel, through which the plasty may be passed without difficulty. In practice, it is virtually impossible to do this without using our special curved rasp. The two orifices of the tunnel are dug approximately 3 cm apart, and the tunnel is completed using the rasp only. However, this

306

instrument is difficult to use and, in particular, attention must be paid not to enlarge the orifice of the tunnel situated at the upper insertion of the medial collateral ligament. It must remain calibrated at 5 mm. If it were inadvertently widened, the plasty would be mobile within it and the method lose all its accuracy.

If an orifice of the tunnel is situated in an area where the bone cortex is relatively fragile, it is wise to hem the edge of the orifice, using a round staple. This precaution avoids possible section of the bone, by the highly stretched plasty, which would obviously interfere with function of the result.

(ii) Strengthening of the transplanted tendon, using carbon fibres

Carbon fibres have the remarkable ability to induce the formation of well-oriented collagen tissue. It strengthens, and may even take over the role of the transplanted tendon. In this area, as in that of biocompatibility, carbon fibres would appear to be superior to all other types of material.

It is experimentally important to avoid dispersal of the fibres. For this reason their inclusion in the tendon selected for transplantation is felt to be necessary. A trocar, 20 cm in length and 2 mm in diameter, is slid to within the thickness of the tendon itself. The manoeuvre is difficult and the trocar can only be advanced very slowly. It is necessary to confirm patiently and constantly that the tendon is not perforated on any of its surfaces. The inserted part of the trocar must go widely beyond the effective zone of the plasty, both above and below. After removal of the introducer, a loop of suture material is inserted into the trocar. This is used to pull through 20 000 carbon fibres, that is, a double 10 000-fibre mesh. A simple withdrawal of trocar leaves the fibres included in the tendon. In our experience, a larger number of fibres is of no value in this case, and may even be harmful. These 20 000 fibres ensure a very marked immediate strengthening and progressively induce the production of a cord of collagen tissue that is highly effective in the support role which the plasty must play.

It is important to avoid the use of large numbers of carbon fibres. The major disadvantage of these fibres is that it is impossible to predict how much collagen tissue will be produced in contact with them. For a given number of fibres, the amount may differ widely from one individual to another. The possible development of an excessively large mass of tissue which it would be necessary subsequently to excise, must be borne in mind. This should lead to great caution in the use of large amounts of fibres.

Ligament Injuries and their Treatment

(d) Restoration of tension to the various parts of the medial collateral ligament and the capsula

In the present state of our knowledge, a plasty cannot hope to replace the medial collateral ligament totally, particularly since, with the exception of certain types of low disinsertion, the lesion of the principal superficial layer is almost always accompanied by a tear in the deep capsular layer, especially in its posteromedial part. The aim of the plasty is to serve as a support, allowing for cautious rehabilitation without waiting for the complete deep healing, that is, 45 days. Good recovery of stability may only result from capsular and ligament healing, in addition to the plasty. Permanent stability is ensured by healing of the structures under appropriate tension. The plasty is designed to provide immediate and temporary stability and to provide subsequent strengthening. This is certainly important, but inadequate alone.

After making a longitudinal incision in the middle of the ligament, and along its whole length, and after having thus identified the scar of the initial lesion, the various capsular structures must be tested in order to find those which are damaged and to assess how tension may be restored to them. By far the commonest case is stretching of the group of structures formed by the medial collateral ligament and the posteromedial capsular layer. This laxity corresponds to poor healing of an upper tear of the medial collateral ligament. The capsuloligamentous layer is detached and pulled upwards and forwards, while the leg is placed in external rotation, thus bringing forwards the tibial insertion of the strong, posterior capsular bundle. In this position, the flap is reinserted with a staple. However, this staple must be inserted very carefully, ensuring that there is no interference with articular range in flexion/extension.

It is much easier to restore tension following a low disinsertion of the ligament, and inserting the staple is then no longer associated with any risk.

At the present time, it is relatively rare to encounter old lesions of the middle part of the ligament. These correspond to a very severe initial lesion with immediate, major medial laxity, almost always associated with rupture of the anterior cruciate ligament and often a lesion of the medial meniscus. This classical triad is now usually treated as a semi-emergency, and residual medial laxity under such circumstances has become rare. However, in old lesions the restoration of tension is quite delicate, since it is necessary to section more or less transversly, within scar tissue only, in order to restore tension by a simple 'overcoat' suture.

15.3.2 PLASTY FOR A TEAR OF THE UPPER PART OF THE MEDIAL COLLATERAL LIGAMENT

This is selected after the initial two stages of all medial plasty procedures. The upper insertion of the ligament is located using a compass. The ligament is then cut lengthwise in order to identify the site of the original lesion (Fig. 15.6). In addition, restoration of tension to the capsulo-ligamentous layer has been prepared. The procedure is as follows.

(1) The tendon of the gracilis muscle is gently separated from that of semitendinosus and is disinserted from the bone. It is strengthened by inclusion of 20 000 carbon fibres, using the technique described. Care must be taken here to insert the trocar as close as possible to the end of the

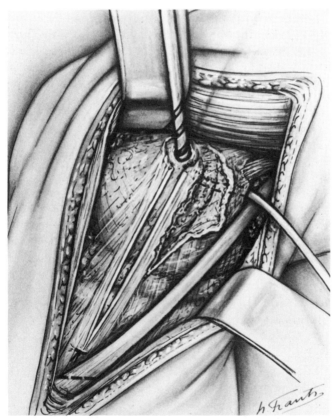

Fig. 15.6 Procedure for a rupture of the medial collateral ligament at its upper part; a bone tunnel is made from the insertion of the medial collateral ligament, located with the dividers, to the insertion of the adductor magnus and the gracilis tendon is divided from its insertion.

tendon (Fig. 15.7a). The useful part of the plasty will be the terminal portion of the tendon.

(2) A tunnel is dug in the bone from the upper insertion of the medial collateral ligament. It must arrive immediately below the insertion of adductor magnus. It is dug taking great care not to widen its anterior orifice.

(3) The plasty is passed from behind forwards, in the bone tunnel, and will lie in the long trench fashioned in the ligament (Fig. 15.7b). It is preferable not to apply excessive traction, since this would distend the musculotendinous junction and cause pain, or even a torn muscle, during rehabilitation. The end of the plasty is attached by a few sutures to the two edges of the trench into the ligament (Fig. 15.8a).

(4) The plasty is then stretched as much as possible, by vigorous traction upwards, exerted on the first part of the tendon before it enters the bone tunnel. During this manoeuvre, the knee must be placed in internal rotation, in order to make the ligament vertical. This tension is fixed by a few sutures attaching the plasty to the tendon of adductor magnus. At this point, it is very important to confirm the precise accuracy of the technique by a few flexion extension movements during which the plasty must remain perfectly stretched.

(5) In order to achieve the required tension in the relaxed capsular ligament complex one staple is used. It is necessary to confirm that these do not limit flexion/extension. With a certain degree of familiarity and a little luck, one staple may transfix the bone tunnel and provide very strong fixation in it for the plasty (Fig. 15.8b).

At any event, it is attached to the adductor tendon and, all along its course in the medial collateral ligament, to both edges of the longitudinal incision, by a series of sutures, taking care when the needle is passed through the plasty to pick up only very little tissue, in order to avoid the inclusion of carbon fibres in the knots. These carbon fibres are very fragile when subjected to torsion and could thus be subjected to serious deterioration if included in a knot.

This upper plasty is the most widely used procedure for ruptures of the medial collateral ligament. It is suitable for more than 90% of cases of medial laxity.

15.3.3 PLASTY FOR A TEAR OF THE LOWER PART OF THE MEDIAL COLLATERAL LIGAMENT

This is a very old technique. The author has been using it since 1970 and published a first description in 1975. However, since that time it has been progressively improved, in particular in 1979, by reinforcement using carbon fibres.

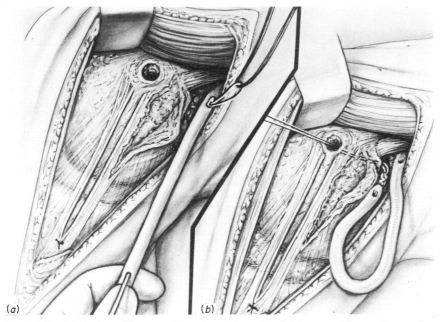

Fig. 15.7 (*a*) Carbon fibres are introduced into the thickness of the tendon, using a trocar. (*b*) The tendon with carbon fibres inserted through the bone tunnel.

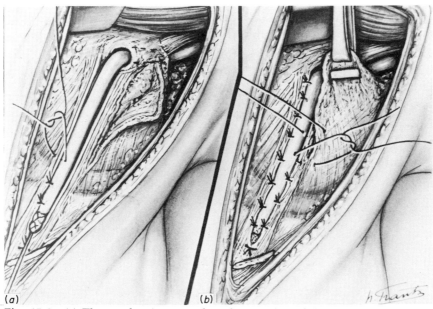

Fig. 15.8 (*a*) The tendon is sutured to the remains of the ligament which are carefully tightened. (*b*) The posterior part of the capsula has been pulled forward and upward and fixed with a staple.

311

It complements the above technique, since it is suitable for those cases where, after the longitudinal incision is made through the middle of the ligament, the fibrous scar appears to be too low to be suitable for treatment under good conditions, using the upper plasty. In practice, it is used for lesions situated below the insertion of the capsular layer onto the periphery of the meniscus, at the level of the joint line.

As always, the beginning of the operation consists of the use of compasses to identify the upper insertion of the ligament, which is then incised along its whole length in order to find the fibrous scar of the initial lesion. This is followed by a review of distended structures to which tension must be restored.

(1) In the upper plasty procedure, restoration of capsuloligamentous tension is best performed at the end of the operation. However, here and by contrast, the ligament must be stretched at the beginning of the operation. If the initial lesion was tibial disinsertion, then the scar is completely freed. It is pulled downwards, the knee being in varus and internal rotation and it is easily fixed in an appropriate position, using a staple. If the scar is at the level of the joint line, or slightly below it, then the ligament should be sectioned, without hesitation, following the oblique transverse scar. Tension is restored to the ligament merely by a series of sutures, just as in the case of a recent lesion.

(2) This plasty, performed from below upwards, will require a very long tendon. It is for this reason that the tendon of semitendinosus must be used, even though this requires functional sacrifice of semitendinosus muscle, which is much more important, particularly in athletes, than the gracilis. The tendon, freed as high as possible, in the muscle itself, is left inserted into the tibia (Fig. 15.9). It will run from below upwards in the trench made within the ligament up to the upper insertion of the ligament. It will be attached in a bone tunnel and will return from below downwards, thereby turning back on itself.

(3) The first stage consists of digging the bone tunnel to be used for anchoring. The upper insertion site, identified using compasses, is gently calibrated to a diameter of 5 mm (Fig. 15.10). The vastus medialis muscle is displaced upwards. The tunnel is fashioned, using drill, gimlet and curved rasp, in the prolongation of the trench made in the ligament. The cortex beneath the vastus medialis is not strong, and in order to protect the bone it is wise to place a round staple, tangent to the lower border of the orifice.

(4) The periosteum is incised between the two orifices of the tunnel, and is extensively detached on each side, using a rugine, thereby creating two flaps which will be used to fix the plasty.

(5) The tendon of semitendinosus is then freed, going as high as

312

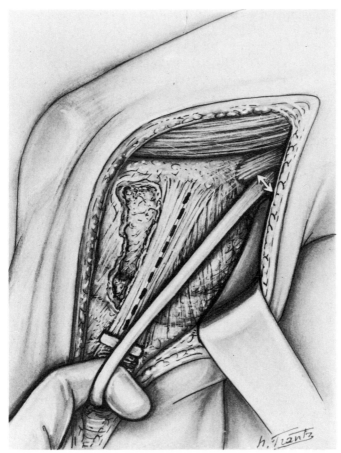

Fig. 15.9 Procedure for a rupture of the lower part of the medial collateral ligament; the remains of the ligament has been tightened and fixed with a staple. The semitendinosus is cut as high as possible, into the muscle, the cut being made the length of the ligament in the middle.

possible. It is strengthened by the inclusion of a mesh of 20 000 carbon fibres. This inclusion should be started as close as possible to the bone insertion onto the tibia.

(6) The plasty is placed into the trench in the ligament. It passes from below upwards in the bone tunnel; it is stretched to the maximum, then brought back down, with the traction maintained (Fig. 15.11).

(7) It is first fixed to the two persiosteal flaps, between the two orifices of the tunnel. It is essential at this time to confirm the precision of the procedure by flexion/extension movements during which the plasty must remain very precisely stretched (Fig. 15.12).

313

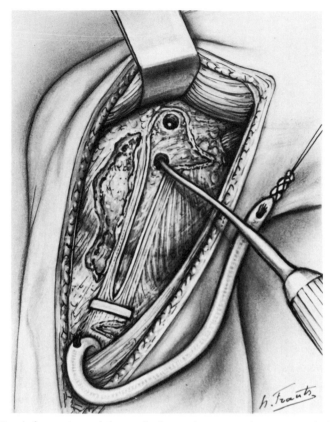

Fig. 15.10 A bone tunnel is made from the upper insertion of the medial collateral ligament placed with the dividers into the femoral cortex under the vastus medialis. Note the carbon fibres included into the tendon.

(8) The terminal portion is fixed to the initial portion and to the two edges of the trench, in order to obtain a very solid final result. This suturing must be made very carefully, first in order not to take up in the sutures the carbon fibres which would be subject to deterioration if the knots were tightened, and secondly, to ensure the coherence of the final result, since there is no other method of fixation.

15.4 Postoperative care

All of these techniques provide immediately a very strong result, requiring no immobilization. However, it is important to be sure that the knee is in extension as soon as the patient recovers from anaesthesia. The later

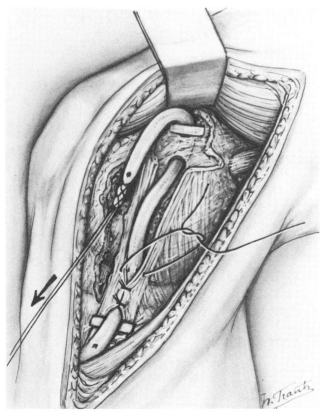

Fig. 15.11 Shows how the tendon has been slipped through the bone tunnel; a staple protects the inferior edge of the superior exit of the tunnel. The tendon when strongly tightened could cut the bone.

such extension is achieved, the more difficult it is to obtain full extension. This is of great importance. By contrast, flexion is always obtained without any great problem, and it is rare that flexion under general anaesthesia is required. However, this is essential if rehabilitation does not result in any progress in flexion, during a 2-week period. If this period is exceeded, then mobilization is more difficult, recovery is more painful and takes longer and is less certain.

In the elderly patient, weight-bearing is allowed as soon as the drain is removed. In the young athletic patient, it is wiser to forbid weight-bearing for 2 weeks, while waiting for healing of the superficial tissues. However, in all cases, from the day following operation, isometric contractions of the quadriceps are begun hourly and for increasingly longer periods.

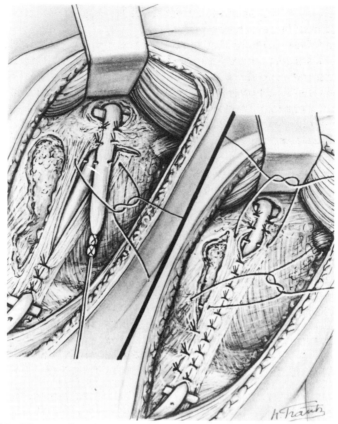

Fig. 15.12 The tendon is sutured to the two parts of the medial collateral ligament. If this is a fresh tear, the capsule is sutured also very carefully.

Crutches are completely eliminated 2 weeks after operation, and walking with weight-bearing presents no difficulty.

Rehabilitation is easy and must be applied rapidly. Long walks should be possible 6 weeks after the operation. Time off work never exceeds 2 months.

15.5 Results

In the short term, results of these ligament reconstruction operations for old lesions are excellent in 60–92% of cases, according to the combinations of lesions present. The best figures are obviously obtained with isolated rupture of one ligament, and the worst in cases involving

316

combined lesions of several ligaments. This is especially true, if the two menisci are to be resected.

With a follow-up period of 4 years, my results remain unchanged, if at the time of surgery, there was not already noteable cartilagenous damage to the femoral condyle. In that case, despite stabilization of the knee, a cartilagenous lesion continues to progress. This is undoubtedly the most important prognostic factor in such operations. Lesions of the cartilage unfortunately develop relatively quickly, and 3 years after the initial accident, instability of the knee is responsible for severe cartilagenous lesion in 50% of cases, especially if the patient attempts to continue with even moderate and intermittent athletic activity.

Thus, stabilization of the knee must be undertaken as soon as possible after the initial accident.

References

Lemaire, M. (1967), Ruptures anciennes du ligament croisé antérieur du genou. *J. Chir. (Paris)*, **93**, 311–20.

Lemaire, M. (1975), Instabilités chroniques du genou. *J. Chir. (Paris)*, **110**, 281–94.

Lemaire, M. and Combelles, F. (1980), Technique actuelle de plastie ligamentaire pour rupture ancienne du L.C.A. *Rev. Chir. Orthop.*, **66**, 523–5.

Lemaire, M. and Miremad, C. (1983(a)), Les instabilités chroniques antérieures et internes du genou. Etude théorique. Diagnostic clinique et radiologique. *Rev. Chir. Orthop.*, **69**, 3–16.

Lemaire, M. and Miremad, C. (1983(b)). Les instabilités chroniques antérieures et internes du genou. Traitement. *Rev. Chir. Orthop.*, **69**, 591–601.

16 Bovine xenografts

WILLIAM C. McMASTER AND NORMAN R. JAFFE

16.1 Introduction

Ligaments and tendons compromised by injury or disease pose difficult surgical dilemmas particularly when prior attempts at reconstruction have failed or when multiple structures require reconstruction. While the use of autogenous structures for such reconstructions is the commonly employed solution, the sacrifice of normal functioning units to act as donors may in itself produce disability. If the procedure utilizing the autologous material fails or is inadequate, the patient may be left with multiple disabilities which may result in a more compromised situation.

Homologous graft tissues prepared by freeze-drying or other preservation and sterilization techniques have been used in the past as an alternative to autogenous structures. Peacock was successful in implanting allograft flexor tendons and their sheaths from cadaver sources with excellent acceptance and clinical function without demonstrating evidence of rejection or immune phenomenon (Peacock and Madden, 1967). Others have replicated this work using various techniques for preservation of the collagenous material with well-documented long-term success in multiple indications and applications (Bright and Green, 1981; Iselin and Pezi, 1976; Salamon et al., 1976). While the apparent clinical success of allograft materials would seem to indicate them as suitable replacements for native structures, there may be difficulty procuring sufficient numbers of donors. The quality of the harvested materials may be inadequate and yield percentages too low for a successful commercial venture. Therefore, most attempts to provide homologous tissues have been on a small-scale individual basis in institutions especially equipped to undertake such an effort.

If one leaves the biological area and considers other materials which might be suitable for such devices, the polymeric materials are a most logical choice. Prosthetic devices intended to augment or substitute for the native or autologous structures have been fabricated from various

319

biocompatible polymers such as dacron, polytetrafluoroethylene (PTFE), polypropylene, and polyethylene. Although these materials have shown promise in bench testing and have often demonstrated high strength, reactivity and deterioration in the *in vivo* environment continues to plague their successful application, particularly in the synovial cavity of the knee joint (Chen and Black, 1980; Noyes, 1981). Carbon filament materials have been broadly used and have seen extensive human experience over the course of time (Alexander *et al.*, 1981; Jenkins *et al.*, 1977). These materials demonstrate high strength in tension and appear to be biocompatible. However, they tend to exhibit extreme brittleness in flexion and fragmentation of the carbon strands is commonplace (Rushton, Dandy and Naylor, 1983). Coating the bare carbon fibre with polylactic acid or collagen to encourage ingrowth and reduce handling problems does not reduce the fragmentation of the material. In sheep, regional lymph node migration of microscopic fragments of the implant has been demonstrated. This has yet to be demonstrated in man or other species. When these materials do fragment intra-articularly, they produce a diffuse staining of articular cartilage and the synovium. What effect this may have on the articular cartilage has not been determined. Parsons *et al* (1983) have postulated that free carbon particles do not alter cartilage mechanics but like talc produce a synovitis which is however less intense. The use of carbon fibre outside the joint space has been successful. Well-documented biological host ingrowth has been described. One problem in these locales is the hypertrophy which occurs and may expand the mass of the original implant up to four times.

These and other problems both real and perceived led to the investigation of xenogeneic sources to provide appropriate tissues of quality and quantity necessary for the fabrication of devices for ligament and tendon reconstruction. The Xenotech Laboratories tendon and ligament bioprostheses are comprised of bovine tendons and ligaments which have been processed in a manner which results in (1) morphologic preservation, (2) conservation of biomechanical characteristics, and (3) biocompatibility. The major component of the bioprostheses is collagen. Collagen, a ubiquitous protein occurring in almost all organisms of the various animal phyla, is to a large part generic in form and function, that is, it invariably serves as the major extracellular structural protein and possesses a chemically similar composition across many distantly related species. It is also one of the unique molecules of the body in that its structure and to some degree function can be conserved long after removal from, or death of, the organism. These characteristics are importantly linked to the success of collagen as a prosthetic material.

16.2 Chemical stabilization of xenografts

The collagen molecule consists of three chains of amino acids bound together in what is commonly referred to as a triple helix. Each of the individual chains comprising the helix is composed of various amino acids, the basic component of all proteins. At both ends of each individual chain of amino acids is a portion which does not participate in the helix resulting in a non-helical extension at each end of the collagen molecule. The significance of these non-helical extensions will become more obvious as we consider how the individual molecules form the larger fibrils.

It is the central helical portion, comprising more than 95% of the molecule, which determines the shape of the molecule and confers its structural and subsequently functional properties. The triple-helical conformation is stabilized by bonds between the three individual peptide chains and by the bonds that hold the chains themselves together, that is, the peptide bonds linking the various adjacent amino acids. These peptide bonds are oriented so that they are buried within the interior of the helix. This unique orientation of the bonds within the triple helix results in the molecule being quite resistant to chemical and enzymatic attack. Finally, and most important with regard to how the individual collagen molecules interact to form the collagen fibril, is the presence of the amino acid lysine in both the helical and non-helical portions of the molecule. As is the case with the other amino acids in the collagen molecule, the part of the lysine molecule participating in the peptide linkage between it and adjacent amino acids is buried within the helix as discussed above; however, the carbon chain, and especially the reactive amine portion of the molecule, are oriented toward the 'outer surface' of the collagen molecule and available for chemical modification and/or reaction.

The collagen fibril is formed by the aggregation or coalescence of individual collagen molecules. How the collagen molecules come to be precisely aligned one next to the other, as it turns out in a staggered fashion, is not completely understood; it is known that during this process the reactive site of a lysine in one molecule reacts with that of another and forms a native or natural crosslink between the two lysine residues. The results of this 'crosslinking' reaction between a lysine residue of another collagen molecule have not been definitively described. The natural crosslink process consists of converting some lysines to aldehyde lysines followed by the reaction of the amine-containing lysine with the converted aldehyde form of lysine.

Figure 16.1 illustrates the coalescence of collagen molecules. The

Ligament Injuries and their Treatment

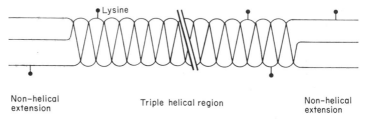

Fig. 16.1 Representation of the collagen molecule illustrating the helical and non-helical regions and lysine extensions; for illustrative purpose the helical region is shown as disproportionate to the non-helical region.

crosslinks are shown as vertical lines and generally occur between the non-helical extension of one molecule and the helical portion of another. The result of this 'polymerization' of the collagen molecules is the formation of the collagen fibril; this is the often-described structure at the electron microscopic level which consists of a single 'fibre-like' structure possessing a characteristic crossbanding pattern. Collagen fibrils represent the mature form of collagen and are the basic structural components of tendons and ligaments.

Once removed from the body, collagenous structures begin to lose their functional properties, most likely as a result of desiccation placed under stress they relinquish their mechanical characteristics as a result of crosslink failure or breakdown without the benefit of repair. These changes occur, albeit slowly, even in those instances where the material which may be destined as a graft is from the recipient's own body.

Since the intermolecular crosslink is the key to the maintenance of collagen's form and function it would seem reasonable to assume that increasing the number of crosslinks should result in a more stable material.

Not all of the lysine residues in the helical portion of the molecule are necessarily involved in native or natural crosslinks. Reasons for this may be that the lysines are not close enough to participate in the crosslinking reaction or that the converted aldehyde form is not available at particular lysine locations. One method by which the lysines may become involved in a crosslinking reaction is by providing a molecule with the proper reactive sites as well as the necessary molecular length to bridge the various distances between lysine residues.

Returning for a moment to the previous discussion concerning natural crosslinks in collagen, it was rather empirically stated that the amine groups of the amino acid lysine have a high affinity for aldehyde groups. In the native state the aldehyde was derived from the modification of another lysine. However, under proper conditions the amine groups of the lysine residues may react with other aldehydes to form molecular species similar, if not identical, to that previously described.

One of the most effective chemicals capable of participating in such a reaction is glutaraldehyde, which has been used effectively as a stabilizing and preserving agent for collagenous bioprostheses for more than a decade. Particular success has been realized in cardiovascular devices as exemplified by the well-documented efficacy of the glutaraldehyde processed porcine and bovine heart valve bioprostheses.

Glutaraldehyde is but one of a rather large class of crosslinking agents known as bifunctional reagents. The term 'bifunctional' refers to the presence of two reactive groups within the molecule. These may or may not necessarily be of the same species, but in the case of glutaraldehyde both reactive groups are aldehydes. Glutaraldehyde consists of five carbon atoms bonded together in a chain fashion; at both ends of the five carbon chain is an aldehyde group (Fig. 16.2).

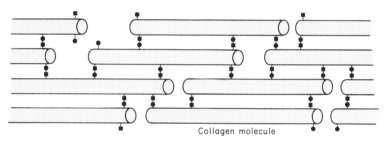

● Lysine
■ Modified lysine

Fig. 16.2 Schematic representation of the 'natural' crosslinking of the collagen molecules in the collagen fibril; each of the 'rods' represent a collagen molecule. The crosslinks are shown restricted to those between a non-helical and helical region of adjacent molecules.

Under some conditions the glutaraldehyde molecules may form polymers. These polymeric chains can be of variable length with each chain terminating at both ends with the reactive aldehyde group. A solution of glutaraldehyde which contains both the monomeric and polymeric forms can result in crosslinks of variable length thereby involving not only crosslinks between closely spaced lysines but between potential crosslink sites that may in molecular terms be quite distant.

With the above information, a model of glutaraldehyde treated collagen can be constructed. This is illustrated in Fig. 16.3 in which glutaraldehyde molecules (G) are shown participating in crosslinks of varying length. Notice that unlike the natural crosslink that usually only occurs

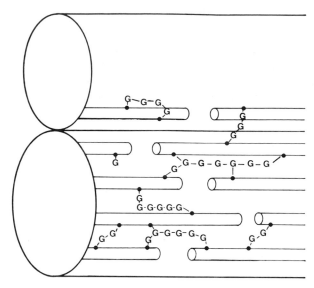

Fig. 16.3 Schematic representation of various glutaraldehyde crosslinks among collagen molecules (small rods) in two adjacent collagen fibrils (large rods); Each 'G' represents a 5-carbon glutaraldehyde molecule.

between two adjacent molecules, the glutaraldehyde crosslink can occur between lysine residues of variably situated molecules, within the same molecule, and even between those occurring in adjacent fibrils.

Collagen stabilized with glutaraldehyde is quite resistant to mechanical, thermal, and chemical modification. However, if the degree of crosslinking is not controlled, the treated material can become both stiff and brittle, characteristics undesirable for tendons and ligaments. This can occur when excess crosslinks are introduced into the collagen matrix or when the balance of the various forms of glutaraldehyde is not controlled. Conversely, if too few crosslinks are present the mechanical stability and resistance to biological modification can be significantly compromised. One of the unique features of the Xenotech Laboratories glutaraldehyde process is that durability and host acceptance are greatly enhanced without sacrificing desirable biomechanic characteristics. This is accomplished by semiquantitative control of the number of sites at which the crosslinking reaction may occur.

In summary, native tendons and ligaments are composed of collagen which has undergone a hierarchical form of organization. The basis of their characteristic properties as collagenous structures is the collagen molecule. The coalescence of the molecules and stabilization of the resulting collagen matrix and anatomic form via the intermolecular crosslink provides the foundation for their functional requirements. Transformation of the tendons and ligaments into bioprotheses is accomplished by further stabilization of the collagen matrix with glutaraldehyde. The conservation of native molecular and anatomical structure without compromise of functional properties is accomplished by controlling the number and nature of the glutaraldehyde crosslinks.

16.3 Animal studies

The investigation of glutaraldehyde fixed and stabilized xenograft material in clinically related animal studies began in 1972. These studies were designed to examine the biocompatibility of the xenograft material, the nature of the healing response, and the effectiveness of the devices in various applications. Early *in vitro* evaluation indicated the glutaraldehyde fixation process rendered the tendon materials stronger (ultimate failure load in tension), slightly stiffer, resistant to crude collagenase digestion, and storable at room temperature (McMaster *et al.*, 1974).

Initial animal implant evaluation included subcutaneous implantation of xenograft materials in rabbit recipients followed up to 1 year. Histological sections of the explants demonstrated unaltered graft material well encapsulated by an organized fibrous scar (Fig. 16.4). Similarly intraperitoneal and intramuscular implants in rats were evaluated by autopsies performed at up to 6 weeks after implantation. Thorough histological survey of brain, kidney, and liver tissue showed no evidence of alteration or neoplastic changes in these tissues.

In order to assess the histological fate of fixed xenograft materials implanted as tendon substitutes, a model of rabbit Achilles tendon replacement was developed in which a segmental resection of Achilles tendon was done and an intercalary implant of xenograft tendon substituted. Evaluation of these grafts up to 1 year after implantation demonstrated maintenance of graft integrity and the ability to provide physiological load transmission. Sections of the graft material demonstrated invasion by host tissues occurring along natural clefts within the graft material. This invasion began early as buds of granulation tissue accompanied by tissue macrophages, fibrocytes and undifferentiated-appearing cells. With time these strands of invading host tissue underwent a maturation in which the cellular elements became fibroblastic in nature. Few foreign body giant cells were seen. Extracellular collagen of host origin was deposited within the invasion areas (McMaster *et al.*, 1974).

To further assess the quantitative properties of the healing response, xenograft tendon was implanted in chicken talons. The chicken talon was

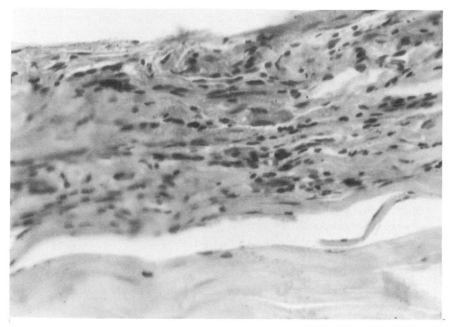

Fig. 16.4 A 1-year implant from the subcutaneous position in the rabbit; the graft material is at the lower border of the slide. The surrounding scar investment is above and appears as mostly collagen with fibroblastic elements.

selected because of the similarity of the talon flexor mechanism to that of the human hand. A segmental resection of the flexor profundus was done and replaced with a xenograft tendon implant. As a control the neighbouring digit underwent a similar procedure in which an autogenous reversal graft was used; 6–0 nylon suture in a simple 90–90 technique was used to produce the anastomosis. It was felt that in subsequent tension studies of the anastomosis site, a 6–0 nylon suture would contribute little to the total strength of the developing scar. The chicken hosts were maintained in a flexed fibreglass cast for 6 weeks. At sacrifice both control and experimental tendons were removed with their investing scar anastomosis. Grossly, the amount and quality of scar tissue surrounding the autogenous reversal graft and the xenograft implant were quite similar. Tensile testing of the distal anastomosis was done in ten consecutive animals. The results of these tests showed that the tensile strengths of the connecting scar were the same for both the xenograft and control group (McMaster, 1975).

A series of animal evaluations were also done to assess the function of xenograft materials in ligamentous positions. The first of these examined the use of the xenograft as a collateral ligament utilizing the rabbit knee as a model. In this study the medial collateral ligament of the knee joint was excised surgically, and replaced with a length of xenograft material which closely approximated the width and mass of the excised collateral ligament. Bone fixation was accomplished by small wire staples fashioned from Kirschner wire. The animals were followed over a period up to 1 year. The graft materials were histologically evaluated by whole knee sections. The results demonstrated that the graft functioned well in stabilizing the knee against valgus deformity; histologically, host tissue ingrowth was noted throughout the substance of the graft material. Host acceptance appeared excellent. Cellular evidence of reactivity was not identified (Fig. 16.5) (McMaster *et al.*, 1975).

To further assess function as a collateral ligament replacement a series of implants was done in dog hosts. The canine medial collateral ligament was surgically excised and replaced with a bovine xenograft appropriately narrowed to duplicate the measurements of the excised canine ligament. Fixation was afforded by stapling. Casts were not used postoperatively. Histological evaluations were done on explants of whole knees up to 1 year implant time. Gross examination of these explants revealed a translucent unremarkable host fibrous tissue covering the graft

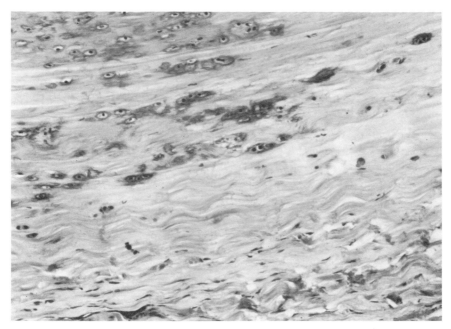

Fig. 16.5 The graft material in this 1-year specimen of a medial collateral replacement in the rabbit adjacent to the bone attachment area demonstrates host ingrowth with some of the host cells undergoing a metaplasia which resembles fibrocartilage with lacunae formation; mineralization is also suggested.

site. Histologically the healing response appeared benign and there was no evidence for collections of reactive or inflammatory tissue. Chronological histological studies revealed that the early healing response consisted of an angioblastic and fibroblastic proliferation of granulation tissue. This early more acute inflammatory process is followed by proliferation of fibroblastic elements and a change of cellular components into a chronic inflammatory phase accompanied by the continued deposition of collagen. This response matures further into a well-organized and vascularized fibrous encapsulation and ingrowth of the graft. No round cell infiltrates, collections of eosinophils or foreign body giant cells were evident (Fig. 16.6).

In a parallel study five animals were used to determine the strength

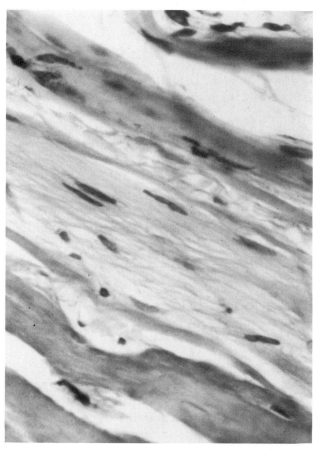

Fig. 16.6 Host ingrowth can be identified in this canine collateral ligament replacement at 6 months; clearly the host fibroblasts are laying down a fine fibrillar collagen.

characteristics of the implanted collateral ligament at an average of 4 months post implant. The fresh harvested knees were held in special jigs on an 1122 Instron. The jigs allowed for alignment of the replaced ligament in parallel with the longitudinal force application of the tensile test. Once set, all other ligament structures were sharply transected and the xenograft implant/bone complex pulled to failure. These tests were performed in the wet state at a strain rate of 50 cm/min. The contralateral limbs were used as controls and were failed under the same testing circumstances. Fixation staples were not removed as they were enveloped by the healing response tissue. Prior to sacrifice, the animals were running and jumping on a regular exercise programme and showed no valgus instability of the knee. Gross inspection of the knees preceding disruptive testing indicated very few degenerative periarticular changes. No meniscus tears were identified. The articular surfaces were well preserved. Results of testing showed an averaged failure at 413 ± 160 N for the xenograft replacement as compared to 760 ± 185 N for the control limbs. All failure of ligament replacement xenografts occurred at fixation sites, no in substance xenograft failures occurred. In the control limbs interstitial failure of the ligament was the mode of failure (McMaster, 1981).

A series of anterior cruciate ligament replacements was done in canine models employing a tendon xenograft with a nominal diameter of 6 mm. Simple resection of the natural anterior cruciate was done surgically. Appropriate bone tunnels were created in the tibia and femur to accommodate the xenograft material which was passed across the knee joint. Attempts were made to place the femoral port high and posterior to avoid a guillotine effect of the intercondylar notch in extension. Fixation was accomplished using barbed staples; proper tension for the graft was determined using the Lachman test with sufficient tension placed on the graft prior to its final fixation to eliminate anterior tibia translation. The fat pad was excised for visualization and to eliminate it as a source of neovascularization for the implanted xenograft material, thereby providing a means to measure host ingrowth from the fixation sites. No cast was used postoperatively and the animals were allowed a free access to activity. The animals were sacrificed at intervals up to 1 year with the knees recovered intact. Visual inspection demonstrated the graft materials to either be partially or totally covered by a synovial investment. The knee joints showed no meniscus tears and minimal evidence of degenerative changes. Occasional marginal osteophytes were noted. No gross disruption of the articular surface was noted. By manual clinical testing the knees were stable. Whole knee sections including the xenograft bone tunnel attachments on both femoral and tibial sides were prepared for histological evaluation. As in the collateral ligament studies

329

host invasion appeared to occur by fibrous ingrowth. Synovial encroachment could be identified surrounding the interarticular portion of the graft material At the extra-articular exit port of the bony tunnels invasion of the graft material, especially at the staple site, could be identified by host elements which were interspersed between the natural clefts within the xenograft (Fig. 16.7). Within the bony tunnels some host tissue ingrowth exhibited a fibrocartilagenous character. In some sections staining characteristics about the developing lacunae suggested mineral deposition. The interarticular portion of the graft showed some evidence of host invasion in the 1 year explants. The grafts were structurally intact and no evidence of gross resorption or replacement of the graft material was noted in this time interval.

Six additional canine subjects were completed employing the surgical techniques in replacing the anterior cruciate ligament. The same postoperative course was followed. One animal was sacrificed soon after surgery due to distemper. Five animals survived and were sacrificed at 4 months. Both knees were removed intact and tested in the fresh state. Failure under tension load was done on an 1122 Instron in special jigs

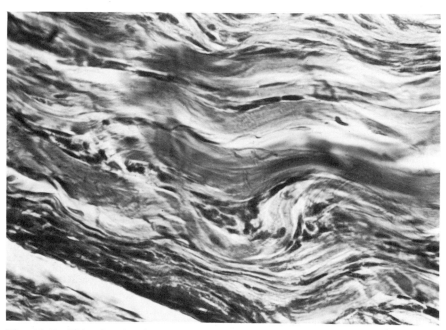

Fig. 16.7 This view is of an anterior cruciate xenograft in the canine model at 6 months and is taken from the tibial tunnel; the typical wavy or crimp pattern of the fixed xenograft can be recognized. It is well infiltrated with host tissue of fibrous nature.

designed to maintain the load application parallel to the direction of the graft fibres at a rate of 1000 cm/min. The non-operated limb served as a control. Failure modes in the control limbs were by bone avulsion, whereas in the experimental knees avulsion of the xenograft from the fixation tunnels occurred, in spite of the clinical stability and excellent function of the operated knees. One animal could not be tested due to failure of the graft at the femoral port. This was due to a stress riser induced through abrasion at the tunnel entrance which was placed inaccurately forward.

The xenograft material used had a nominal diameter of 6 mm and registered a maximal failure load in bench testing of 314 ± 57 N. In the test animals the failure of control anterior cruciates was 1004.5 ± 605.6 N. The experimental replaced complex demonstrated failure at 286.6 ± 137.5 N. There are basic problems in these comparisons; the control limb certainly gives an accurate assessment of the canine anterior cruciate/bone complex under tensile load, however, the experimental series is more of a test of fixation at this early time than of the ligament material and indicates that significant healing of the implant material has not yet occurred. In spite of the low loads recorded at failure, the replacement complex maintained clinical stability of the knees under physiological load conditions.

The series of animal studies has demonstrated that the xenograft implant materials are accepted by host animals and provide a functional link for transmission of force and maintenance of joint stability. Histological examination showed the grafts invaded by host tissue transitioning from an immediate or acute inflammatory profile to a chronic inflammatory response and finally a fibrous stage mimetic of a normal healing response. Recent preliminary studies investigating the ultrastructural nature of the fibrotic tissue ingrowth have demonstrated interdigitation of host collagen fibrils with the xenograft fibrils.

16.3.1 BIOMECHANICAL CHARACTERIZATIONS

Bench testing of xenograft implants for clinical use has been carried out by the Cleveland Research Institute (Berg et al., 1983). Well aware of the known problems of testing ligament and tendon materials in the fresh state, in particular those associated with grip slippage and stress riser creation, special roller grips were developed to grasp the specimens. Although these grips worked satisfactorily they did not eliminate the problems entirely. Failures in tension testing commonly occurred near the grips. Thus, the data derived from these tests contain a bias due to these problems and it is felt the figures for ultimate load and tensile strength represent minimums. This has been confirmed recently by additional testing using cryogrips where the ends of the biomaterials are more securely held without crushing; results with these grips were up to three times those recorded with the mechanical grips.

The conditions for standard testing in tension to failure were immersion in saline at 37°C and extension at 100%/sec. Testing was done on MTS equipment. Strains were recorded with an online mechanical extensiometer attached directly to the test specimen. This technique does produce some bias as the material undergoing testing may well not fail uniformly or within the confines of the extensiometer. Additionally, recent studies have shown that there even may be regional differences within a given collagenous structure when strains are recorded segmentally. The same experimental problems may plague the more sophisticated video strain techniques if the area under surveillance does not contribute wholly to the failure site.

The CLR (8 mm xenograft tendon) material demonstrated a maximum tensile load of 1066 ± 145 N, a tensile strength of 33 ± 5 MPa, an elastic modulus of 2007 ± 721 MPa and a strain of 3 ± 1%. The LR (broad ligament xenograft) material demonstrated a maximum tensile load of 451 ± 131 N, a tensile strength of 14 ± 4 MPa, an elastic modulus of 390 ± 195 MPa, and a strain of 4 ± 1%. The GR (6 mm tendon xenograft) material demonstrated a maximum load of 596 ± 166 N, a tensile strength of 32 ± 5 MPa, an elastic modulus of 1356 ± 217 MPa, and a strain of 7 ± 1%. The GR (4 mm tendon xenograft) material demonstrated a maximum load of 314 ± 57 N, a tensile strength of 32 ± 5 MPa, an elastic modulus of 792 ± 157 MPa, and a strain of 7 ± 2%. Although it is difficult to compare these results to figures reported in the literature for native human tissues because of different test conditions, strain rates and grip techniques etc., these figures do suggest that the xenograft materials exhibit similar properties to the structures they are to replace. Most importantly, the values obtained for the xenografts are not lower than those of comparably tested human structures by any of the parameters tested.

Fatigue testing of biological materials is a difficult task. Fatigue testers have been developed for some biological materials such as heart valve leaflets. The results from such tests indicate that these leaflets ought to fail within 2 years. However, in clinical experience this is not supported. Thus, the data derived from such tests may be misleading. In addition, the time required for such tests using available equipment is a problem particularly in view of the special circumstances when working with biological materials, such as the strains required and the recovery time necessary when testing a viscoelastic material. Cyclic testing of xenograft material has been done up to 50 000 cycles. Fatigue failures were not observed in these specimens. Destructive tensile testing of the cycled materials demonstrated excellent preservation of properties. Permanent strains recorded were: $0.3 \pm 0.5\%$ for LR, 0% for CLR, and $1 \pm 0.4\%$ for the GR material after 50 000 cycles.

Returning to the concepts of stabilization of the collagen molecule with glutaraldehyde, the chemical bond which results as a consequence of the glutaraldehyde with the collagen is of the covalent type. The increased crosslinking is expressed in the mechanical property figures by increased tensile strength and elevated modulus. It is felt that the stiffness which is present will not be deleterious and negatively affect the performance of these biomaterials.

In general, the xenograft materials exhibit excellent bench mechanical characteristics. However, such testing is fraught with many pitfalls including biological variation in the materials, mechanical problems in the test equipment, and the ability to reliably reproduce test parameters. Even more difficult is the ability to compare results to those of other authors or materials because of the lack of consensus on uniformity of testing. *In vivo* experience will probably provide the ultimate accurate assessment of their biomechanical suitability. However, as it would be foolish to utilize a material which demonstrated obviously inferior performance under bench conditions, these tests provided a sounding of the general adequacy of the mechanical properties of the materials.

16.4 Clinical results

Human clinical trials with bovine xenografts were initiated in Europe in December 1980. Shortly thereafter, initial clinical trials began under IDE regulations of the Food and Drug Administration. Currently 45 clinical centres throughout the United States are functioning with broad spectrum application of xenograft implants including flexor tendon grafts and ligament replacement materials in and about multiple joints. There has been particular interest in application of these materials to problems in and about the knee joint. Any implant device must be judged from many facets when one considers its usefulness to the surgeon and patient recipient. Safety of the device is an overriding concern. Implantation of the device must not result in carcinogenic developments, allergic phenomenon, or acute morbidity which will affect the well being of the patient. Implantation of such a device should not be directly responsible for mortality. Most of these questions can be answered within implant times of 1 year, although certainly more extended implant times may be necessary to answer other concerns. It is our feeling that most of the major safety concerns have been clearly viewed and these materials have demonstrated short-term safety when implanted in human subjects. Another aspect of a new biomaterial has to do with efficacy. Short-term efficacy of these biomaterials has been demonstrated. They can be fixed within bony tunnels and can be stapled, sutured, or trapped under bony flaps. They do not have a handling problem which compromises their integrity at the time of insertion, and they can be well adapted to the surgical techniques of fixation commonly employed by the experienced surgeon. In addition, they will provide the stability required, and, over the period of time clinical assessment has been followed so far, stability and integrity of the material has not proved to deteriorate with time. However, long-term function of these biomaterials has not been established by the current clinical follow-up studies. Only after a much larger group of patients has been followed for a period of 3–5 years in the cruciate position, for instance, will one have the authority to make a statement on long-term function.

To put the clinical application of these biomaterials into perspective a risk classification has been developed. The classification is based on a combination of factors which can have significant impact on the clinical outcome of the implant procedure. These factors are characteristic of the procedure and/or certain adjunct activities and are exclusive of the use of the xenograft as part of the total procedure. These include the type of procedure, the technique dependency of the procedure, infection risk associated with the duration and type of procedure, and the relationship of the postoperative management to the procedure.

In instances where a material is utilized in a soft tissue bed as a non-gliding, static, low force-bearing implant, the major risks are associated with anatomical compatibility and secondarily, with the 'tacking down' or appropriate fixation to the surrounding tissue. In these procedures the major function desired of the graft is that of a suitable filler or matrix; the absence of repetitive loading forces lessen the importance of those aspects of technique associated with graft placement. Also in these procedures the rehabilitative postoperative management is not as susceptible to complications as in those instances where the management regimen must be carefully monitored with regard to weight-bearing and motion.

The transmission of forces as in extensor and flexor applications is primarily dependent on the adequacy of the proximal and distal fixation, the resistance or susceptibility of the graft to adhesions with the surrounding tissue bed, and the existence of adequate sheathing structures. These procedures, in the absence of infection, are not generally associated with complications other than those that might be related to the functional adequacy of the repair.

Procedures involving the replacement or repair of intra-articular or extra-articular ligamentous structures are extremely sensitive to accurate positioning and tensioning of the grafted material. Malposition can lead to the creation of stress risers and result in mechanical damage to the graft

(Landon, Mikosz and Andriacchi, 1983). Also excessive slack or tension applied to the graft prior to fixation can result in inadequate stabilization or restricted joint motion.

The sensitivity and fragility of the synovium make it particularly susceptible to irritation and injury resulting in an inflammatory response most frequently diagnosed as non-specific reactive synovitis. The exposure of the synovium to mechanical disruption during surgery, a failed synovial healing response, or any pre-existing acute or chronic synovial involvement with the patient's condition contribute to an increased risk of synovial inflammation during various intra-articular procedures. Reinjury of a placed graft or mechanical disruption associated with or exclusive of the surgical procedures involving the exposure and/or manipulation of intra-articular synovial tissue have an inherent added risk exclusive of other conditions.

Postoperative management of orthopaedic procedures which are particularly sensitive to the onset, duration, and degree of weight-bearing and active range of motion must be carefully regimented and monitored. Early movement can result in various complications associated with adequate healing and fixation of materials within bony structures and with the formation of tracts. If partial or full weight-bearing is begun concomitant with premature movement the risk of a complication occurring can be significantly increased because of the possibility of failure of the procedure. This is of especial significance in intra-articular stabilization because of the probable involvement of the synovium and synovial fluid.

Based on the above considerations, the following risk classification has been developed for assessing the clinical outcome of the surgical procedures.

16.4.1 RISK CLASS

I. Device used in a situation where no significant active or passive forces are applied to the material. This involves the use of the device in a non-stabilizing situation, for example, as a spacer or filler. Level one does not include use of the graft as an interpositional material, that is, within the joint.

II. Device used in a situation where the major functional requirements are the transference of muscle forces as in extensor/flexor repairs or in muscle transfer procedures.

III. Device used to stabilize a joint extra-articularly. This does not include any use of the graft within a synovial space or cavity.

IV. Device used to stabilize a joint intra-articularly. This involves situations in which any portion of the graft resides within a synovial space or cavity or is in contact with the synovial membrane. The manner in which the device gains entrance to the synovial cavity may vary. Also included are intra-articular uses of the device which do not result in joint stabilization, for example, use as an interpositional resurfacing material.

Clinical assessment of outcome in various risk categories are somewhat varied at this time and are skewed heavily towards knee instability problem management. Anterior cruciate replacement requirements are probably one of the more stringent requirements in terms of function and stability any synthetic ligament material will face. In evaluating the outcome of anterior cruciate procedures, we have developed a scoring method comparing preoperative evaluations with scores similarly obtained at 6 and 12 months postoperatively. The following six clinical tests were performed as part of the data collection system for evaluation of Xenotech bioprostheses: Lachman, anterior drawer, anterior lateral rotational instability, anterior medial rotational instability, pivot shift, and effusion. For each test a score of 0 would indicate no measurable instability or difference from the opposite limb, if uninjured; a score of 4 would represent the maximum instability by comparison. A combined functional score is then determined. A score of 0 would indicate no measurable instability or insufficiency compared to the uninjured control limb, whereas a score of 24 would represent the worst case of instability.

The following is a compilation of all implants done by various clinical centres within the United States under IDE FDA guidelines and is part of the required data retrieval system established to provide adequate longitudinal follow-up on all bioprostheses. These assessments were all completed by August 1983, and are part of a in–progress submission report to the FDA with regards to the ongoing clinical study. The data were collected from 16 clinical centres, 96 patients were involved, 27 were female and 69 were male. The number of implants involved from all classes equalled 100 implants and a mean implant time in all classes was 8.1 months (Tables 16.1, 16.2 and 16.3)

As can be seen in class 4 indications there was a total of 48 patients who had been followed out to the 1 year point. The preoperative mean score for the entire population as well as for patients who had completed the 6-month evaluation and patients who had been followed through the 12-month subset was ten. There are fewer number of patients in the 12-month subset. All patients in the 12-month subset are included in the 6-month subset. Comparing preoperative and postoperative scores, the 6-month subset showed a postoperative score of 1 compared to 10 preoperatives; the 12-month subset had a mean score of 2 compared to 11 preoperatively. If one breaks down the various components of the functional test score and similarly compares the preoperative and

336

Table 16.1 Anterior cruciate ligament clinical follow-up: USA combined functional score

| | | Preoperative | | Postoperative | |
	Total population	6-month subset	12-month subset	6 Months	12 Months
Number of patients	48	30	16	30	16
Population score	474	313	169	38	38
Mean score	10	10	11	1	2

Table 16.2 Anterior cruciate ligament clinical follow-up: Lachman test (0–4+)

| | | Preoperative | | Postoperative | |
	Total population	6-Month subset	12-Month subset	6 months	12 Months
Number of patients	48	30	16	30	16
Population score	116	76	42	14	11
Mean score	2.4	2.5	2.6	0.5	0.7

Table 16.3 Anterior cruciate ligament clinical follow-up: anterior drawer (0−4+)

| | | Preoperative | | Postoperative | |
	Total population	6-Month subset	12-Month subset	6 Months	12 Months
Number of patients	45	28	16	28	16
Population score	103	70	41	9	13
Mean score	2.3	2.5	2.6	0.3	0.8

postoperative data in 6-month and 12-month subsets, one can see the similar improvement in score and maintenance.

Earlier clinical experiences began in Europe (Abbink, 1983) the sample was 104 patients, average age 34 years with a range of 16–73 years; 120 grafts were implanted in all risk classifications. The mean implant time in all classifications was 13.2 months with a range of 3–26 months. A clinical summarization is provided for those patients included in this study who received risk class 3 and 4 devices. A total of 104 patients with 120 implants are included. The variance between numbers of patients and implants occurs because in many cases of complex knee instability; two or more grafts were utilized. Follow-up on this group of patients was quite good with only one patient not available for follow-up at the time of the most recent assessment. The same objective group of tests was used to evaluate these patients as has been described for United States patients. In summary, the mean preoperative score for patients with a 6-month minimum follow-up was 8.1 and postoperatively the score had decreased to 0.4. Similarly, a group of patients with a maximum 12-month follow-up had a preoperative mean score of 8.6 with a drop to 0.5 at 6 months and 0.5 at 12 months. Some patients had a follow-up assessment at 24 months by the time of going to press. The preoperative mean score for those patients was 10 with a postoperative 6-month score of 0.5 which was maintained throughout the 24-month follow-up period. Similarly, if one breaks the combined score into its component tests and looks at these assessments a similar maintenance of improvement is demonstrated (Tables 16.4, 16.5 and 16.6).

Table 16.4 Anterior cruciate ligament clinical follow-up, Europe: combined functional score

		Number of patients	Population total score	Mean score
All patients with minimum	Preoperative	45	363	8.1
6-months follow-up	6 month	45	19	0.4
Subset of patients with maxi-	Preoperative	19	163	8.6
mum follow-up 12 months	6 month	19	9	0.5
	12 month	19	10	0.5
Subset of patients with maxi-	Preoperative	2	20	10
mum follow-up 24 months	6 month	2	1	0.5
	12 month	2	1	0.5
	24 month	2	1	0.5

Table 16.5 Anterior cruciate ligament clinical follow-up: Lachman (0−4+)

		Number of patients	Population total score	Mean score
All patients with minimum 6	Preoperative	46	102	2.2
month follow-up	6 month	46	7	0.2
Subset of patients with maxi-	Preoperative	19	43	2.3
mum follow-up 12 months	6 month	19	3	0.2
	12 month	19	4	0.2
Subset of patients with maxi-	Preoperative	2	5	2.5
mum follow-up 24 months	6 month	2	0	0
	12 month	2	0	0
	24 month	2	0	0

Table 16.6 Anterior cruciate ligament clinical follow-up: anterior drawer (0−4+)

		Number of patients	Population total score	Mean score
All patients with minimum 6	Preoperative	55	81	1.5
month follow-up	6 month	55	5	0.1
Subset of patients with maxi-	Preoperative	23	35	1.5
mum follow-up 12 months	6 month	23	3	0.1
	12 month	23	2	0.1
Subset of patients with maxi-	Preoperative	2	3	1.5
mum follow-up 24 months	6 month	2	0	0
	12 month	2	0	0
	24 month	2	0	0

16.5 Complications

Data concerning complications has been meticulously collected and analysed for the United States study group.

16.5.1 INFECTION

Bacterial infection developed postoperatively in eight patients necessitating graft removal. All cases of infection occurred in class 4 procedures. In seven cases the organisms were identified as species generally considered to be common hospital contaminants (*Staphylococcus sp.* − four cases, *Pseudomonas aeruginosa* − one case, *Streptococcus viridans* − one case,

Enterobacter cloacae – one case), indicating that the infections were acquired in the hospital environment, most likely during surgery, and not related to graft sterility. The patient with the *Streptococcus viridans* infection was positive for the organism prior to surgery. A *Chlamydia* infection developed in one individual apparently as a consequence of an unresolved sepsis prior to surgery. Death rate kinetic studies have verified that the device sterilant effectively eliminates the organisms identified in all the reported cases in a very short time.

In management of infection, several precepts have been developed. As a consequence of the nature of the graft material, it is obvious the graft will be colonized. The only means by which systemic antibiotics could enter the graft immediately after implant is by diffusion, making it unlikely that satisfactory levels of antibiotics within the graft material can be achieved. It is therefore felt that in the face of infection the graft material should be removed with thorough debridement of the wound and irrigation with 10l of saline solution. Appropriate aerobic and anaerobic cultures should be taken and antibiotics used which are specific against those strains identified from the intraoperative cultures. Intravenous antibiotic use should continue for a minimum of 2 weeks. Following this an oral antibiotic regimen should be maintained for a minimum of 1 month or until all clinical signs and appropriate laboratory tests are normal. It is interesting to note in the United States series that the surgical procedures associated with infection occurred early in the investigation and appeared to be related to excessive or improper handling of the graft and extended operating time. Instances of infection were restricted to three investigational centres. Three of the infections occurred in a facility with a 10% clean operative infection rate. At the time of this writing no additional infections have been reported since the initial eight cases.

16.5.2 SYNOVITIS

Synovitis, as evidenced by swelling and/or effusion, has been reported in 16 patients. Twelve cases resulted in graft removal. In eight of the cases the onset of the inflammatory synovitic response occurred and persisted throughout the early postoperative period. In four cases the patients presented with acute swelling at approximately 24 weeks. This was transient. Spontaneous resolving effusion in the absence of any specific diagnosis has been reported in two cases. Recurrent, unresolved effusion has been reported in two cases. All cases of synovitis occurred in class 4 procedures involving anterior cruciate reconstruction.

Eight of the cases which resulted in seven explants occurred in one centre and were associated with an aggressive rehabilitation programme without plaster immobilization involving early weight-bearing and active range of motion activity. The procedures were done arthroscopic-assisted and although the majority of patients were chronically unstable with complex instability, a simplistic approach to management using only an anterior cruciate ligament replacement without secondary procedures was done. This would seem predestined to failure. Premature mobilization, active range of motion, and weight-bearing possibly resulted in inadequate incorporation of the graft within the bony tunnels and inhibition of the synovial investment of the intra-articular portion of the graft. Movement of the graft within the bony tunnels can lead to the development of stress risers which may result in fraying or total rupture of the graft with concomitant irritation of the synovium.

The remaining eight cases occurred in two centres in patients immobilized in plaster for 6–8 weeks. In five cases resulting in graft explant the acute onset and persistence of the inflammatory response appeared to be associated with disruption of the graft as a consequence of failure of the graft to become incorporated and fixed in the bony tunnels. Bony tunnels of too large a diameter can result in inadequate fixation and the possible formation of a tract between the intra-articular and extra-articular compartments. This may result in a localized sterile inflammatory response as a consequence of synovial fluid tracking through the bony tunnels. A subcutaneous collection of synovial fluid can be irritating, producing a localized inflammatory response and even local skin reactivity such as blistering or the development of a fistula. Also, malposition of the bony tunnels is known to produce stress risers that usually result in graft damage or failure with synovitis – a consequence of the irritative process caused by the broken or frayed graft in the synovial cavity. The importance of surgical technique and adherence to an appropriate postoperative and rehabilitation regimen are important.

In those instances where synovial tissue was obtained either as a consequence of synovectomy or biopsy the pathological findings were consistent with chronic non-specific synovitis.

16.6 Summary

The need for an appropriate ligament replacement graft material has been well documented. Several prototypes of various materials are currently available and are in various stages of investigational development in human subjects. Continued interest in these materials and their clinical outcome by the orthopaedic surgical community speaks for itself in regard to the perceived need. The xenograft biomaterials have proven to be effective and functional in several series of long-term animal

Ligament Injuries and their Treatment

evaluations. The early clinical assessment of patients with complex instability, particularly in the anterior cruciate position, indicates the xenograft bioprosthesis as a useful adjunct in the reconstruction surgical procedures designed to manage these problems. One, of course, understands that these instability problems are managed by a combination of intra-articular and extra-articular procedures which are highly technique-dependent and require the careful management of a skilled and learned knee surgeon; naive technical errors in the use of such materials can potentially compromise the long-term results.

References

Abbink, E. P. (1983), Preliminary report on the use of xenografts in knee instability problems. *Orthop. Trans.*, **7**, 84.

Alexander, H., Parson, J. R., Strauchler, I. D., Corcoran, S. F., Gona, O., Mayott, C. and Weiss, A. B. (1981), Canine patella tendon replacement. *Orthop. Rev.*, **10**, 41–51.

Berg, W. S., Stahurski, T. M., Moran, J. M. and Greenwald, A. S. (1983), Mechanical properties of bovine xenografts. *Orthop. Trans.*, **7**, 279–80.

Bright, R. and Green, W. (1981), Freeze dried fascia lata allografts: a review of 47 cases. *J. Ped. Orthop.*, **1**, 13–22.

Chen, E. H., Black, J. (1980), Materials design analysis of the prosthetic anterior cruciate ligament. *J. Biomed. Mat. Res.*, **14**, 567–86.

Iselin, F. and Pezi, W. (1976), Use of chemically present tendon allografts in hand surgery. *Hand*, **8**, 167–72.

Jenkins, D., Forster, I., McKibbins, B. *et al.* (1977), Induction of tendon and ligament formation by carbon implants. *J. Bone Joint Surg.*, **59B**, 53–7.

Landon, G. C., Mikosz, R. and Andriacchi, T. P. (1983), The influence of attachment position of the force displacement characteristics of the anterior cruciate ligament. *Orthop. Trans.*, **7**, 247–8.

McMaster, W. (1975), Tendon grafting with glutaraldehyde fixed material. *Proceedings of the 7th International Biomaterials Symposium*, Clemson, S. C., 28 April.

McMaster, W. C. (1981), Histologic evaluation of a xenograft medial collateral ligament implant. *Orthop. Trans.*, **5**, 257.

McMaster, W., Liddle, S., Anzel, S. *et al.* (1974), Evaluation of buffered glutaraldehyde fixed tendon as a graft material. *Proceedings of the 6th International Biomaterials Symposium*, Clemson, S. C., 22 April.

McMaster, W., Liddle, S., Anzel, S. *et al.* (1975), Medial collateral ligament replacement in the rabbit: a preliminary report. *Am. J. Sports Med.*, **3**, 271–6.

Noyes, F. (1981), Knee ligaments injury and treatment. *Clinical Biomechanics*, Presented at AAOS, Las Vegas, Nevada, 26 February to 3 March.

Parsons, J. R., Byhani, S., Alexander, H. and Weiss, A. B. (1983), Carbon fiber debris within the synovial joint: time-dependent mechanical and histologic studies. *Trans ORS*, **March**.

Peacock, E. E. and Madden, J. W. (1967), Human composite flexor tendon allografts. *Am Surg.*, **166**, 624–9.

Rushton, N., Dandy, D. J. and Naylor, C. P. E. (1983), The clinical, arthroscopic, and histological findings after replacement of the anterior cruciate ligament with carbon fibre. *J. Bone Joint Surg.*, **65B**, 308–9.

Salamon, A., Balint, J., Hamori, J. *et al.* (1976), Collagen synthesis, studies by submicroscopic methods in beta-propiolactone and in tendon homografts preserved by gamma radiation. *Magy, Traumatol. Orthop*, **19**, 272–83.